Clinical Cases in Dermatology

Series Editor

Robert A. Norman, Tampa, FL, USA

This series of concise practical guides is designed to facilitate the clinical decision-making process by reviewing a number of cases and defining the various diagnostic and management decisions open to clinicians.

Each title is illustrated and diverse in scope, enabling the reader to obtain relevant clinical information regarding both standard and unusual cases in a rapid, easy to digest format. Each focuses on one disease or patient group, and includes common cases to allow readers to know they are doing things right if they follow the case guidelines.

More information about this series at https://link.springer.com/bookseries/10473

Anna Waśkiel-Burnat • Roxanna Sadoughifar
Torello M. Lotti • Lidia Rudnicka

Editors

Clinical Cases in Scalp Disorders

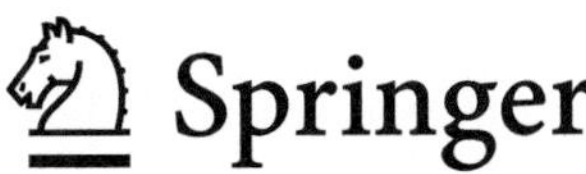

Editors
Anna Waśkiel-Burnat
Department of Dermatology
Medical University of Warsaw
Warsaw, Poland

Torello M. Lotti
Dermatology
Marconi University
Rome, Roma, Italy

Roxanna Sadoughifar
Dermatology
Marconi University
Rome, Roma, Italy

Lidia Rudnicka
Department of Dermatology
Medical University of Warsaw
Warszawa, Poland

ISSN 2730-6178   ISSN 2730-6186   (electronic)
Clinical Cases in Dermatology
ISBN 978-3-030-93425-5   ISBN 978-3-030-93426-2   (eBook)
https://doi.org/10.1007/978-3-030-93426-2

This Springer imprint is published by the registered company Springer Nature Switzerland AG
The registered company address is: Gewerbestrasse 11, 6330 Cham, Switzerland

Contents

Chapter 1
A 72-Year-Old Woman with a Diffuse Erythema, Scaling on the Scalp and Coexisting Hair Loss

Magdalena Jasińska, Adriana Rakowska, Joanna Czuwara,
Mateusz Kamiński, Patrycja Gajda-Mróz, Małgorzata Olszewska,
and Lidia Rudnicka

A 72-year-old woman was admitted to the Department of Dermatology due to diffuse erythematous and poikilodermic lesions on the trunk and extremities associated with diffuse hair loss and scaling on the scalp. The first lesions appeared on the trunk one year ago. Since then, gradual progression of the disease was observed. Hair loss and scaling were observed for four months. The patient denied general symptoms such as fever or weight loss as well as subjective symptoms related to the affected skin. The history of dermatological and non-dermatological diseases was negative.

On physical examination mild erythema and scaling on the scalp were detected (Fig. 1.1). Moreover, diffuse erythematous and poikilodermic patches on the skin under the breasts, on the abdomen, lumbosacral area, armpits, groins and thighs were detected. No peripheral lymphadenopathy was presented. Trichoscopy revealed numerous pili torti, eight-shaped hairs, visible anagen bulbs, yellow dots, clustered white and yellowish scales as well as follicular spicules-like scaling in some areas of the scalp. Moreover, irregular linear blood vessels in a perifollicular distribution were detected (Fig. 1.2).

A histopathological examination showed epidermis with hyperkeratosis, miniaturization of the hair follicles and many atypical, enlarged lymphocytes tagging the dermoepidermal junction and hair follicular epithelia. A superficial perivascular lymphohistiocytic infiltrate in the dermis was observed. The collagen fibers at the papillary dermis were thicker indicating the chronicity of the process (Fig. 1.3). Immunohistochemical staining showed decreased expression of CD2+, CD3+ (<50%) and CD7+ T cells (<10%). Laboratory tests were within normal limits.

M. Jasińska (✉) · A. Rakowska · J. Czuwara · M. Kamiński · P. Gajda-Mróz · M. Olszewska
L. Rudnicka
Department of Dermatology, Medical University of Warsaw, Warsaw, Poland
e-mail: adriana.rakowska@wum.edu.pl; joanna.czuwara@wum.edu.pl;
patrycja.gajda@wum.edu.pl; lidia.rudnicka@wum.edu.pl

© The Author(s), under exclusive license to Springer Nature
Switzerland AG 2022
A. Waśkiel-Burnat et al. (eds.), *Clinical Cases in Scalp Disorders*, Clinical
Cases in Dermatology, https://doi.org/10.1007/978-3-030-93426-2_1

Fig. 1.1 A 72-year-old woman with a mild erythema and scaling on the scalp

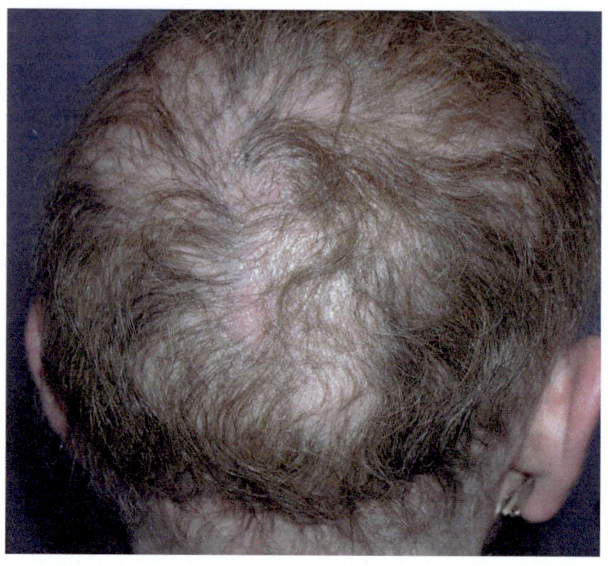

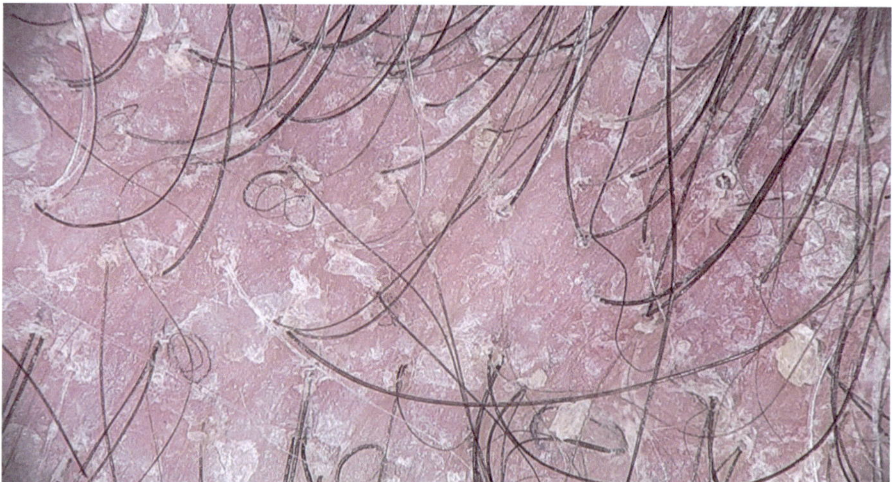

Fig. 1.2 Trichoscopy shows eight-shaped hairs, white and yellowish scales (×20)

Chest X-ray and abdominal ultrasound were normal. Peripheral lymph nodes ultrasound showed oval and spindle-shaped lymph nodes without signs of increased flow in both groins.

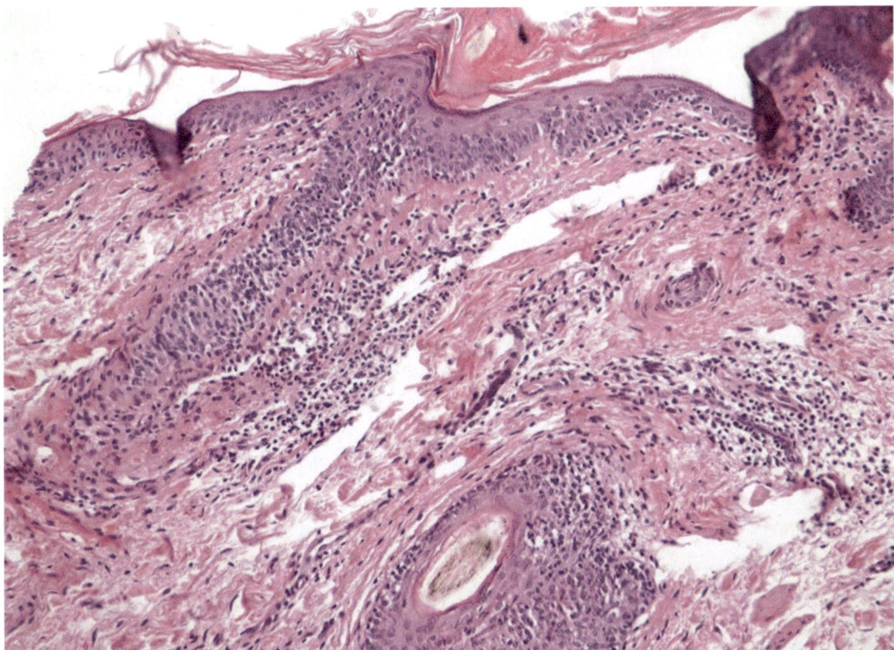

Fig. 1.3 A histopathological examination shows epidermis with hyperkeratosis, miniaturization of the hair follicles and many atypical, enlarged lymphocytes tagging the dermoepidermal junction and hair follicular epithelia. A superficial perivascular lymphohistiocytic infiltrate in the dermis is observed. The collagen fibers at the papillary dermis are thicker indicating the chronicity of the process (H&E)

Based on the case description and the photographs, what is your diagnosis?

Differential Diagnoses
1. Mycosis fungoides.
2. Allergic contact dermatitis.
3. Psoriasis.
4. Seborrheic dermatitis.

Diagnosis
Mycosis fungoides.

Discussion

Mycosis fungoides is the most common primary cutaneous T-cell lymphoma. It accounts for 4% of all non-Hodgkin lymphoma cases. The pathogenesis of mycosis fungoides remains unclear. However, the role of genetic predisposition, environmental, occupational and infectious factors has been suggested. The condition is most common in adults over 50 years of age. A male predominance is observed [1]. The clinical presentation of mycosis fungoides varies with the stage of the disease. In the earliest, patchy stage, single or multiple, various in diameter, erythematous, or brownish scaly patches are localized most commonly on the gluteal region and proximal thighs. The plaque stage is characterized by the presence of annular or horseshoe-shaped lesions with an infiltrated base, raised, well-defined edges and asymmetrical distribution. The face and scalp may be also affected. In the tumor stage, erythematous-purplish papules or nodules of larger diameter are observed. Less common clinical variants of mycosis fungoides include bullous, purpuric, poikilodermatous, hypopigmented, follicular and Pagetoid reticulosis [2]. The hair loss is observed in 2.5% of patients with mycosis fungoides. It is more common in women compared to men. Hair loss in the course of mycosis fungoides is mainly patchy (84%). However, alopecia totalis or universalis may occur. Hair loss in patients with mycosis fungoides is characterized by two clinical patterns. In same patients, areas of hair loss with normal skin or mild erythema and scaling are observed. In others, hair loss is associated with patchy, plaque or follicular lesions. Diagnosis of mycosis fungoides requires a combination of clinical, pathologic, and molecular features. In histopathological examination, superficial lymphoid infiltrate, epidermotropism and lymphoid atypia are the predominant features. In immunohistochemical examination, decreased expression of CD2+,CD3+ (<50%), and CD7+ (<10%) T cells is characteristic [1, 3]. Dermoscopy may be useful to establish initial diagnosis. Dermoscopic features of mycosis fungoides are white-pinkish structureless areas, orange-yellowish patchy areas, dotted and linear irregular vessels [4, 5]. Moreover, in trichoscopy, pili torti, eight-shaped hairs, thick white interfollicular bands, color heterogeneity of the background and perifollicular arrangement of vessels are observed [6]. Treatment of mycosis fungoides depends on the disease's stage. In early-stages, topical corticosteroids, topical nitrogen mustards, topical bexarotene, imiquimod, psoralen-ultraviolet therapy or ultraviolet B therapy are usually recommended. Local radiation and total skin electron beam therapy may be also useful. For more extensive disease, combinations of skin-directed therapies and systemic therapies are used. The various systemic options available include retinoids, methotrexate, interferons, targeted immunotherapy and polychemotherapy [1].

The scalp involvement in mycosis fungoides should be differentiated with psoriasis, contact dermatitis and seborrheic dermatitis.

Seborrheic dermatitis is a chronic inflammatory dermatologic condition. It presents as well-delimited erythematous plaques with greasy-looking, yellowish scale. Itching sensation is usually presented [7]. Seborrheic dermatitis is characterized by a seasonal pattern, presenting more frequently during winter, and improving usually during summer. Hair loss is rarely presented [8].

Allergic contact dermatitis is an inflammatory eczematous skin disease. The disease is rarely presented on the scalp area, because of the great thickness of the epidermis in this region. In the case of application of irritants or allergens on the scalp symptoms are usually observed on the face or neck area. Clinically, contact dermatitis presents as erythema with scaling and coexisted itch. In acute disease, vesicles or pustules may be present. Hair loss is rarely observed [9].

Scalp psoriasis is characterized by red, thickened plaques with silver-white scale, either contained within the hairline, or extending onto the forehead, ears, and posterior neck. In many cases, severe itch occurs. Hair loss is rarely observed [10].

In the presented patient, the diagnosis of mycosis fungoides was established. Treatment with subcutaneous methotrexate (15 mg once a week) and topical clobetasol propionate 0.05% cream (once a day) was initiated.

Key Points

- Hair loss affects 2.5% of patients with mycosis fungoides and includes patchy, totalis or universalis pattern.
- In mycosis fungoides, hair loss with normal skin or associated with patchy, plaque or follicular lesions may be observed.

References

1. Vaidya T, Badri T. Mycosis fungoides. Treasure Island (FL): StatPearls; 2020.
2. Larocca C, Kupper T. Mycosis fungoides and Sézary syndrome: an update. Hematol Oncol Clin North Am. 2019;33(1):103–20.
3. Cerroni L. Mycosis fungoides-clinical and histopathologic features, differential diagnosis, and treatment. Semin Cutan Med Surg. 2018;37(1):2–10.
4. Lallas A, Apalla Z, Lefaki I, Tzellos T, Karatolias A, Sotiriou E, et al. Dermoscopy of early stage mycosis fungoides. J Eur Acad Dermatol Venereol. 2013;27(5):617–21.
5. Sławińska M, Sokołowska-Wojdyło M, Sobjanek M, Golińska J, Nowicki RJ, Rudnicka L. The significance of dermoscopy and trichoscopy in differentiation of erythroderma due to various dermatological disorders. J Eur Acad Dermatol Venereol. 2021;35(1):230–40.
6. Rakowska A, Jasińska M, Sikora M, Czuwara J, Gajda-Mróz P, Warszawik-Hendzel O, et al. Cutaneous T-cell lymphoma in erythrodermic cases may be suspected on the basis of scalp examination with dermoscopy. Sci Rep. 2021;11(1):282.
7. Borda LJ, Wikramanayake TC. Seborrheic dermatitis and dandruff: a comprehensive review. J Clin Investig Dermatol. 2015;3(2).
8. Clark GW, Pope SM, Jaboori KA. Diagnosis and treatment of seborrheic dermatitis. Am Fam Physician. 2015;91(3):185–90.
9. Rozas-Muñoz E, Gamé D, Serra-Baldrich E. Allergic contact dermatitis by anatomical regions: diagnostic clues. Actas Dermosifiliogr. 2018;109(6):485–507.
10. Blakely K, Gooderham M. Management of scalp psoriasis: current perspectives. Psoriasis (Auckl). 2016;6:33–40.

Chapter 2
A 25-Year-Old Man with Suppurative Nodules of the Scalp

Karolina Kozera-Wojtan and Adriana Rakowska

A 25-year-old man was presented with suppurative nodules of the scalp since two years. Patient did not complain of any symptoms. There was a history of usage of anabolic steroids for recreational performance enhancement.

Physical examination revealed boggy, suppurative nodules with coexisted hair loss on the vertex and the occipital areas of the scalp (Fig. 2.1). On palpation, pustular and hemorrhagic discharge was presented. Additionally, acne conglobata of the face was noticed. On trichoscopy, yellow dots, 3D yellow dots, black dots and yellow structureless areas were observed (Fig. 2.2).

Histopathology showed neutrophilic, mixed-cell perifollicular infiltration in the dermis.

Based on the case description and the photographs, what is your diagnosis?

Differential Diagnoses
1. Folliculitis decalvans.
2. Acne keloidalis.
3. Dissecting cellulitis.
4. Furunculosis.

Diagnosis
Dissecting cellulitis.

K. Kozera-Wojtan (✉) · A. Rakowska
Department of Dermatology, Medical University of Warsaw, Warsaw, Poland
e-mail: karolina.kozera-wojtan@wum.edu.pl; adriana.rakowska@wum.edu.pl

A. Waśkiel-Burnat et al. (eds.), *Clinical Cases in Scalp Disorders*, Clinical Cases in Dermatology, https://doi.org/10.1007/978-3-030-93426-2_2

Fig. 2.1 A 25-year-old man with, suppurative nodules with coexisted hair loss on the vertex and the occipital areas of the scalp

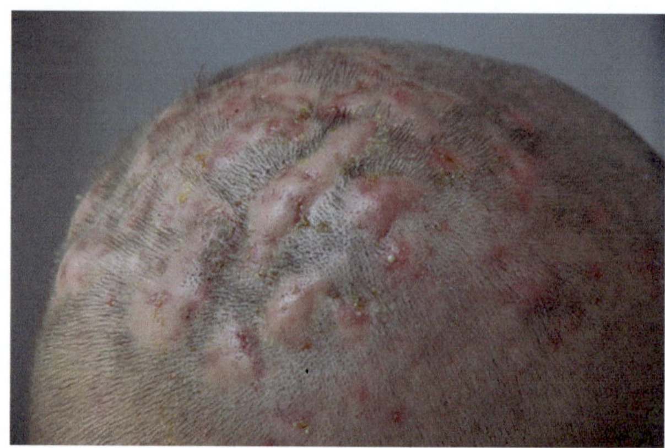

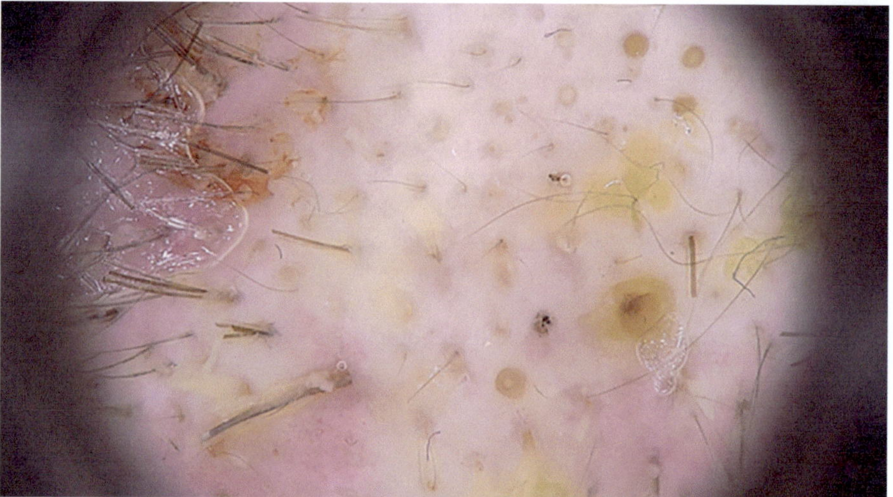

Fig. 2.2 Trichoscopy shows yellow dots, 3D yellow dots, black dots and yellow structureless areas (×20)

Discussion

Dissecting cellulitis is a chronic inflammatory disease classified as a primary neutrophilic cicatricial alopecia [1, 2]. The precise pathogenesis of dissecting cellulitis is unknown. However the role of hyperkeratosis, follicular occlusion and subsequent inflammation has been described [2, 3]. The role of androgens has been also suggested [3]. Dissecting cellulitis occurs almost exclusively in young men of African descent. Clinically, multiple firm, violaceous papules which coalesce to form plaques and nodules are observed. Abscesses and sinus tracts with pustular or hemorrhagic fluid are also presented. Hypertrophic scars and keloids may appear.

The vertex and occipital areas are most commonly affected. The course of the disease is usually chronic with periodic flares. Diagnosis of dissecting cellulitis is mainly based on the clinical and histopathological features. Trichoscopy can be useful to avoid scalp biopsy. The trichoscopic findings differs depending on the stage and activity of the disease. In the early stages of the disease black and yellow dots predominate. In the advanced stages yellow structureless areas and 3D yellow (soap bubble) dots are seen. The end-stages show ivory-white or white areas without follicular openings [4]. A histopathological examination is characterized by the presence of a lymphocytic infiltrate in the lower dermis extending into the subcutis. Other findings include abscesses consisting of neutrophils, lymphocytes, and plasma cells as well as granulomatous foreign body reactions [5]. In patients with dissecting cellulitis, bacterial and fungal cultures are usually negative. However, secondary superinfection may occur (*Staphylococcus aureus*, *Pseudomonas aeruginosa*, anaerobic bacterias). The treatment options include topical or intralesional corticosteroids, topical antibiotics, systemic antibiotics (ciprofloxacin, clindamycin, rifampin, and trimethoprim/sulfamethaxole) and isotretinoin. Systemic corticosteroids and tumor necrosis factor inhibitors may be also useful [1–3].

Differential diagnoses for the presented included folliculitis decalvans, acne keloidalis and furunculosis.

Folliculitis decalvans most commonly occurs in young to middle-aged men. The disease is initially characterized by follicular papules and pustules. Subsequently, tufted hairs, erosions, hemorrhagic crusts, and nodules are detected. Lesions are most commonly localized in the vertex, parietal and occipital areas of the scalp. Moreover, folliculitis decalvans may be noted in other locations, including the face, neck, axillae and pubic region [6].

Acne keloidalis nuchae, also known as folliculitis keloidalis nuchae, affects mainly young man of African descent. Clinically, it is characterized by the presence of single or multiple smooth dome-shaped, firm, follicular papules and pustules progressing to keloid–like plaques associated with hair loss. In chronic, recurrent disease abscesses and purulent fistulas may be observed. Lesions mainly occur on the neck and occipital area [7].

Furunculosis is a deep infection of the hair follicle that leads to abscess formation with accumulation of pus and necrotic tissue. The most common infectious agent is *Staphylococcus aureus*, but other bacteria may also be causative. Clinically, furuncles present as red, swollen, and tender nodules of varying size and at times with an overlying pustule. If several adjacent follicles are infected they may coalesce and form a larger nodule, known as a carbuncle. The lesions can appear on any hair-bearing area. However, lower extremities are most commonly affected. Scarring can appeared after skin lesions healing [8].

In the presented patient, based on the clinical presentation, trichoscopic examination and histopathology, the diagnosis of dissecting cellulitis was established. The patient was treated with oral isotretinoin at the dose 20 mg per day with good tolerance, achieving clinical improvement within a few weeks.

Key Points
- Dissecting cellulitis is a primary neutrophilic cicatricial alopecia.
- It presents as multiple firm, violaceous papules which coalesce to form plaques and nodules; abscesses and sinus tracts with pustular or hemorrhagic fluid may be also observed.

References

1. Guo W, Zhu C, Stevens G, Silverstein D. Analyzing the efficacy of izotretinoin in treating dissecting cellulitis: a literature review and meta-analysis. Drugs R&D. 2021;21(1):29–37.
2. Sung K, Lee S, Jeong Y, Lee S. Dissecting cellulitis of the scalp: a diagnostic challenge. Arch Plast Surg. 2020;47(6):631–2.
3. Kurtzman DJB, Alexander CE. Image gallery: dissecting cellulitis of the scalp following anabolic steroid use. Br J Dermatol. 2017;177(4):e160.
4. Melo DF, Lemes RD, Pirmez R, Duque-Estrada B. Trichoscopic stages of dissecting cellulitis: a potential complementary tool to clinical assessment. An Bras Dermatol. 2020;95(4):514–7.
5. Uchiyama M, Harada K, Tobita R, Irisawa R, Tsuboi R. Histopathologic and dermoscopic features of 42 cases of folliculitis decalvans: a case series. J Am Acad Dermatol. 2020;S0190-9622(20):30515–6.
6. Bolduc C, Sperling LC, Shapiro J. Primary cicatricial alopecia: other lymphocytic primary cicatricial alopecias and neutrophilic and mixed primary cicatricial alopecias. J Am Acad Dermatol. 2016;75(6):1101–17.
7. East-Innis ADC, Stylianou K, Paolino A, Ho JD. Acne keloidalis nuchae: risk factors and associated disorders – a retrospective study. Int J Dermatol. 2017;56(8):828–32.
8. Ibler KS, Kromann CB. Recurrent furunculosis – challenges and management: a review. Clin Cosmet Investig Dermatol. 2014;7:59–64.

Chapter 3
A 28-Year-Old Male with a Giant Lesion on the Scalp

Katarzyna Borowska and Piotr Brzeziński

A 28-year-old man presented with a slowly growing congenital lesion on the scalp. The dermatological examination revealed an yellowish verrucous plaque (6 cm × 3 cm) on the scalp (Fig. 3.1). The lesion was present at birth, slowly enlarged with age, and grew most rapidly during the pubertal hormonal surge. He had no other growth or developmental abnormalities. Histology showed epidermal hyperplasia as well as hyperplasia and malpositioning of the sebaceous glands.

Based on the case description and the photograph, what is your diagnosis?

Differential Diagnoses
1. Seborrheic keratosis.
2. Epidermal nevus.
3. Nevus sebaceus of Jadassohn.
4. Juvenile xanthogranuloma.

Diagnosis
Nevus sebaceus of Jadassohn.

K. Borowska (✉)
Department of Histology and Embryology with Experimental Cytology Unit, Medical University of Lublin, Lublin, Poland

P. Brzeziński
Department of Physiotherapy and Medical Emergency, Faculty of Health Sciences, Pomeranian Academy, Słupsk, Poland

Department of Dermatology, Provincial Specialist Hospital in Slupsk, Ustka, Poland

© The Author(s), under exclusive license to Springer Nature Switzerland AG 2022
A. Waśkiel-Burnat et al. (eds.), *Clinical Cases in Scalp Disorders*, Clinical Cases in Dermatology, https://doi.org/10.1007/978-3-030-93426-2_3

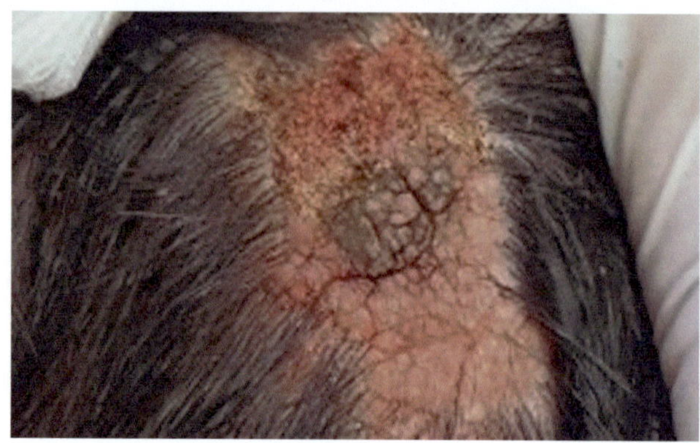

Fig. 3.1 A 28-year-old man with a yellowish, verrucous lesion on the scalp

Discussion

Nevus sebaceus is a congenital malformation, first described in 1895 by Josef Jadassohn, with an estimated incidence of less than 1/100,000 [1, 2]. It is a relatively uncommon hamartoma involving not only the pilosebaceus follicle but also the epidermis and often other adnexal structures [3]. Nevus sebaceus occurs without sex predilection [4]. Nevus sebaceus is most commonly located on the scalp (59.3%), but it has been described on other areas such as the face, neck or oral mucosa [5, 6]. Nevus sebaceus tends to evolve through three stages [7]. During infancy, nevus sebaceus typically appears as a smooth or velvety yellow-orange well-circumscribed plaque. Histologically, a paucity of underdeveloped sebaceous glands and hair follicles is noticed. At puberty, hormonal changes cause proliferation and hyperplasia of the lesion and lead to a larger and more verrucous appearance. The final stage is characterized by the appearance of nodules or tumors, with the presence of thin telangiectasias [8]. Light microscopy shows masses of hypertrophic sebaceous glands, with possible papillomatosis and hyperkeratosis of the overlying epidermis. In the third (late adult life), nevus sebaceus has a well-documented neoplastic potential [9]. The clinical signs suggesting neoplastic transformation include rapid enlargement or development of a nodularity or an ulceration [10]. Various types of appendegeal tumors, malignant and/or benign, such as basal cell carcinoma, syringocystadenoma papilliferum, trichoblastoma, and hidradenoma may develop secondarily within nevus sebaceus [11]. While multiple neoplasms may occasionally arise within the same lesion it is rare for four or more neoplasms to occur simultaneously [12]. A meta-analysis of 4900 cases of nevus sebaceus found that secondary tumors developed in 24% of patients; most commonly benign basaloid proliferations such as trichoblastomas [13].

The timing of surgical intervention is controversial. No definitive consensus on surgical intervention versus close observation exists. While smaller lesions may be technically easier to excise, younger patients may not be amenable to anesthesia. Secondary tumor transformation seems to be seen almost exclusively in adults patients.

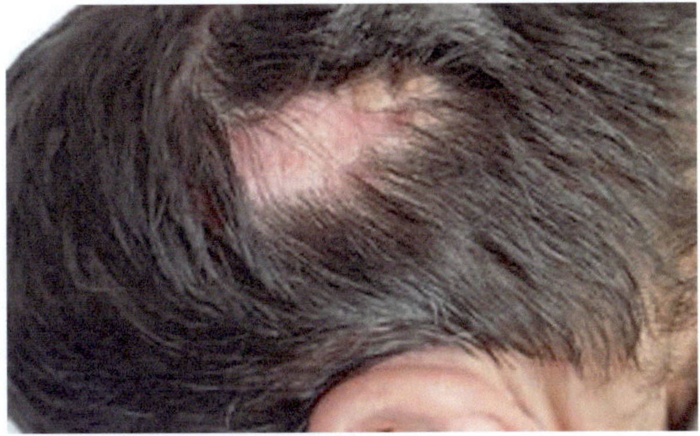

Fig. 3.2 The lesion after carbon dioxide laser therapy

In the presented patients, diagnosis of nevus sebaceus of Jadassohn was established. The patient did not consent to surgical therapy. He underwent a two series of carbon dioxide laser treatment with good effect (Fig. 3.2).

Key Points
- The differential diagnosis of nevus sebaceus depends on the stage of development.
- Generally, nevus sebaceus follows a benign course.
- The clinical signs suggesting neoplastic transformation include rapid enlargement or development of a nodularity or an ulceration.
- The progression and frequency of secondary tumors increases with age of the patient.
- The timing of surgical intervention is controversial.

References

1. Laino L, Steensel MA, Innocenzi D, Camplone G. Familial occurrence of nevus sebaceus of Jadassohn: another case of paradominant inheritance? Eur J Dermatol. 2001;11:97–8.
2. Weyers W. Josef Jadassohn—an appreciation on the occasion of his 150th birthday. Am J Dermatopathol. 2013;35:742–51.
3. West C, Narahari S, Kwatra S, Feldman S. Autosomal dominant transmission of nevus sebaceus of Jadassohn. Dermatol Online J. 2012;18:17.
4. Happle R, Konig A. Familial naevus sebaceus may be explained by paradominant transmission. Br J Dermatol. 1999;141:377.
5. Morency R, Labelle H. Nevus sebaceus of Jadassohn: a rare oral presentation. Oral Surg Oral Med Oral Pathol. 1987;64:460–2.
6. Al Hammadi A, Lebwohl MG. Nevus sebaceus. 2014. http://emedicine.medscape.com/article/1058733-overview. Accessed 20 May 2015.
7. Mehregan A, Pinkus H. Life history of organoid nevi. Special reference to nevus sebaceus of Jadassohn. Arch Dermatol. 1965;91:574–88.
8. Kim NH, Zell DS, Kolm I, Oliviero M, Rabinovitz HS. The dermoscopic differential diagnosis of yellow lobularlike structures. Arch Dermatol. 2008;144:962.

9. Jaqueti G, Requena L, Sánchez Yus E. Trichoblastoma is the most common neoplasm developed in nevus sebaceus of Jadassohn: a clinicopathologic study of a series of 155 cases. Am J Dermatopathol. 2000;22:108–18.
10. Miller CJ, Ioffreda MD, Billingsley EM. Sebaceous carcinoma, basal cell carcinoma, trichoadenoma, trichoblastoma, and syringocystadenoma papilliferum arising within a nevus sebaceus. Dermatol Surg. 2004;30:1546–9.
11. Elder DE, Elenitsas R, Johnson BL, Murphy GF. Lever's histopathology of the skin. 9th ed. Philadelphia: Lippincott Williams & Wilkins; 2005.
12. Stavrianeas NG, Katoulis AC, Stratigeas NP, Karagianni IN, Patertou-Stavrianea M, Varelzidis AG. Development of multiple tumors in a sebaceous nevus of Jadassohn. Dermatology. 1997;195:155–8.
13. Groesser L, Herschberger E, Ruetten A, et al. Postzygotic HRAS and KRAS mutations cause nevus sebaceous and Schimmelpenning syndrome. Nat Genet. 2012;44(7):783–8.

Chapter 4
A 2-Month-Old Boy with a Pigment Lesion on the Scalp

Anna Waśkiel-Burnat, Olga Warszawik-Hendzel, Małgorzata Olszewska, and Lidia Rudnicka

A two-month-old boy was consulted by a dermatologist to assess a dark-brown lesion on the scalp which was presented at birth. No dermatological on non-dermatological diseases were reported. There was no family history of similar skin lesion.

A physical examination revealed dark brown plaque on the right side of occipital area (Fig. 4.1). On dermoscopy, dark brown and brown structureless areas were observed (Fig. 4.2).

Based on the case description and the photographs, what is your diagnosis?

Differential Diagnoses
1. Mongolian spot.
2. Congential melanocytic nevus.
3. Nevus spilus.
4. Café-au-lait spots.

Diagnosis
Congenital melanocytic nevi.

Discussion

Congenital melanocytic nevi are melanocytic nevi that have their onset at birth or during the first two years of life [1]. They result from in-utero somatic mutations concerning genes that play a role in the mitogen-activated protein kinase (MAPK)

A. Waśkiel-Burnat (✉) · O. Warszawik-Hendzel · M. Olszewska · L. Rudnicka
Department of Dermatology, Medical University of Warsaw, Warsaw, Poland
e-mail: anna.waskiel@wum.edu.pl; olga.warszawik-hendzel@wum.edu.pl;
malgorzata.olszewska@wum.edu.pl; lidia.rudnicka@wum.edu.pl

A. Waśkiel-Burnat et al. (eds.), *Clinical Cases in Scalp Disorders*, Clinical Cases in Dermatology, https://doi.org/10.1007/978-3-030-93426-2_4

Fig. 4.1 A 2-month-old boy with a dark brown plaque on the right side of occipital area

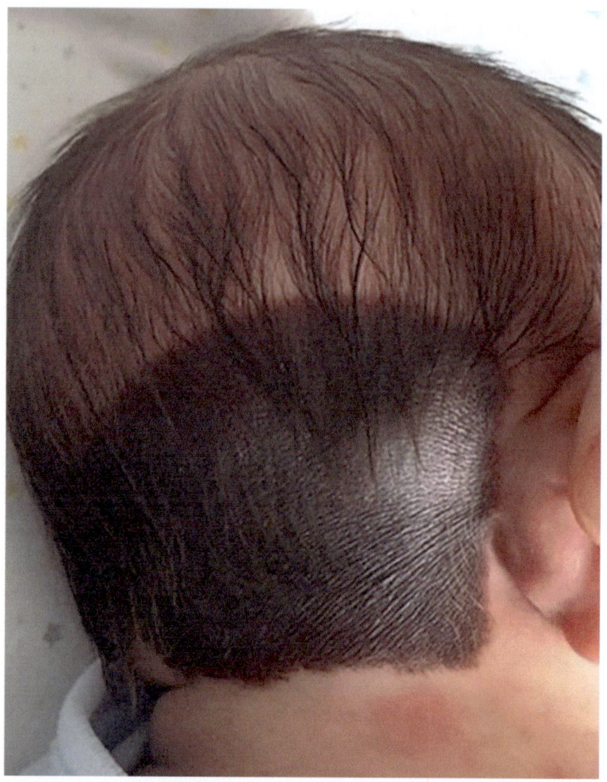

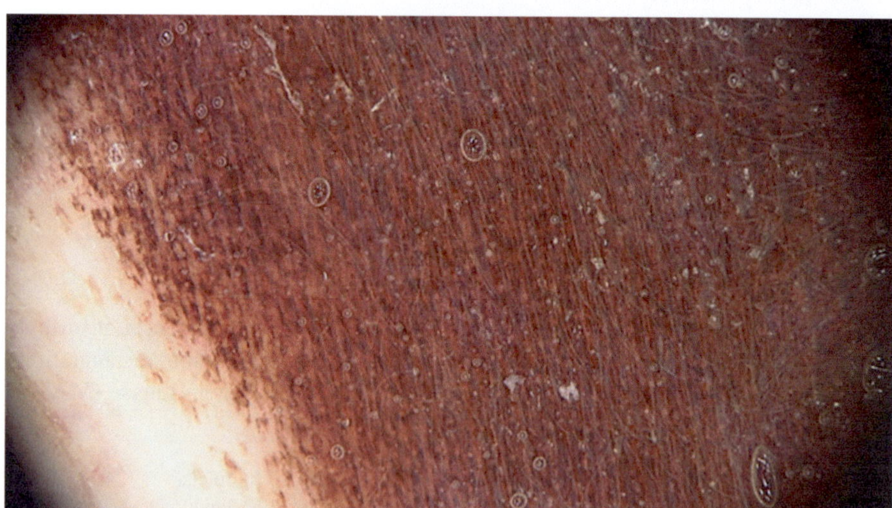

Fig. 4.2 Dermoscopy shows brown and dark brown structureless areas (×20)

pathway [2]. Congenital melanocytic nevi are relatively common with an incidence among newborns ranging between 0.2% and 6% [2]. There is a female predominance. Congenital melanocytic nevi initially present as pigmented macules or slightly raised oval papules or plaques. They usually darken over time and become raised or verrucous. Congenital melanocytic can display a wide variety of colors ranging from light brown to black. Hypertrichosis is commonly observed. Congenital melanocytic nevi usually grows proportionally with the child [1, 3]. Although often asymptomatic, larger lesions may have clinical features of xerosis, ulceration, pruritis, or skin erosions. Furthermore, the unsightly aesthetic appearance may cause significant psychosocial impacts on children and parents [1]. Congenital melanocytic nevi are classified according to their estimated adult size as small (<1.5 cm), medium (1.5–20 cm), large or giant (>20 cm) [3]. Giant nevi occasionally show satellite smaller lesions. Congenital melanocytic nevi may be associated with melanocyte proliferation in the central nervous system. In this case, neurological symptoms, including seizures, cranial nerve dysfunction, or signs and symptoms of increased intracranial pressure may be observed [3]. Moreover, large lesions have a higher risk of melanoma development. Congenital melanocytic nevi are usually diagnosed based on the clinical appearance. Dermoscopy or punch biopsy for histopathological examination may be used in cases of diagnostic doubt. Dermoscopy is characterized by the globular, structureless, reticular, or mixed patterns. A histopathological examination shows nevomelanocytes or nevus cells in the epidermis in well-ordered clusters as well as in the dermis as cords, sheets, or nests [3]. Treatment options may be divided into surgical and non-surgical. Non-surgical therapeutic options include dermal abrasion, chemical peels, cryotherapy, electrosurgery, and ablative lasers. These methods reduce pigmentation and improve the cosmetic appearance without fully removing nevi cell [3].

Differential diagnoses for the presented patient included Mongolian spot, nevus spilus and café-au-lait spots.

Mongolian spots are congenital birthmarks most commonly presented over the lumbosacral area. They are bluish-green to black in color and oval to irregular in shape. They most commonly affect individuals of African or Asian descent [4].

Nevus spilus presents as a well-circumscribed tan macule or patch with many smaller dark brown macules or papules scattered throughout the hyperpigmented background. Most commonly the lesions are acquired during infancy or childhood. The trunk and extremities are most commonly affected [5].

Café-au-lait spots present as uniform tan-brown round or oval macules with distinct margins and variable border. These lesions tend to enlarge in proportion to general body growth during the first several years of life and then stabilize. Regress in later years may be observed [6].

In the presented patient, based on the clinical and dermoscopic findings the diagnosis of congenital melanocytic nevi was established.

Key Points
- Congenital melanocytic nevi are melanocytic nevi that have their onset at birth or during the first two years of life.
- They present as pigmented macules or slightly raised oval papules or plaques. They usually darken over time and also become raised or verrucous.

References

1. Macneal P, Patel BC. Congenital melanocytic nevi. Treasure Island (FL): StatPearls; 2020.
2. Zayour M, Lazova R. Congenital melanocytic nevi. Clin Lab Med. 2011;31(2):267–80.
3. Navarro-Fernandez IN, Mahabal G. Congenital nevus. Treasure Island (FL): StatPearls; 2020.
4. Gupta D, Thappa DM. Mongolian spots: how important are they? World J Clin Cases. 2013;1(8):230–2.
5. Vaidya DC, Schwartz RA, Janniger CK. Nevus spilus. Cutis. 2007;80(6):465–8.
6. Taïeb A, Boralevi F. Hypermelanoses of the newborn and of the infant. Dermatol Clin. 2007;25(3):327–36. viii

Chapter 5
A 30-Year-Old Man of African Descent with Keloid-Like Plaques on the Nape of the Neck

Enechukwu Nkechi Anne

A 30-year-old man of African descent presented with a two-year history of progressively growing skin lesions on the nape of the neck. The patient complained of itching and burning sensation which increased after the haircuts. Moreover, occasional bleeding and pustular discharge were reported. The patient reported having frequent closely shaven haircuts. There was no fever, bone pain, or discharging swellings in the axilla. No history of acne vulgaris was reported. There was no family history of a similar condition.

A physical examination revealed firm keloid-like plaques with hairs loss on the nape of the neck (Fig. 5.1). On trichoscopy, peripheral hyperpigmentation and white areas with the absence of hair follicle openings in the central part of the keloidal plaques were observed (Fig. 5.2).

Based on the case description and the photographs, what is your diagnosis?

Differential Diagnoses
1. Folliculitis keloidalis nuchae.
2. Dissecting cellulitis of the scalp.
3. Follicultis decalvans.
4. Kerion.

Diagnosis
Folliculitis keloidalis nuchae.

E. N. Anne (✉)
Department of Dermatology and Venereology, Nnamdi Azikiwe University,
Nnewi, Anambra State, Nigeria
e-mail: na.enechukwu@unizik.edu.ng

© The Author(s), under exclusive license to Springer Nature
Switzerland AG 2022
A. Waśkiel-Burnat et al. (eds.), *Clinical Cases in Scalp Disorders*, Clinical
Cases in Dermatology, https://doi.org/10.1007/978-3-030-93426-2_5

Fig. 5.1 A 30-year-old man with keloid-like plaques on the nape of the neck

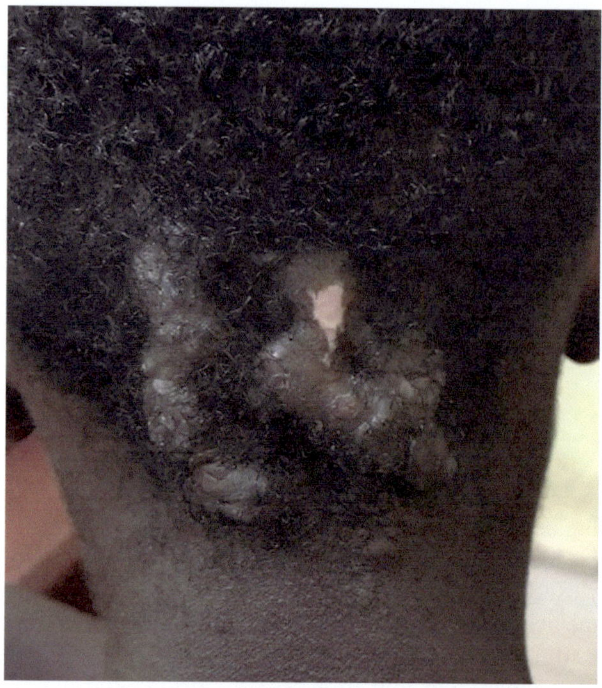

Fig. 5.2 Trichoscopy with the presence of peripheral hyperpigmentation and central white areas with the absence of hair follicle openings (×20)

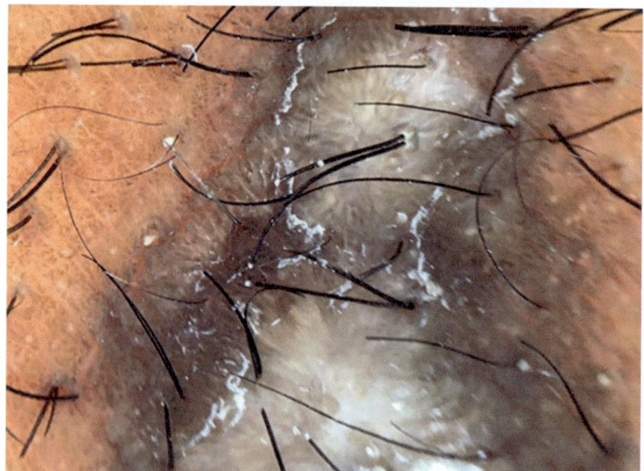

Discussion

Acne keloidalis nuchae, also known as folliculitis keloidalis nuchae, is a recurrent chronic follicular inflammation subsequently resulting in scarring alopecia [1]. The etiopathogenesis remains unclear. The role of androgens, obesity and genetic predisposition is hypothesized. Ingrown hair, trauma, infections, close shave haircuts, friction from collars and helmets are suggested as trigger factors [1–3]. Young men of African descent with tightly curled hair are most commonly affected. Clinically, in the early stages acne keloidalis nuchae is characterized by the presence of single or multiple smooth dome-shaped, firm, follicular papules and pustules progressing to keloid-like plaques associated with hair loss in later stages. In chronic, recurrent disease abscesses and purulent fistulas may be observed. Lesions occur mainly on the neck and occipital area of the scalp [4]. Pain, itching and burning sensation as well as bleeding are reported. Diagnosis of acne keloidalis nuchae is usually established based on clinical presentation. Trichoscopy at the early stage shows perifollicular pustules with peripilar white halo and dome-shaped often hyperpigmented papules while in advanced stages tufted hairs, loss of follicular openings and fibrotic white areas are seen. In histological examination, nonspecific granulation tissue with histiocytes, giant cells, and plasma cells are detected [5]. Traditional management of acne keloidalis nuchae focuses on preventing disease progression with avoidance of mechanical irritation and the use of antimicrobial cleansers to prevent secondary infection [6]. Pharmacological therapy includes topical and intralesional corticosteroids, topical and systemic antibiotics and retinoids. Severe and recalcitrant lesions may be amenable to surgery with or without postsurgical radiotherapy, electro- and cryosurgeries and laser therapy [6].

The differential diagnoses for the presented patient included folliculitis decalvans, dissecting cellulitis and tinea capitis profunda.

Folliculitis decalvans is a type of primary neutrophilic cicatricial alopecia [5]. It is commonly seen among middle-aged men of African descent but the disease also occurs in Caucasians [7]. Clinically, the disease is characterized by follicular papules and pustules with tufted hairs. Subsequently scarring is observed [8]. In folliculitis decalvans, lesions are not restricted to the occipital area and they are commonly observed on the vertex region. Moreover, other hair bearing areas such as beard, neck, axillary and pubic region may be affected [5].

Dissecting cellulitis is a primary neutrophilic scarring hair loss which almost exclusively occurs in young men of African descent [5]. The disease may occur alone or as a component of the follicular occlusion tetrad (hidradenitis suppurativa, acne conglobate, dissecting cellulitis and pilonidal cyst) [8]. Dissecting cellulitis presents as follicular papules and pustules which progress to form deep seated fluctuant nodules, abscesses and large sinuses leading to scarring alopecia. The vertex and occipital areas are most commonly affected [8].

Kerion is a form of inflammatory tinea capitis mainly observed in the prepubertal population [9]. It presents as a painful, crusty carbuncle-like boggy plaque with subsequent scarring. It usually occurs as a solitary lesion, most commonly on the occipital area [10].

Based on the patient's history and clinical presentation, the diagnosis of acne keloidalis nuchae was established. The patient was treated with intralesional corticosteroids and oral doxycycline. The avoidance of frequent close hair shaving, tight collars and helmets was recommended.

Key Points
- Acne keloidalis nuchae occurs mainly in young men of African descent.
- The disease is characterized by the presence of follicular papules and pustules progressing to keloid-like plaques associated with hair loss.
- The neck and occipital area are most commonly affected.

References

1. Ogunbiyi A. Acne keloidalis nuchae: prevalence, impact, and management challenges. Clin Cosmet Investig Dermatol. 2016;9:483–9.
2. Ogunbiyi A, Adedokun B. Perceived aetiological factors of folliculitis keloidalis nuchae (acne keloidalis) and treatment options among Nigerian men. Br J Dermatol. 2015;173(Suppl 2):22–5.
3. Matsunaga AM, Tortelly VD, Machado CJ, Pedrosa LR, Melo DF. High frequency of obesity in acne keloidalis nuchae patients: a hypothesis from a Brazilian study. Skin Appendage Disord. 2020;6(6):374–8.
4. East-Innis ADC, Stylianou K, Paolino A, Ho JD. Acne keloidalis nuchae: risk factors and associated disorders – a retrospective study. Int J Dermatol. 2017;56(8):828–32.
5. Kanti V, Rowert-Huber J, Vogt A, Blume-Peytavi U. Cicatricial alopecia. J Dtsch Dermatol Ges. 2018;16(4):435–61.
6. Maranda EL, Simmons BJ, Nguyen AH, Lim VM, Keri JE. Treatment of acne keloidalis nuchae: a systematic review of the literature. Dermatol Ther. 2016;6(3):363–78.
7. Ross EK, Vincenzi C, Tosti A. Videodermoscopy in the evaluation of hair and scalp disorders. J Am Acad Dermatol. 2006;55(5):799–806.
8. Fanti PA, Baraldi C, Misciali C, Piraccini BM. Cicatricial alopecia. G Ital Dermatol Venereol. 2018;153(2):230–42.
9. Stein LL, Adams EG, Holcomb KZ. Inflammatory tinea capitis mimicking dissecting cellulitis in a postpubertal male: a case report and review of the literature. Mycoses. 2013;56(5):596–600.
10. John AM, Schwartz RA, Janniger CK. The kerion: an angry tinea capitis. Int J Dermatol. 2018;57(1):3–9.

Chapter 6
A 30-Year-Old Man with Recurrent Scaling and Itching of the Scalp

Agnieszka Kaczorowska and Anna Waśkiel-Burnat

A 30-year-old man presented with a four-year history of a recurrent scaling on the scalp and greasy hair. Moreover, he complained of an intensive itch. The condition tended to intensify during winter and improve during summer, especially after sun exposure. He denied connection between symptoms and certain shampoos, hair conditioners, hair dyes, hairstyling products or headgears. Patient had suffered from depression for ten years. No family history of dermatological diseases was reported.

A physical examination of the scalp revealed a diffuse erythema with yellowish, greasy scales (Fig. 6.1). On trichoscopy, a yellowish, diffuse scaling and thin arborizing vessels were detected (Fig. 6.2).

Based on the case description and the photographs, what is your diagnosis?

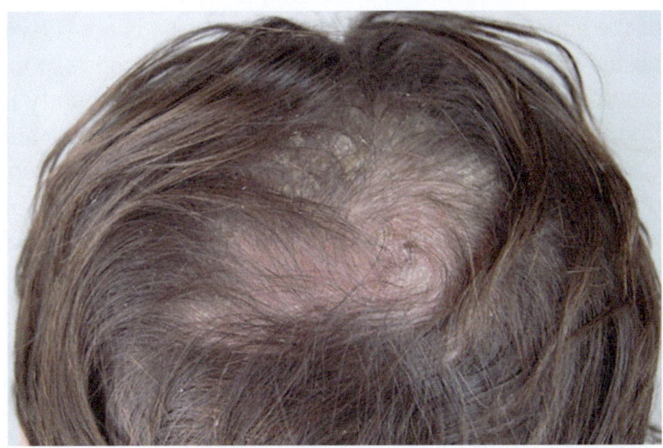

Fig. 6.1 A 30-year-old man with a diffuse erythema and yellowish, greasy scales on the scalp

A. Kaczorowska (✉) · A. Waśkiel-Burnat
Department of Dermatology, Medical University of Warsaw, Warsaw, Poland
e-mail: agnieszka.kaczorowska@wum.edu.pl; anna.waskiel@wum.edu.pl

© The Author(s), under exclusive license to Springer Nature Switzerland AG 2022
A. Waśkiel-Burnat et al. (eds.), *Clinical Cases in Scalp Disorders*, Clinical Cases in Dermatology, https://doi.org/10.1007/978-3-030-93426-2_6

Fig. 6.2 Trichoscopy with the presence of yellowish scaling (×20)

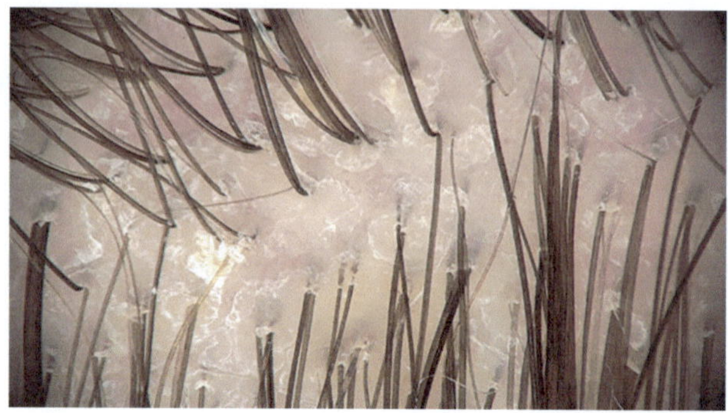

Differential Diagnoses

1. Psoriasis.
2. Seborrheic dermatitis.
3. Tinea capitis.
4. Contact dermatitis.

Diagnosis

Seborrheic dermatitis.

Discussion

Seborrheic dermatitis is a chronic, inflammatory skin disorder which affects 3–10% of the general population. The pathogenesis is not fully understood. It has been suggested that the condition is caused by an altered response to *Malassezia* yeasts and their metabolites. Seborrheic dermatitis occurs mainly in infants (usually within the first three months of life), adolescents, young adults and the elderly. Men are more commonly affected compared to women [1]. The condition is more frequently reported in immunocompromised patients (organ transplant recipients, patients with HIV/AIDS or chronic alcoholic pancreatitis), patients with neurological and psychiatric diseases (Parkinson's disease, depression, epilepsy) and patients with Down syndrome [2]. It is characterized by the presence of erythematous plaques with greasy, yellowish scales and no hair loss [2]. Usually, a mild itch is present. Lesions are located in areas with a high concentration of sebaceous glands, such as the scalp (mainly the vertex and parietal areas), nasolabial folds, ears, eyebrows, chest, back, axilla and groin [2, 3]. Seborrheic dermatitis tends to intensify with stress and in winter months and to improve in summertime. The diagnosis of seborrheic dermatitis is usually established clinically. In case of ambiguity trichoscopy and histopathology can be helpful. The most characteristic trichoscopic features of seborrheic dermatitis include an increased number of thin, arborizing vessels and yellowish scales [4]. A histopathological examination shows acanthosis, focal spongiosis and parakeratosis [1]. In the treatment of scalp seborrheic dermatitis, shampoos containing selenium sulfide, zinc pyrithione, coal tar or antifungal agents are commonly used. In case of more severe inflammation, topical corticosteroids can be beneficial. If seborrheic dermatitis is particularly widespread or refractory, an oral treatment with antifungal agents or isotretinoin may be added [5].

Differential diagnoses for the presented case included psoriasis, tinea capitis and contact dermatitis.

Psoriasis is the main differential diagnosis. The condition affects mainly the extensor surfaces of the elbows and knees, scalp, and lower back. Scalp psoriasis is characterized by the presence of red, thickened plaques with a silvery-white scale, along with the hairline or extending onto the forehead, ears, and posterior neck. The frontal and occipital areas are most commonly affected. Itch may be reported [6]. The term 'sebopsoriasis' corresponds to an overlap between seborrheic dermatitis and psoriasis [4].

Another differential diagnosis is tinea capitis, a fungal infection of the scalp that affects mainly children. The disease is characterized by the presence of hair loss areas with coexisting scaling, inflammation or pustules [7]. Itch is usually reported [4].

Contact dermatitis is an inflammatory eczematous skin disease. The disease is rarely present on the scalp area, because of great thickness of the epidermis in this region. In case of application of irritants or allergens on the scalp, symptoms are usually observed on the face or neck. Clinically, contact dermatitis presents as an erythema with scaling and coexisting itch [8]. In acute disease, vesicles or pustules may be present.

In the presented patient, the diagnosis of seborrheic dermatitis was established based on the clinical picture. Treatment with ketoconazole shampoo and topical mometasone furoate twice a week was recommended. Resolution of skin lesions was achieved.

Key Points
- Seborrheic dermatitis is a common inflammatory condition of the scalp.
- It presents as an erythema with a yellowish scaling and coexisting itch.

References

1. Naldi L, Diphoorn J. Seborrhoeic dermatitis of the scalp. BMJ Clin Evid. 2015;2015:1713.
2. Borda LJ, Wikramanayake TC. Seborrheic dermatitis and dandruff: a comprehensive review. J Clin Investig Dermatol. 2015;3(2) https://doi.org/10.13188/2373-1044.1000019.
3. Tucker D, Masood S. Seborrheic dermatitis. Treasure Island (FL): StatPearls; 2020.
4. Rudnicka L, Olszewska M, Rakowska A. Atlas of trichocopy: dermoscopy in hair and scalp disease. London: Springer; 2012.
5. Borda LJ, Perper M, Keri JE. Treatment of seborrheic dermatitis: a comprehensive review. J Dermatolog Treat. 2019;30(2):158–69.
6. Blakely K, Gooderham M. Management of scalp psoriasis: current perspectives. Psoriasis (Auckl). 2016;6:33–40.

7. Adesiji YO, Omolade FB, Aderibigbe IA, Ogungbe O, Adefioye OA, Adedokun SA, et al. Prevalence of tinea capitis among children in Osogbo, Nigeria, and the associated risk factors. Diseases. 2019;7(1):13.
8. Rozas-Muñoz E, Gamé D, Serra-Baldrich E. Allergic contact dermatitis by anatomical regions: diagnostic clues. Actas Dermosifiliogr. 2018;109(6):485–507.

Chapter 7
A 32-Year-Old Woman with an Intense Pruritus of the Scalp

Sylwia Chrostowska, Joanna Golińska, and Aleksandra Wielgoś

A 32-year-old woman presented with a few-week history of intense pruritus of the scalp. The patient was a kindergarten teacher for the year. No personal history of dermatological and non-dermatological conditions was reported. The patient's sister suffered from seborrheic dermatitis.

A physical examination revealed excoriations, erythema and mild scaling on the scalp and posterior neck. Moreover, nits and lice were observed. On trichoscopy, lice, brown and translucent ovoid eggs attached to the hair shaft were detected (Figs. 7.1 and 7.2).

Based on the case description and the photographs, what is your diagnosis?

Differential Diagnoses
1. Pediculosis capitis (head lice).
2. Tinea capitis.
3. Psoriasis.
4. Seborrheic dermatitis.

Diagnosis
Pediculosis capitis (head lice).

Discussion

Head lice are obligate ectoparasites that infect the scalp area. Pediculosis capitis is found worldwide with no limitations based upon age, sex, race, or socioeconomic class. The main route of transmission is direct head-to-head contact. Head lice are

S. Chrostowska (✉) · J. Golińska · A. Wielgoś
Department of Dermatology, Medical University of Warsaw, Warsaw, Poland
e-mail: sylwia.chrostowska@wum.edu.pl; joanna.golinska@wum.edu.pl

A. Waśkiel-Burnat et al. (eds.), *Clinical Cases in Scalp Disorders*, Clinical Cases in Dermatology, https://doi.org/10.1007/978-3-030-93426-2_7

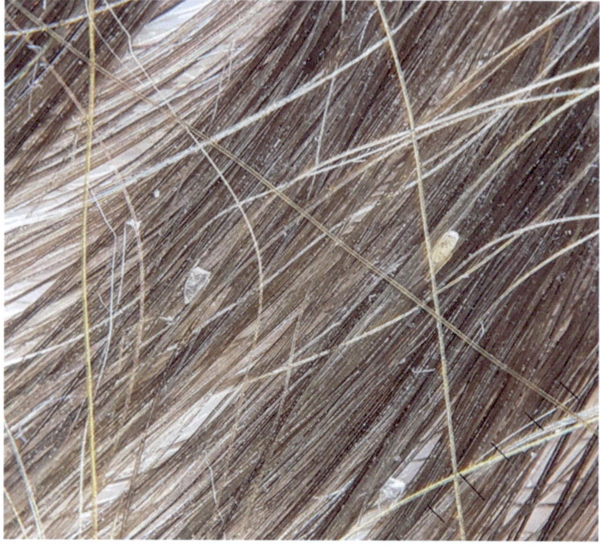

Fig. 7.1 Trichoscopy with brown and translucent ovoid eggs attached to the hair shaft (×10)

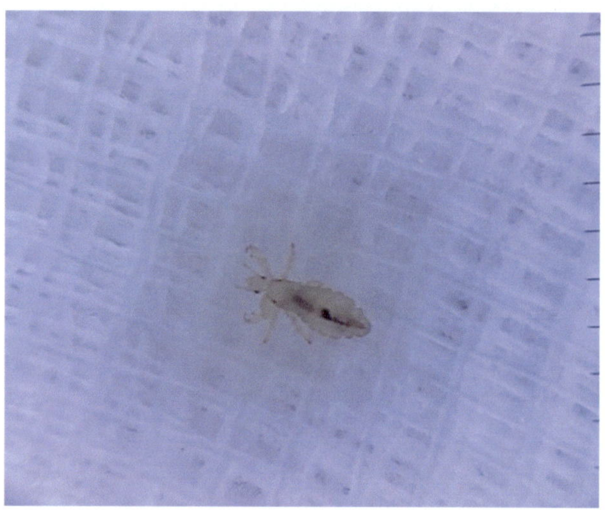

Fig. 7.2 Trichoscopy shows a louse (×10)

approximately 2–3 mm long parasites that feed on the human blood approximately every four to six hour. The female louse lives for 30 days, during which time she lays between five and ten eggs a day on hair shafts. Pediculosis capitis most commonly affects children between three and 11 years of age. It is characterized by the presence of excoriations, erythema and scaling on the scalp and posterior neck. Itching and burning sensation are reported. In case of secondary bacterial infection, a low-grade fever and local lymphadenopathy may occur. Diagnosis is made by the identification of nits and/or lice on the scalp hair. Viable eggs are usually tan to brown in color, while hatched eggs are clear to white. Dermoscopy may help to better visualize nits and lice. In treatment of pediculisis capitis, pyrethrins synergized with piperonyl butoxide or permethrin cream/lotion are commonly used. Benzyl alcohol lotion, dimethicone, spinosad cream rinse and ivermectin solution are also recommended. Another therapeutic option for head lice is oral ivermectin [1].

In the presented patient, tinea capitis, psoriasis and seborrheic dermatosis were included in the differential diagnosis.

Tinea capitis is a fungal infection of the scalp that affects mainly children. The disease is characterized by the presence of hair loss areas with coexisted scaling, inflammation or pustules. Itch is usually reported [2].

Scalp psoriasis is characterized by the presence of red, thickened plaques with a silver-white scale, either contained within the hairline, or extending onto the forehead, ears, and posterior neck. The frontal and occipital areas are most commonly affected. Itch may be reported [3].

Seborrheic dermatitis presents as well-delimited erythematous plaques with greasy-looking, yellowish scales [4]. Itching sensation is usually presented [5]. Seborrheic dermatitis is characterized by a seasonal pattern, presenting more frequently during winter, and improving usually during summer [5].

In the presented patient, based on clinical presentation and the presence of nits on hair shafts, the diagnosis of pediculosis capitis was established. The patient was successfully treated with permethrin lotion.

Key Points
- Pediculosis capitis is a common parasite infection of the scalp.
- It is characterized by the presence of excoriations, erythema and scaling on the scalp and posterior neck with coexisted pruritus.

References

1. Bolognia JL, et al. Dermatology. 4th ed. Elsevier, Section 12, Chapter 84 Infection, Infestations and Bites; 2018. p. 1507–9.
2. Adesiji YO, Omolade FB, Aderibigbe IA, Ogungbe O, Adefioye OA, Adedokun SA, et al. Prevalence of tinea capitis among children in Osogbo, Nigeria, and the associated risk factors. Diseases. 2019;7(1):13.
3. Blakely K, Gooderham M. Management of scalp psoriasis: current perspectives. Psoriasis (Auckl). 2016;6:33–40.
4. Clark GW, Pope SM, Jaboori KA. Diagnosis and treatment of seborrheic dermatitis. Am Fam Physician. 2015;91(3):185–90.
5. Borda LJ, Wikramanayake TC. Seborrheic dermatitis and dandruff: a comprehensive review. J Clin Investig Dermatol. 2015;3(2).

Chapter 8
A 32-Year-Old Woman with Itching and Burning Sensation of the Scalp

Anna Waśkiel-Burnat, Małgorzata Olszewska, and Lidia Rudnicka

A 32-year-old woman presented with a six-month history of itching and burning sensation of the occipital area of the scalp. No personal history of dermatologic diseases was reported. The patient had depression since three years.

A physical examination revealed hair loss area on the occipital region with the presence of broken hair at the same level above the scalp. Moreover, an erosion with surrounding fibrosis was detected (Fig. 8.1). On trichoscopy uniform in length broom hairs were presented (Fig. 8.2). Moreover, an erosion surrounded by white areas lacking of follicular openings was observed.

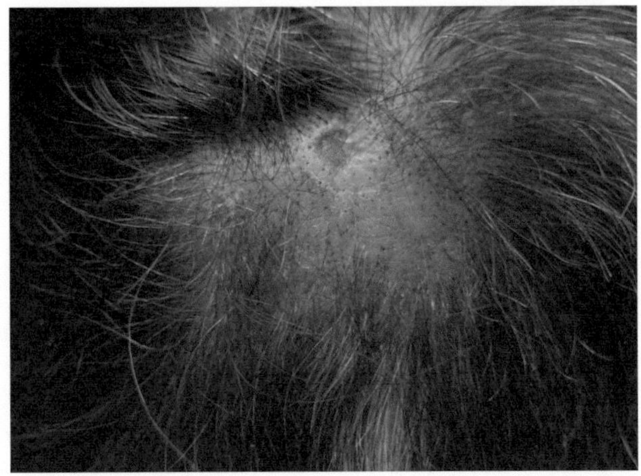

Fig. 8.1 A 32-year-old woman with localized hair loss on the occipital area. Broken hair at the same level above the scalp and an erosion surrounded by fibrosis is presented

A. Waśkiel-Burnat (✉) · M. Olszewska · L. Rudnicka
Department of Dermatology, Medical University of Warsaw, Warsaw, Poland
e-mail: anna.waskiel@wum.edu.pl; malgorzata.olszewska@wum.edu.pl;
lidia.rudnicka@wum.edu.pl

A. Waśkiel-Burnat et al. (eds.), *Clinical Cases in Scalp Disorders*, Clinical Cases in Dermatology, https://doi.org/10.1007/978-3-030-93426-2_8

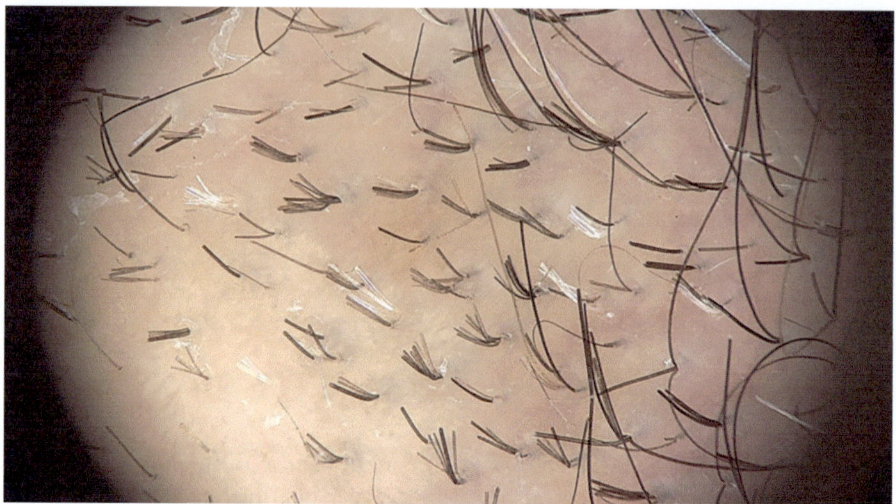

Fig. 8.2 Trichoscopy with the presence of uniform in length broom hairs (×20)

Based on the case description and the photographs, what is your diagnosis?

Differential Diagnoses
1. Scalp dysesthesia.
2. Tinea capitis.
3. Trichotillomania.
4. Lichen planopilaris.

Diagnosis
Scalp dysesthesia.

Discussion

Scalp dysesthesia is a syndrome characterized by abnormal sensations (such as burning, stinging or itching) of the scalp in the absence of any objective dermatological findings [1]. Pathogenesis of scalp dysesthesia is not fully described. However, it has reported that symptoms can be exacerbated by psychological or physical stress; may be manifestations of an underlying psychiatric disorder; or may represent a type of chronic pain syndrome [1]. Scalp dysesthesia is more commonly described in patients with cervical spine abnormalities [1]. The condition more commonly affects women compared to men [3]. The signs of scalp dysesthesia are a consequences of repeated rubbing and scratching (trichoteiromania) [2]. The vertex area is most commonly affected [2]. The diagnosis of scalp dysesthesia is mainly established based on clinical picture. Trichoscopy can be helpful to confirm diagnosis. Characteristic trichoscopic markers of scalp dysesthesia are uniform in length broom hairs, block hairs and short hairs with trichorrhexis nodosa [2]. Topical corticosteroids and oral antihistamines are most commonly used for scalp dysesthesia treatment. Pregabalin, gabapentin and low-dose antidepressants may be effective [1, 3].

In the presented case, tinea capitis, trichotillomania and lichen planopilaris were included into differential diagnosis.

Lichen planopilaris presents as cicatricial alopecia with the presence of perifollicular erythema and follicular hyperkeratosis and the periphery. It predominantly affects the vertex or parietal areas of the scalp [3]. The disease is mostly diagnosed in women between 40 and 60 years of age.

Tinea capitis is a cutaneous fungal infection or dermatophytosis of the scalp [4]. It is the most commonly observed in children between three and seven years of age [5]. Clinically, it presents as hair loss areas with coexisted scaling, inflammation or pustules [6].

Trichotillomania (hair-pulling disorder) is defined as hair loss from a patient's repetitive self-pulling of hair [7]. Clinically, it presents as non-scarring hair loss area with the presence of different length hair. The parietal area is most commonly affected. Trichotillomania beyond the scalp may also involve eyebrows, eyelashes, and pubic hairs [7].

The patient was diagnosed with scalp dysesthesia. Treatment with topical mometasone furoate once a day was initiated.

Key Points
- Scalp dysesthesia is characterized by abnormal sensations of the scalp (such as burning, stinging or itching).
- The dermatologic signs of scalp dysesthesia are a consequences of repeated rubbing and scratching (trichoteiromania).

References

1. Laidler NK, Chan J. Treatment of scalp dysesthesia utilising simple exercises and stretches: a pilot study. Australas J Dermatol. 2018;59(4):318–21.
2. Rakowska A, Olszewska M, Rudnicka L. Trichoscopy of scalp dysesthesia. Adv Dermatol Allergol Postępy Dermatologii i Alergologii. 2017;34(3):245–7.
3. Kinoshita-Ise M, Shear NH. Diagnostic and therapeutic approach to scalp dysesthesia: a case series and published work review. J Dermatol. 2019;46(6):526–30.
4. Fuller LC, Barton RC, Mohd Mustapa MF, Proudfoot LE, Punjabi SP, Higgins EM. British Association of Dermatologists' guidelines for the management of tinea capitis 2014. Br J Dermatol. 2014;171(3):454–63.
5. Michaels BD, Del Rosso JQ. Tinea capitis in infants: recognition, evaluation, and management suggestions. J Clin Aesthet Dermatol. 2012;5(2):49–59.
6. Adesiji YO, Omolade FB, Aderibigbe IA, Ogungbe O, Adefioye OA, Adedokun SA, et al. Prevalence of tinea capitis among children in Osogbo, Nigeria, and the associated risk factors. Diseases. 2019;7(1):13.
7. Sah DE, Koo J, Price VH. Trichotillomania. Dermatol Ther. 2008;21(1):13–21.

Chapter 9
A 33-Year-Old Woman with Brain Metastases of Unknown Origin and a Melanotic Lesion on the Scalp

Małgorzata Maj, Olga Warszawik-Hendzel, Małgorzata Olszewska, and Lidia Rudnicka

A 33-year-old woman with brain metastases of unknown origin was consulted in the Department of Dermatology. There was no personal of family history of skin cancer.

A physical examination of the scalp revealed an atypical pigmented skin lesion (5 cm × 5 cm) with irregular borders, nodules and multiple, variable colors (black, brown, grey, white, pink, purple and yellow) located on the right temporal area (Fig. 9.1). On dermoscopy, multiple brown and black dots, irregular structures, blue-white veil, pseudopods, scar-like depigmentation, irregular linear vessels as well as hairpin and dotted vessels were observed (Fig. 9.2).

Based on the case description and the photographs, what is your diagnosis?

Differential Diagnoses
1. Melanoma.
2. Pigmented basal cell carcinoma.
3. Seborrheic keratosis.
4. Melanotic nevus.

Diagnosis
Melanoma.

M. Maj (✉) · O. Warszawik-Hendzel · M. Olszewska · L. Rudnicka
Department of Dermatology, Medical University of Warsaw, Warsaw, Poland
e-mail: malgorzata.maj@wum.edu.pl; olga.warszawik-hendzel@wum.edu.pl; malgorzata.olszewska@wum.edu.pl; lidia.rudnicka@wum.edu.pl

© The Author(s), under exclusive license to Springer Nature Switzerland AG 2022
A. Waśkiel-Burnat et al. (eds.), *Clinical Cases in Scalp Disorders*, Clinical Cases in Dermatology, https://doi.org/10.1007/978-3-030-93426-2_9

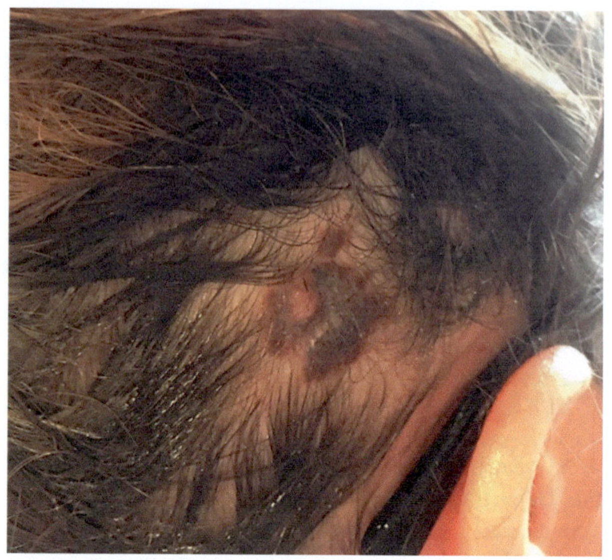

Fig. 9.1 A 33-year-old woman with an typical pigmented skin lesion with irregular borders, nodules and multiple, variable colors located on the right temporal area

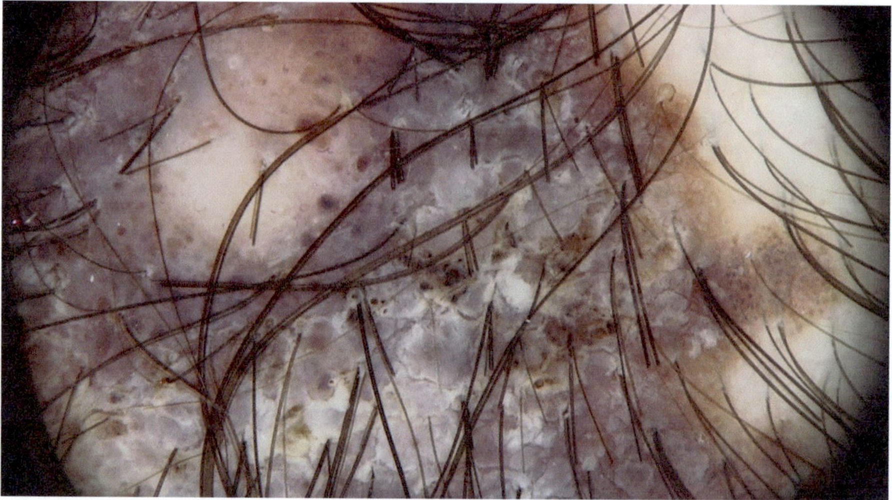

Fig. 9.2 Dermoscopy with the presence of black dots, irregular structures, blue-white veil and scar-like depigmentation (×20)

Discussion

Melanoma is the most fatal form of skin cancer [1]. Older age, low Fitzgerald skin phototypes, multiple (100) nevi, personal and family history of skin cancer, and personal history of intense ultraviolet exposure are the most critical risk factors for melanoma development [1–3]. Melanoma most commonly affects the elderly.

However, it is the third most common cancer in adolescents and young adults ages 15–39 years [4]. The typical cutaneous melanoma occurs as an asymmetric macule or nodule with irregular borders, frequently with variations in color within the lesion. It may also presents as a pink or red lesion (amelanotic melanoma) [1]. Based on the growth pattern melanoma is classified into superficial spreading, nodular, lentigo maligna, and acral. Histopathology is a gold standard diagnostic method in melanoma. Dermoscopy is helpful to establish initial diagnosis. Characteristic dermoscopic features of cutaneous melanoma include atypical pigment network, angulated lines, negative network, atypical streaks and atypical dots/globules. Blue-white veil, atypical blotches, regression structures, peripheral tan structureless areas, shiny white structures and atypical vascular structures are also melanoma-specific findings [5]. In histopathological examination, nests of atypical melanocytes within the epidermis and/or dermis are observed [2]. Atypical melanocytes may be detected higher up in the epidermis, termed, pagetoid spread. There may be also continuous atypical melanocytes along the dermal-epidermal junction, termed lentiginous proliferation. Markers for melanocytic differentiation, used to highlight melanocytes include HMB-45, Melan-A/Mart 1, MITF, and Sox-10. In histopathology, the invasion depth (Breslow thickness) should be evaluated as it considered to be the most important prognostic indicator which guides treatment [3]. In melanoma wide local excision is recommended. Melanoma in-situ should be excised with margins of 5 mm–1 cm, melanoma <1 mm thick with 1 cm margins, melanoma 1 mm–2 mm thick with 1–2 cm margins and melanoma >2 mm thick with 2 cm margins.

Scalp melanomas account for 7% of all melanomas [6]. Hair loss, chronic sun damage and history of skin cancer are well-recognized risk factors for developing the scalp melanoma. Similarly, to cutaneous melanoma on the other areas, the scalp melanoma occurs mostly in the elderly, with average age ranging from 50 to 67 years. Men are more commonly affected compared to women [7]. The scalp melanoma is characterized by more aggressive biologic behavior and is often diagnosed at a late stage. Indeed, patients with the scalp melanoma have poorer outcome and are in particularly high risk of brain metastasis compared to patients with melanoma on other head and neck areas [6]. Similarly to melanoma in other areas, wide local excision is recommended. Scalp melanoma in situ should be excised with 5 mm margins, melanoma <1 mm thick with 1 cm margins, melanoma 1–4 mm thick with 2 cm margins and melanoma >4 mm thick with 3 cm margins [6].

Differential diagnoses for the presented patient included pigmented basal cell carcinoma, seborrheic keratosis and melanotic nevus.

Basal cell carcinoma is the most common type of skin malignancy. The incidence rate of the disease increases with age. Basal cell carcinoma presents as a tiny, hardly visible papule, growing into a nodule or a plaque that is sometimes ulcerated. The face, scalp or neck areas are most commonly affected. Basal cell carcinoma on the scalp tends to present more pigmented compared to other body sites [8].

Seborrheic keratosis results from benign clonal expansion of epidermal keratinocytes. It is most common in the middle-aged and elderly, however it may also present in young adults. Typical lesion is sharply demarcated, round or oval-shaped, elevated and stuck on the skin with a verrucous, dull, uneven, or punched-out surface. The color of the lesions varies from skin color, yellowish, light to dark brown, grey, and black. Seborrheic keratosis may present as an isolated or multiple lesions. The chest, back, scalp (mainly the temporal areas) and neck are most commonly affected [9].

The scalp is an anatomical location for nevi with site-related atypia, a subset of melanocytic nevi that share histologic features with melanoma but are benign. The clinical patterns of the scalp melanocytic nevi are solid brown, solid pink, eclipse and cockade. The lesions are most commonly presented on the vertex and parietal areas [10].

Based on patient's history, clinical and dermoscopic findings initial diagnosis of melanoma was established. The patient was referred for surgical removal of the lesion. A histopathological examination confirmed clinical diagnosis of melanoma with pT3a, Breslow 2.3 mm and BRAF V600 mutation.

Key Points
- Scalp melanomas account for 7% of all melanomas.
- Scalp melanoma presents as an asymmetric macule or nodule with irregular borders, frequently with variations in color within the lesion; it may also presents as pink or red lesion.
- Scalp melanoma is characterized by more aggressive biologic behavior and is often diagnosed at a late stage.

References

1. Kibbi N, Kluger H, Choi JN. Melanoma: clinical presentations. Cancer Treat Res. 2016;167:107–29.
2. Leonardi GC, Falzone L, Salemi R, Zanghì A, Spandidos DA, McCubrey JA, et al. Cutaneous melanoma: from pathogenesis to therapy (review). Int J Oncol. 2018;52(4):1071–80.
3. Hartman RI, Lin JY. Cutaneous melanoma-a review in detection, staging, and management. Hematol Oncol Clin North Am. 2019;33(1):25–38.
4. O'Neill CH, Scoggins CR. Melanoma. J Surg Oncol. 2019;120(5):873–81.
5. Marghoob NG, Liopyris K, Jaimes N. Dermoscopy: a review of the structures that facilitate melanoma detection. J Am Osteopath Assoc. 2019;119(6):380–90.
6. Saaiq M, Zalaudek I, Rao B, Lee Y, Rudnicka L, Czuwara J, et al. A brief synopsis on scalp melanoma. Dermatol Ther. 2020;33(4):e13795.
7. Terakedis BE, Anker CJ, Leachman SA, Andtbacka RH, Bowen GM, Sause WT, et al. Patterns of failure and predictors of outcome in cutaneous malignant melanoma of the scalp. J Am Acad Dermatol. 2014;70(3):435–42.
8. Marzuka AG, Book SE. Basal cell carcinoma: pathogenesis, epidemiology, clinical features, diagnosis, histopathology, and management. Yale J Biol Med. 2015;88(2):167–79.
9. Hafner C, Vogt T. Seborrheic keratosis. J Dtsch Dermatol Ges. 2008;6(8):664–77.
10. Tcheung WJ, Bellet JS, Prose NS, Cyr DD, Nelson KC. Clinical and dermoscopic features of 88 scalp naevi in 39 children. Br J Dermatol. 2011;165(1):137–43.

Chapter 10
A 34-Year Man with Verrucous Lesion on the Scalp

Paulina Chmielińska, Aleksandra Wielgoś, and Agnieszka Kaczorowska

A 34-year old man presented with an elevated solitary lesion on the scalp. The lesion occurred at birth and was slowly growing during puberty. The patient reported occasional bleeding from the lesion that usually occurs after hair brushing. Family history of dermatological diseases was negative.

A physical examination of the scalp revealed a 3 cm × 1.5 cm verrucous, yellowish lesion with coexisted hair loss on the occipital area (Fig. 10.1). On dermoscopic examination, yellowish globules aggregated in clusters on the erythematous background were observed (Fig. 10.2).

Based on the case description and the photographs, what is your diagnosis?

Differential Diagnoses
1. Juvenile xanthogranuloma.
2. Nevus sebaceous of Jadassohn.
3. Verrucous epidermal nevus.
4. Basal cell carcinoma.

Diagnosis
Nevus sebaceous of Jadassohn.

Discussion

Nevus sebaceous of Jadassohn is congenital hamartomatous lesion with an epithelial and adnexal origin presents in 0.3% of the general population [1]. Women and men are equally affected. The lesion is usually located on the head and neck areas.

P. Chmielińska (✉) · A. Wielgoś · A. Kaczorowska
Department of Dermatology, Medical University of Warsaw, Warsaw, Poland
e-mail: agnieszka.kaczorowska@wum.edu.pl

A. Waśkiel-Burnat et al. (eds.), *Clinical Cases in Scalp Disorders*, Clinical Cases in Dermatology, https://doi.org/10.1007/978-3-030-93426-2_10

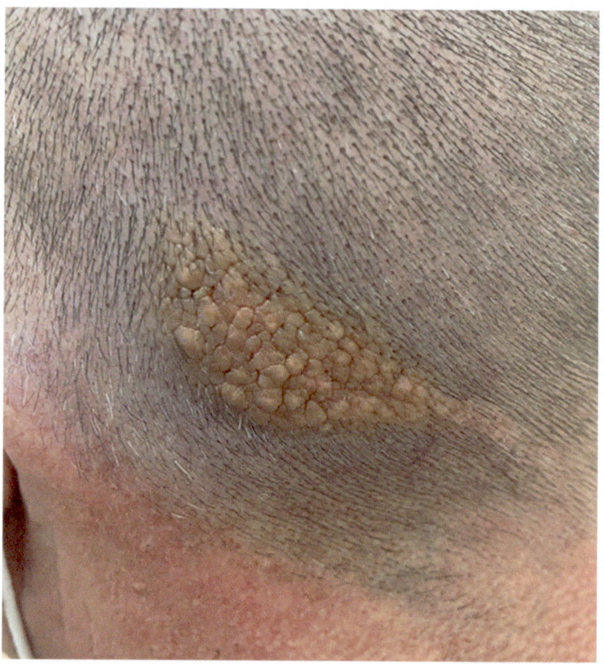

Fig. 10.1 A 34-yer-old man with a verrucous, yellowish lesion with coexisted hair loss on the occipital area

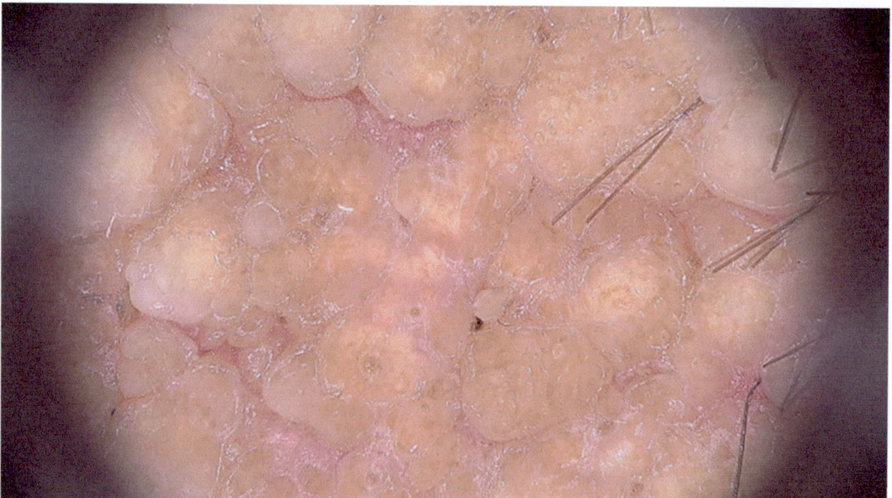

Fig. 10.2 Dermoscopy with the presence of yellowish globules aggregated in clusters on the erythematous background (×20)

On the scalp, the parietal and vertex areas are most commonly affected. Three clinically distinct stages of nevus sebaceous are observed [2]. At birth or in an early infancy, nevus sebaceous appears as a hairless, solitary, linear or round, slightly raised, pinkish, yellow or orange plaque, with a smooth surface. During puberty, the lesion grows and becomes verrucous and nodular. The growth of the nevus sebaceous results from development of sebaceous and apocrine glands associated with hormonal changes. Later, in life, in 20–30% of cases neoplastic transformation may occur. Both, benign and malignant neoplasms such as trichoblastoma, sebaceoma, eccrine poroma, syringocystadenoma papilliferum, tricholemmoma, hidradenoma and hidrocystoma, basal cell carcinoma, squamous cell carcinoma, apocrine and adnexal carcinoma, and melanoma arising in nevus sebaceous have been reported. Nevus sebaceous is most commonly diagnosed based on the clinical manifestation. In cases of ambiguity dermoscopy and punch biopsy with histopathological examination may be useful. Most characteristic dermoscopic features of naevus sebaceous include brown globules aggregated in clusters on a yellowish background [3]. In histopathological examination, acanthosis, papillomatosis and hyperkeratosis are observed. The presence of immature sebaceous glands with the absence of terminal hair follicles are usually presented [4]. Due to the risk of neoplastic transformation, surgical removal of the lesion is commonly recommended. However, there is no consensus when the lesion should be prophylactically removed. Some dermatologists suggest regular physical and dermoscopic evaluation instead of prophylactic excision of the lesion [2].

Differential diagnoses for the presented patient were juvenile xantogranuloma, verrucous epidermal nevus and basal cell carcinoma.

Juvenile xanthogranuloma is a type of non-Langerhans cell histiocytosis that represents less than 1% of all neoplasms arising from lymph nodes and connective tissue. It predominantly occurs in infants and young children and is more common in men. The condition presents as reddish to yellowish papule, plaque, or nodule. The head and neck areas are most commonly affected. Contrary to nevus sebaceous, juvenile xanthogranuloma is a self-healing condition [5].

Verrucous epidermal nevus is a benign, noninflammatory malformation usually present at birth or occurring within the first years of life. Clinically, it appears as skin-colored to brown, sharply demarcated, papillomatous papules coalescing into plaques. The lesion may be located anywhere, including the head, trunk, or extremities [6].

Basal cell carcinoma is the most common type of skin malignancy that mainly affects elderly population. Basal cell carcinoma presents as a tiny, hardly visible papule, growing into a nodule or a plaque that is sometimes ulcerated. The face, scalp or neck areas are most commonly affected [7].

In the presented patient, based on clinical and dermoscopic findings, the diagnosis of nevus sebaceous was established. The patient refused surgery. Regular physical and dermoscopic evaluation was recommended.

Key Points

- Nevus sebaceous of Jadassohn is a congenital benign skin lesion that commonly affects the scalp area.
- Nevus sebaceous appears at birth or in an early infancy as a hairless, solitary, linear or round, slightly raised, pinkish, yellow or orange plaque, with a smooth surface. During puberty, the lesion grows and becomes verrucous and nodular.
- In 20–30% of cases neoplastic transformation may occur.

References

1. Lopez AS, Lam JM. Nevus sebaceous. CMAJ. 2019;191(27):E765.
2. Moody MN, Landau JM, Goldberg LH. Nevus sebaceous revisited. Pediatr Dermatol. 2012;29(1):15–23.
3. Kelati A, Baybay H, Gallouj S, Mernissi FZ. Dermoscopic analysis of nevus sebaceus of Jadassohn: a study of 13 cases. Skin Appendage Disord. 2017;3(2):83–91.
4. Robinson AJ, Brown AP. Malignant melanoma arising in sebaceous naevus (of Jadassohn): a case report. J Plast Surg Hand Surg. 2016;50(4):249–50.
5. Hernandez-Martin A, Baselga E, Drolet BA, Esterly NB. Juvenile xanthogranuloma. J Am Acad Dermatol. 1997;36(3 Pt 1):355–67. quiz 368-9
6. Asch S, Sugarman JL. Epidermal nevus syndromes. Handb Clin Neurol. 2015;132:291–316.
7. Marzuka AG, Book SE. Basal cell carcinoma: pathogenesis, epidemiology, clinical features, diagnosis, histopathology, and management. Yale J Biol Med. 2015;88(2):167–79.

Chapter 11
A 36-Year-Old Man with Inflammatory Lesions and Crusts on the Scalp

Adriana Rakowska

A 36-year-old man presented with a one-year history of inflammatory lesions and crusts on the scalp. The first painful pustules appeared eight years ago. Since then, gradual progression of the disease was observed. The patient complained of pain and burning sensation. He was previously treated with short course of doxycycline with temporal improvement.

On physical examination, a diffuse scalp erythema with the presence of pustules and an area of scarring alopecia on the vertex were observed. Moreover, tufted hairs were presented (Fig. 11.1). Trichoscopy revealed tufted hairs, perifollicular pustules, starburst pattern hyperplasia, linear vessels and milky-read areas lacking of follicular openings (Fig. 11.2).

Based on the case description and the photographs, what is your diagnosis?

Differential Diagnoses
1. Kerion.
2. Folliculitis decalvans.
3. Lichen planopilaris.
4. Psoriasis.

Diagnosis
Folliculitis decalvans.

A. Rakowska (⊠)
Department of Dermatology, Medical University of Warsaw, Warsaw, Poland
e-mail: adriana.rakowska@wum.edu.pl; dermatologia@wum.edu.pl

© The Author(s), under exclusive license to Springer Nature Switzerland AG 2022
A. Waśkiel-Burnat et al. (eds.), *Clinical Cases in Scalp Disorders*, Clinical Cases in Dermatology, https://doi.org/10.1007/978-3-030-93426-2_11

Fig. 11.1 A 36-year-old man with a diffuse scalp erythema, pustules and an area of scarring alopecia on the vertex. Moreover tufted hairs are presented

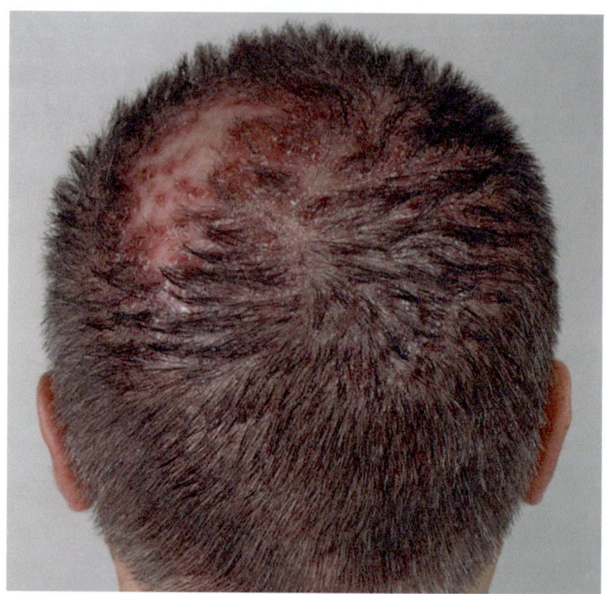

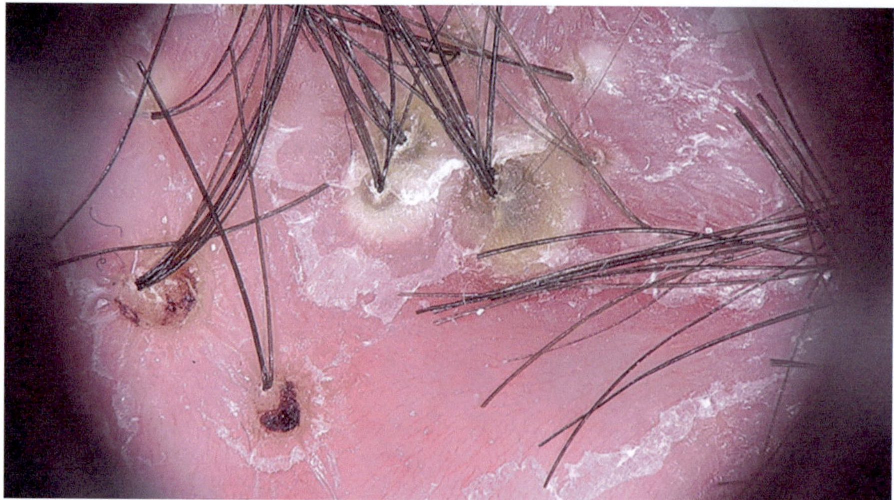

Fig. 11.2 Trichoscopy shows tufted hairs, perifollicular pustules, perifollicular scaling, linear vessels and red areas lacking of follicular openings (×40)

Discussion

Folliculitis decalvans is a rare type of neutrophilic cicatricial alopecia [1]. It comprises 2.8% of all cases of hair loss and 10.7%–11.2% of all cases of cicatricial alopecias [2]. The etiopathogenesis of the disease remains unclear. It may result from a complex combination of a bacterial infection (particularly *Staphylococcus aureus*), a hypersensitivity reaction to "superantigens," and a defect in host cell–mediated immunity regulation. Folliculitis decalvans most commonly occurs in young to middle-aged men of African descent [3]. The disease is characterized by the presence of follicular papules and pustules. With progression, tufted hairs, erosions, hemorrhagic crusts, and nodules are detected [2]. Tufted hairs correspond to the multiple hair shafts (five–twenty) emerging from one single dilated follicular opening and comprise characteristic feature of folliculitis decalvans [4]. They are formed by the clustering of adjacent follicular units as result of fibrosis and retention of telogen hairs within the involved follicles [4]. In late stages of the disease, irregularly shaped patches of cicatricial alopecia occur [4]. The lesions are associated with pain, itching and burning sensation. Lesions are most commonly localized on the vertex (55%–91%), parietal, and occipital areas of the scalp [5, 6]. Moreover, folliculitis decalvans may be noted in other locations, including the face, neck, axillae, and pubic region. The diagnosis of folliculitis decalvans is established based on the clinical manifestation and histopathological examination. Trichoscopy may be useful to avoid scalp biopsy. The most characteristic trichoscopic features of folliculitis decalvans are tufted hairs surrounded by a band of yellowish scales and perifollicular epidermal hyperplasia, which may be arranged in a starburst pattern (starburst sign). Other trichoscopic features are yellowish tubular scaling, follicular pustules, and yellow discharge. In longstanding disease, white and milky-red areas lacking of follicular openings are observed. The initial histopathologic features of folliculitis decalvans are comedo-like dilatation of follicular ostium with intra- and perifollicular neutrophilic infiltration [1, 2]. In advanced disease, several hairs from separate roots merging into a single infundibulum with a dilated ostium (tufted hairs) are detected [1]. The infiltrate consists of neutrophils, lymphocytes, and plasma cells and extends into the adventitial dermis [2]. Hair shaft granulomas with foreign body reaction are observed [2]. In end-stage lesions, follicular and interstitial dermal fibrosis and hypertrophic scarring are detected [2] Bacterial and fungal cultures should always be obtained [1]. Mild to moderate growth of *Staphylococcus aureus* in bacterial culture is reported in 20%–75% of patients with folliculitis decalvans [7]. The first-line treatment for folliculitis decalvans usually consists of oral tetracyclines. In severe cases or ineffectiveness of tetracyclines, combination of rifampicin and clindamycin is recommended [1]. Isotretinoin can be also useful [1]. Additionally to systemic treatment, topical antiseptic agents and antibiotics or topical and intralesional corticosteroids can be used. Other treatment option include dapsone, first-generation cephalosporin, systemic steroids, topical calcineurin inhibitors, photodynamic therapy and surgical treatment [1].

Differential diagnoses for the presented patient included kerion, lichen planopilaris and scalp psoriasis.

Kerion is a form of inflammatory tinea capitis that is mainly observed in the prepubertal population [8]. It presents as a painful, crusty carbuncle-like boggy plaque with subsequent scarring. It usually occurs as a solitary lesion, most commonly on the occipital area [9].

Lichen planopilaris, the most common cause of cicatricial alopecia, is mainly observed in women, between 40 and 60 years of age. Typically, the vertex and parietal areas are involved. The disease presents as hair loss area with the presence of perifollicular erythema and follicular hyperkeratosis at the periphery [1]. The lesions are commonly associated with itching, burning sensation and scalp tenderness.

Scalp psoriasis is characterized by red, thickened plaques with a silver-white scale, either contained within the hairline, or extending onto the forehead, ears, and posterior neck. The lesions may cause itching [10].

In the presented patient, based on the clinical presentation and trichoscopic findings, the diagnosis of folliculitis decalvans was established. The patient was treated with combination of oral clindamycin 300 mg twice daily and rifampicin 300 mg twice daily with clinical improvement. After inflammatory process was decreased, therapy and oral isotretinoin (0.5 mg/kg/day) was started.

Key Points
- Folliculitis decalvans is a rare form of neutrophilic cicatricial alopecia which affects mainly the scalp area.
- It is characterized by the presence of follicular papules, pustules, tufted hairs, erosions, hemorrhagic crusts, and nodules.

References

1. Kanti V, Rowert-Huber J, Vogt A, Blume-Peytavi U. Cicatricial alopecia. J Dtsch Dermatol Ges. 2018;16(4):435–61.
2. Wu WY, Otberg N, McElwee KJ, Shapiro J. Diagnosis and management of primary cicatricial alopecia: part II. Skinmed. 2008;7(2):78–83.
3. Ross EK, Vincenzi C, Tosti A. Videodermoscopy in the evaluation of hair and scalp disorders. J Am Acad Dermatol. 2006;55(5):799–806.
4. Rudnicka L, Olszewska M, Rakowska A. Atlas of trichoscopy: dermoscopy in hair and scalp disease. London: Springer; 2012.
5. Miguel-Gomez L, Rodrigues-Barata AR, Molina-Ruiz A, Martorell-Calatayud A, Fernandez-Crehuet P, Grimalt R, et al. Folliculitis decalvans: Effectiveness of therapies and prognostic factors in a multicenter series of 60 patients with long-term follow-up. J Am Acad Dermatol. 2018;79(5):878–83.
6. Bunagan MJ, Banka N, Shapiro J. Retrospective review of folliculitis decalvans in 23 patients with course and treatment analysis of long-standing cases. J Cutan Med Surg. 2015;19(1):45–9.
7. Chanasumon N, Sriphojanart T, Suchonwanit P. Therapeutic potential of bimatoprost for the treatment of eyebrow hypotrichosis. Drug Des Devel Ther. 2018;12:365–72.
8. Stein LL, Adams EG, Holcomb KZ. Inflammatory tinea capitis mimicking dissecting cellulitis in a postpubertal male: a case report and review of the literature. Mycoses. 2013;56(5):596–600.
9. John AM, Schwartz RA, Janniger CK. The kerion: an angry tinea capitis. Int J Dermatol. 2018;57(1):3–9.
10. Blakely K, Gooderham M. Management of scalp psoriasis: current perspectives. Psoriasis (Auckl). 2016;6:33–40.

Chapter 12
A 38-Year-Old Woman with Nodular Lesions and a Persistent Pruritus of the Scalp

Patrycja Gajda-Mróz, Adriana Rakowska, Joanna Czuwara, Mariusz Sikora, Małgorzata Olszewska, and Lidia Rudnicka

A 38-year-old woman was presented with several nodules on the occipital and parietal areas of the scalp with coexisted pruritus. The first violaceus nodules on the occipital area appeared seven years ago and then spontaneously resolved after a few months. Progressively increasing nodular lesions on the occipital and parietal areas have been developing since three years. The patient was treated with topical corticosteroids and cryotherapy with no clinical improvement.

No personal history of non-dermatological conditions was reported.

On physical examination a number of nodular lesions were found on the occipital and parietal areas (Fig. 12.1). Severe bleeding after mechanical irritation was observed. Trichoscopy showed a homogenous pink areas. No hair shaft abnormalities were observed (Fig. 12.2).

In complete blood count eosinophilia (1.0 G/l, 8%) was observed. No abnormalities in the chest X-ray and ultrasound of the abdominal cavity and the minor pelvis were described. A histopathological examination revealed clusters of proliferating capillaries and cellular infiltrate, localized around the blood vessels and composed mainly of lymphocytes and large number of eosinophils.

Based on the case description and the photographs, what is your diagnosis?

P. Gajda-Mróz (✉) · A. Rakowska · J. Czuwara · M. Olszewska · L. Rudnicka
Department of Dermatology, Medical University of Warsaw, Warsaw, Poland
e-mail: patrycja.gajda@wum.edu.pl; adriana.rakowska@wum.edu.pl; joanna.czuwara@wum.edu.pl; mariusz.sikora@wum.edu.pl; malgorzata.olszewska@wum.edu.pl; lidia.rudnicka@wum.edu.pl

M. Sikora
National Institute of Geriatrics, Rheumatology and Rehabilitation, Warsaw, Poland
e-mail: mariusz.sikora@spartanska.pl

A. Waśkiel-Burnat et al. (eds.), *Clinical Cases in Scalp Disorders*, Clinical Cases in Dermatology, https://doi.org/10.1007/978-3-030-93426-2_12

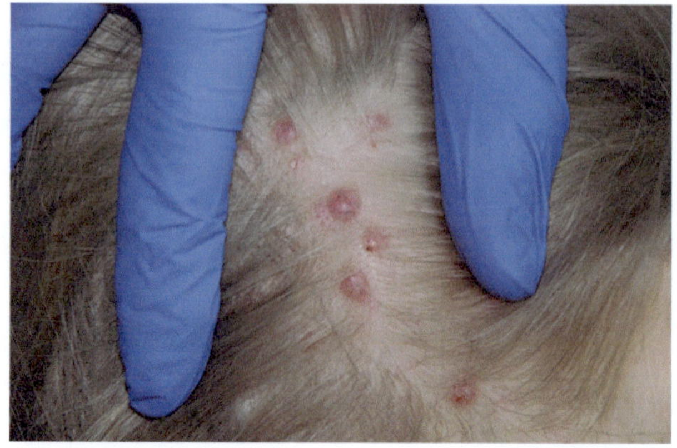

Fig. 12.1 A 38-year-old woman with nodules on the occipital and parietal areas

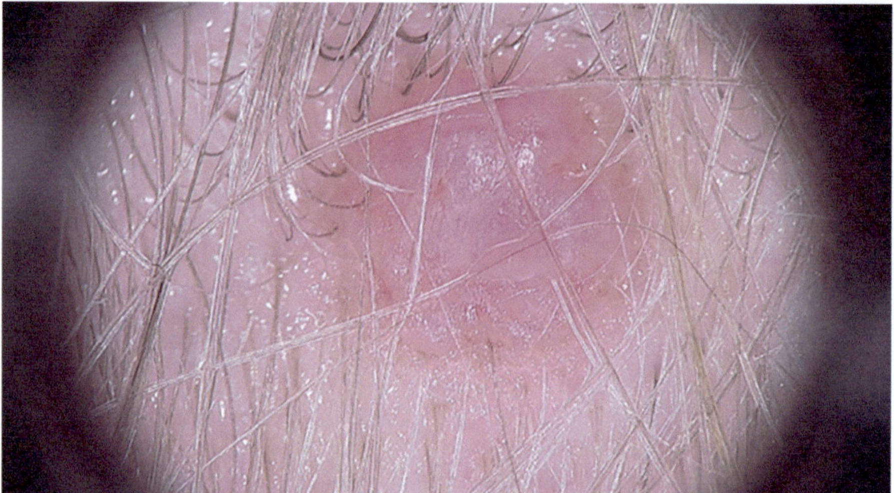

Fig. 12.2 Trichoscopy with the presence of pink, homogenous area (×20)

Differential Diagnoses
1. Pyogenic granuloma.
2. Kimura's disease.
3. Scalp metastases.
4. Angiolymphoid hyperplasia with eosinophilia.

Diagnosis
Angiolymphoid hyperplasia with eosinophilia.

Discussion

Angiolymphoid hyperplasia with eosinophilia is an uncommon benign vascular and inflammatory disorder. It is not clear whether the disease is primarily a vascular neoplasm, a lymphoproliferative process or hypersensitivity reaction [1]. The role of mechanical injury and hormonal factors (hypothyroidism, pregnancy) was suggested. Angiolymphoid hyperplasia with eosinophilia typically affects adults. It presents as a single nodule or a group of several red-brown or violaceous papules or small nodules. The periauricular area (36.3%), face (28.2%), and scalp (17.3%) are mainly affected. Other locations such as trunk, extremities or genitalia are rarely involved [2]. Pruritis and bleeding may occur. Extracutaneous manifestation has been described on oral mucosa, parotid gland, orbit, colon and bones [3]. Regional lymphadenopathy is presented in 5–10% of patients with angiolymphoid hyperplasia with eosinophilia. Peripheral blood eosinophilia is described in 10–20% of cases while the serum IgE level is usually within normal limits [1]. Diagnosis of angiolymphoid hyperplasia with eosinophilia is based on clinical findings and histopathological examination. Dermoscopy may comprise additional diagnostic method. Dermoscopic findings of angiolymphoid hyperplasia with eosinophilia are vascular structures (lacunes, vessels and reddish background) and brown dots. Histologically, the condition is characterized by the presence of a vascular proliferation with epithelioid endothelial cells with surrounding lymphocytic and eosinophilic infiltrate [1]. Considering the high recurrence risk, there is no the best therapeutic option for angiolymphoid hyperplasia with eosinophilia. Many approaches have been tried. Conventional therapies include corticosteroids (local and systemic), methotrexate, pentoxifylline, propranolol, isotretinoin, cryotherapy, thalidomide, phototherapy, or surgical excision [2].

Angiolymphoid hyperplasia with eosinophilia should be differentiated from Kimura's disease, pyogenic granuloma and scalp metastases.

Kimura's disease is a benign lymphoproliferative disorder that mainly occurs in young men of Asian descent. It presents as nodular lesions usually localized subcutaneously in the periauricular and submandibular areas. In contrast to angiolymphoid hyperplasia with eosinophilia, Kimura's disease is typically associated with peripheral blood eosinophilia, an increased serum level of IgE, lymphadenopathy and salivary gland hypertrophy [4].

Pyogenic granuloma is a benign vascular tumor of the skin or mucous membranes characterized by rapid growth. Children and young adults are usually affected. Pyogenic granuloma typically occurs on the trunk or extremities as a single red papule [5].

Scalp metastases constituted 6.9% of all cutaneous metastases from various visceral malignancies. Typically they present as isolated dermal nodules with superficial discoloration or changes in the texture [6].

In the presented patient, based on clinical and histopathological features the diagnosis of angiolymphoid hyperplasia with eosinophilia was established. Treatment with intralesional injection with acetonide triamcinolone (ten mg/ml) every four–six weeks was started. Reduction of the pruritus and partial resolution of skin lesions was achieved.

Key Points
- In the case of papular or nodular lesions on the scalp angiolymphoid hyperplasia with eosinophilia should be considered in differential diagnosis.
- The disease is characterized by the presence of a single nodule or a group of several red-brown or violaceous papules or small nodules.

References

1. Bahloul E, Amouri M, Charfi S, Boudawara O, Mnif H, Boudawara T, Turki H. Angiolymphoid hyperplasia with eosinophilia: report of nine cases. Int J Dermatol. 2017;56(12):1373–8. https://doi.org/10.1111/ijd.13800. Epub 2017 Oct 23
2. Adler BL, Krausz AE, Minuti A, Silverberg JI, Lev-Tov H. Epidemiology and treatment of angiolymphoid hyperplasia with eosinophilia (ALHE): a systematic review. J Am Acad Dermatol. 2016;74(3):506–512.e11.
3. Busquets AC, Sanchez JL. Angiolymphoid hyperplasia with eosinophilia induced by trauma. Int J Dermatol. 2006;45(10):1211–4.
4. Gupta A, Shareef M, Lade H, Ponnusamy SR, Mahajan A. Kimura's disease: a diagnostic and therapeutic challenge. Indian J Otolaryngol Head Neck Surg. 2019;71(Suppl 1):855–9. https://doi.org/10.1007/s12070-019-01601-5.
5. Kissou A, Hassam BE. Dermoscopy of pyogenic granuloma. Pan Afr Med J. 2017;27:110. https://doi.org/10.11604/pamj.2017.27.110.12278.
6. Mayer JE, Maurer MA, Nguyen HT. Diffuse cutaneous breast cancer metastases resembling subcutaneous nodules with no surface changes. Cutis. 2018 Mar;101(3):219–23.

Chapter 13
A 3-Year-Old Boy with an Erythematous, Infiltrated Plaque on the Occipital Area

Marta Kurzeja, Małgorzata Olszewska, and Lidia Rudnicka

A three-year-old boy was presented with a two-week history of a erythematous, infiltrated plaque on the occipital area of the scalp. There was no fever reported. No other family member was affected. No personal history of dermatological or non-dermatological diseases was reported.

A physical examination revealed an erythematous plaque partially covered with purulent exudate and hemorrhagic crusts on the occipital area (Fig. 13.1). Cervical lymphadenopathy was detected. On trichoscopy, maroon yellow areas with whitish clouds and yellow areas with extravasations were detected (Fig. 13.2). No hair shaft abnormalities were observed.

In laboratory tests an increased white blood cell count with neutrophilia and an elevated C-reactive protein were detected. In bacterial culture *Staphylococcus aureus* was found. A Wood lamp and mycological examination were negative.

Based on the case description and the photographs, what is your diagnosis?

Differential Diagnoses
1. Kerion.
2. Impetigo.
3. Pemphigus vulgaris.
4. Seborrheic dermatitis.

Diagnosis
Impetigo.

M. Kurzeja (✉) · M. Olszewska · L. Rudnicka
Department of Dermatology, Medical University of Warsaw, Warsaw, Poland
e-mail: marta.kurzeja@wum.edu.pl; malgorzata.olszewska@wum.edu.pl; lidia.rudnicka@wum.edu.pl

A. Waśkiel-Burnat et al. (eds.), *Clinical Cases in Scalp Disorders*, Clinical Cases in Dermatology, https://doi.org/10.1007/978-3-030-93426-2_13

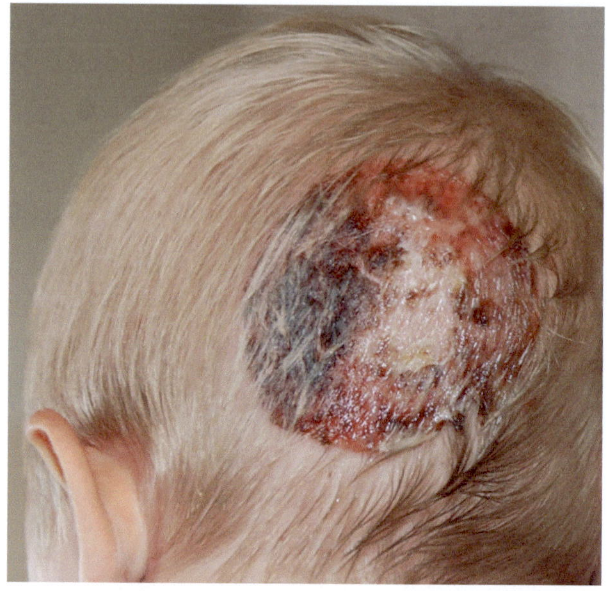

Fig. 13.1 A 3-year-old boy with an erythematous plaque partially covered with purulent exudate and hemorrhagic crusts on the occipital area

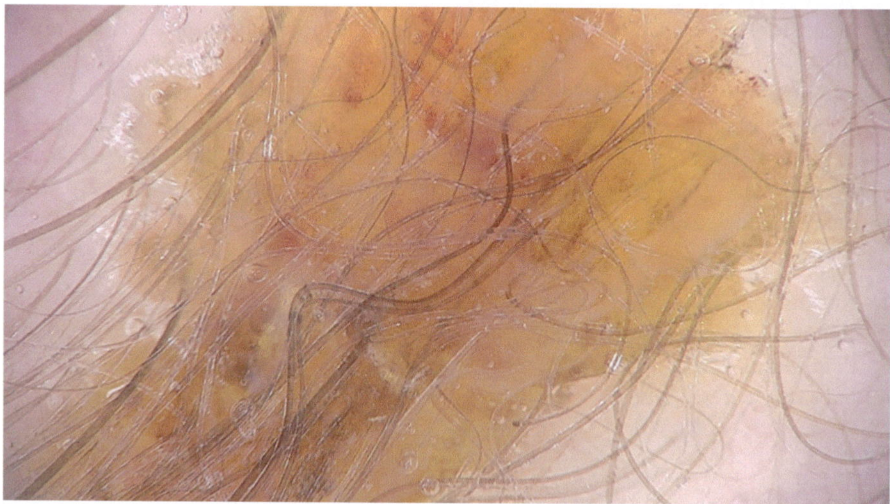

Fig. 13.2 Trichoscopy shows yellow areas with extravasations. No hair shaft abnormalities are observed (×70)

Discussion

Impetigo is an acute bacterial infection. It is most commonly observed in children, between two and five years of age. The disease is highly contagious and primarily caused by *Staphylococcus aureus* or *Streptococcus pyogenes*. Impetigo is distinguished as either non-bullous (70% of all cases) and bullous (30% of cases) [1]. Nonbullous impetigo is characterized by honey-colored crusts on erythematous background localized most commonly on the face and extremities. Mild regional lymphadenopathy commonly occurs, but systemic symptoms are rarely observed. Mucous membranes are not affected. Bullous impetigo is characterized by the presence of small vesicles, which becomes flaccid bullae. They contain a clear or yellow fluid which eventually progresses to become purulent or dark. Once the bullae rupture, an erythematous base with a rim of scale is observed [1–3]. Bullous impetigo tends to be less contagious. Lesions besides the face and extremities, are localized on the armpits, trunk, and perianal region [1]. Buccal mucous membranes may be also affected. Regional lymphadenopathy is rarely presented. Systemic symptoms, such as fever, are more common compared to nonbullous impetigo [2]. Complications of impetigo are rare. Glomerulonephritis occurs in 5% of patients with impetigo [2]. The diagnosis of impetigo is usually based on the clinical picture. A bacterial culture from the lesion may be necessary if the lesion is resistant to treatment, but it is not required prior to initial therapy. In case of widespread impetigo, an increased white blood cell count with neutrophilia and an elevated C-reactive protein may be observed [2, 3]. Impetigo is most commonly treated with topical antibiotics such as mupirocin, retapamulin, and fusidic acid [4]. Systemic antibiotics should be recommended for all cases of bullous impetigo and cases of non-bullous impetigo with more than three lesions, scalp or deep tissue involvement, systemic signs of infection, lymphadenopathy or lesions in the oral cavity [1, 2]. Beta-lactamase-resistant antibiotics such as cephalosporins, amoxicillin-clavulanate, dicloxacillin are recommended [2].

Differential diagnoses for the presented case included kerion, pemphigus vulgaris and seborrheic dermatitis.

Kerion is a form of inflammatory tinea capitis mainly observed in the prepubertal population [5]. It presents as a painful, crusty carbuncle-like boggy plaque with subsequent scarring. It usually occurs as a solitary lesion, most commonly on the occipital area [6]. On trichoscopy, hair shaft abnormalities are presented.

Pemphigus vulgaris is a form of an autoimmune bullous disease affecting the skin and mucous membranes. Women between 50 and 60 years of age are most commonly affected [3]. Skin involvement is characterized by flaccid blisters and erosions localized mainly on the flexural areas, face, scalp, and extremities [7].

Seborrheic dermatitis is an inflammatory skin disorder characterized by the presence of erythematous plaques with greasy, yellowish scales. Mild itch is usually presented. No hair loss is observed. The scalp (mainly the vertex and parietal areas) is most commonly affected. However, the disease can be also observed on the face, chest, back, axilla and groin areas [8].

Based on the clinical features the patient was diagnosed with impetigo. He was treated with intravenous and then oral amoxicillin with clavulonic acid for 14 days. Additionally, topical antiseptics were used. Complete resolution of skin lesion was observed.

Key Points
- Impetigo is an acute, bacterial skin infection which may affect the scalp area.
- The disease presents as honey-colored crusts (nonbullous impetigo) or small vesicles, which becomes flaccid bullae (bullous impetigo).

References

1. Pereira LB. Impetigo – review. An Bras Dermatol. 2014;89(2):293–9.
2. Nardi NM, Schaefer TJ. Impetigo. Treasure Island (FL): StatPearls; 2020.
3. Cole C, Gazewood J. Diagnosis and treatment of impetigo. Am Fam Physician. 2007;75(6):859–64.
4. Koning S, van der Sande R, Verhagen AP, van Suijlekom-Smit LW, Morris AD, Butler CC, et al. Interventions for impetigo. Cochrane Database Syst Rev. 2012;1(1):Cd003261.
5. Stein LL, Adams EG, Holcomb KZ. Inflammatory tinea capitis mimicking dissecting cellulitis in a postpubertal male: a case report and review of the literature. Mycoses. 2013;56(5):596–600.
6. John AM, Schwartz RA, Janniger CK. The kerion: an angry tinea capitis. Int J Dermatol. 2018;57(1):3–9.
7. Kridin K. Pemphigus group: overview, epidemiology, mortality, and comorbidities. Immunol Res. 2018;66(2):255–70.
8. Borda LJ, Wikramanayake TC. Seborrheic dermatitis and dandruff: a comprehensive review. J Clin Investig Dermatol. 2015;3(2) https://doi.org/10.13188/2373-1044.1000019.

Chapter 14
A 41-Year-Old Man with a Solitary Lesion on the Right Temporal Area

Leszek Blicharz, Alina Graczyk, Monika Łukiewicz, and Joanna Czuwara

A 41-year-old man presented with a four-year history of a progressing lesion localized on the scalp. He also complained of fatigue. The patient had been treated with topical corticosteroids and adapalene without significant improvement.

A physical examination revealed an irregular, annular red-brown plaque on the right temporal area (7 cm × 7 cm) (Fig.14.1). On trichoscopy, yellowish-orange structureless areas with the presence of irregular linear and thin arborising vessels were observed. Moreover, whitish areas with loss of follicular openings were detected (Fig. 14.2). No hair shaft abnormalities were presented.

Laboratory tests were normal. A mycological examination was negative. A histopathological examination revealed "naked" granulomas surrounded by lymphocytic inflammatory infiltrate located in the dermis (Fig.14.3). In computed tomography of the chest bilateral hilar lymphadenopathy and disseminated parenchymal changes in the form of micronodules were detected.

Based on the case description and the photographs, what is your diagnosis?

Differential Diagnoses
1. Sarcoidosis.
2. Psoriasis.
3. Tinea capitis.
4. Tuberculosis.

Diagnosis
Sarcoidosis.

L. Blicharz (✉) · A. Graczyk · M. Łukiewicz · J. Czuwara
Department of Dermatology, Medical University of Warsaw, Warsaw, Poland
e-mail: leszek.blicharz@wum.edu.pl; joanna.czuwara@wum.edu.com

A. Waśkiel-Burnat et al. (eds.), *Clinical Cases in Scalp Disorders*, Clinical
Cases in Dermatology, https://doi.org/10.1007/978-3-030-93426-2_14

Fig. 14.1 A 41-year-old man with an irregular, annular red-brown plaque on the right temporal area

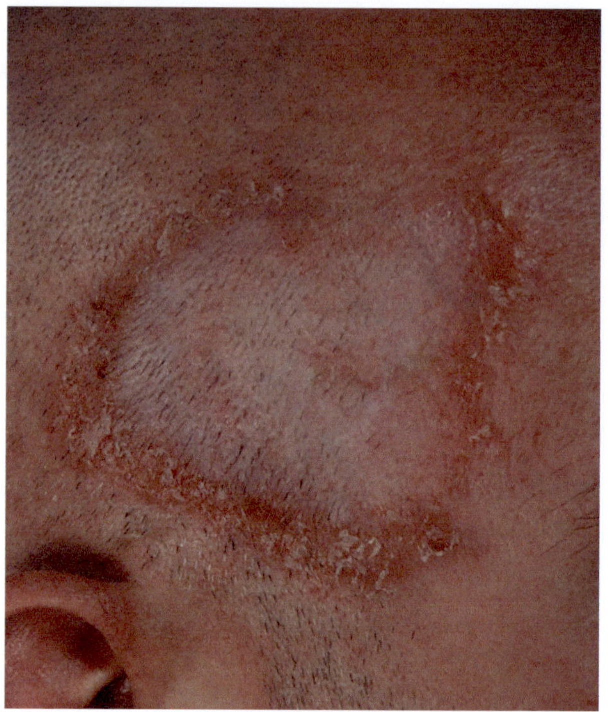

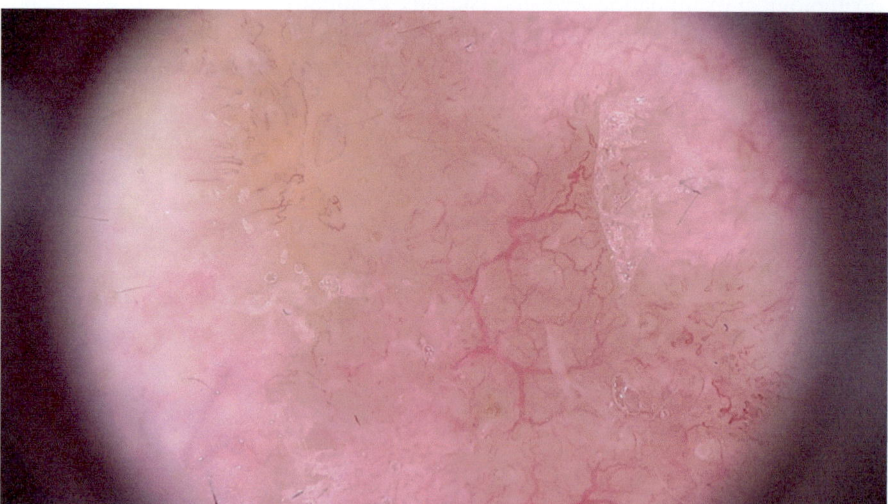

Fig. 14.2 Trichoscopy with the presence of yellowish-orange structureless areas and linear and thin arborizing vessels. Whitish areas with loss of follicular openings are also present (×20)

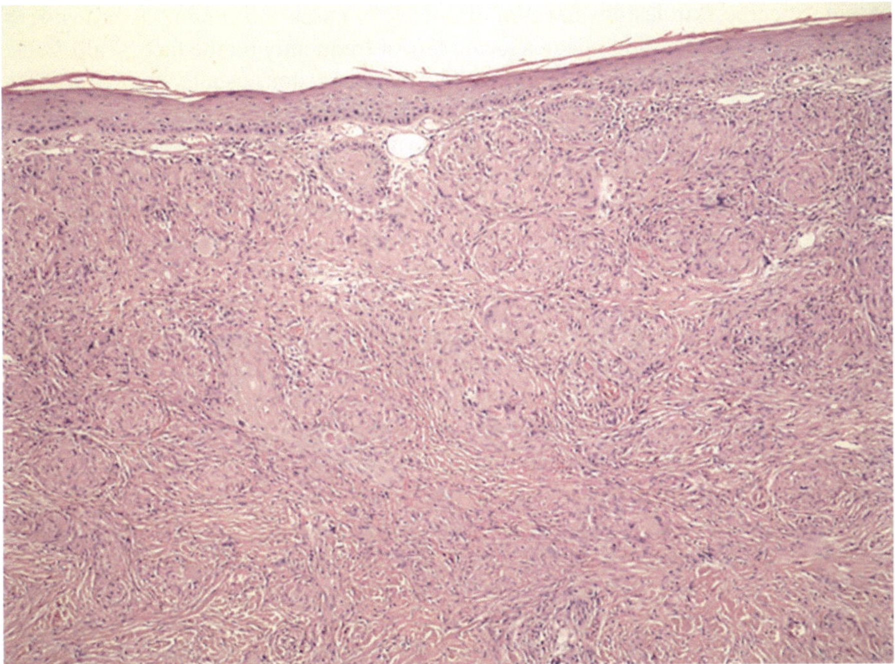

Fig. 14.3 A histological examination with "naked granulomas" consisting of the collection of epithelioid histiocytes with multinucleate giant cells and a sparse infiltrate of the lymphocytes at the periphery

Discussion

Sarcoidosis is a systemic disease associated with the formation of non-caseating granulomas in various organs, including the lung, heart, lymph nodes, and skin [1]. The etiopathology of sarcoidosis remains unclear. It has been suggested that granulomas are a result of excessive immune response triggered by environmental factors in genetically predisposed individuals [2]. The incidence of sarcoidosis is estimated at 2.3–11.5 in 100,000 per year with a slight female predominance. The average age of onset is between 47 and 51 years [3]. The clinical course of sarcoidosis is heterogeneous. In the initial phase, patients are most frequently present with persistent cough, skin and ocular involvement, lymphadenopathy, and fatigue. In most cases, the disease spontaneously resolves during the first two years (acute sarcoidosis), but the symptoms may also persist for >three–five years (chronic sarcoidosis) [1]. Skin manifestations are found in 20–30% of patients. The lesions have a highly variable presentation and may be divided into nonspecific and specific [4]. The most common nonspecific cutaneous manifestations include erythema nodosum and lupus pernio. Specific skin lesions develop in 9–15% of cases and present as brown-reddish papules, nodules, and plaques located most frequently on the face, scalp, back, and extensor surfaces of the extremities. The papular lesions usually resolve without scarring. Plaques can be associated with central fibrosis. If located on the scalp, they may occasionally cause scarring alopecia. Dermoscopy of specific cutaneous lesions typically shows yellowish-orange structures or areas ("apple jelly"), irregular linear vessels and whitish areas in the case of a long-standing disease course [5]. In histopathological examination, non-necrotising granulomas with a central area composed of macrophages, epithelioid cells, multinucleated giant cells, and lymphocytes surrounded by fibrosis are detected. The diagnosis of sarcoidosis is based on three criteria: (1) clinical and radiological presentation, (2) evidence of non-caseating granulomas, and (3) evidence of no alternative diseases [1]. Radiologic signs typically include bilateral hilar lymphadenopathy or micronodular pulmonary infiltration associated with a typical lymphatic distribution [6, 7]. There is no commonly accepted treatment algorithm for sarcoidosis. In the case of isolated cutaneous involvement, topical or intralesional corticosteroids are preferred. Oral antimalarials or tetracyclines may also prove successful [4]. Systemic treatment with corticosteroids or immunosuppressants should be administered in the case of pulmonary, cardiac, or neurological system involvement, symptomatic hypercalcemia, or lack of response to topical treatment in the ocular disease [1]. Systemic corticosteroids (e.g. prednisone) remain the first-line therapy. Methotrexate is regarded as the second-choice drug. Other treatment options involve azathioprine or leflunomide [1, 7].

Sarcoidosis may clinically resemble other dermatological entities [4]. Differential diagnoses for the presented case included psoriasis, tinea capitis and cutaneous tuberculosis.

Scalp psoriasis is characterized by the presence of red, thickened plaques with a silver-white scale. The frontal and occipital areas are most commonly affected. Other typically affected areas are the extensor surface of elbows and knees, and the lower back [8]. No pulmonary changes are observed.

Tinea capitis is a fungal infection of the scalp that affects mainly children. The disease is characterized by the presence of hair loss areas with coexistent scaling, inflammation or pustules [9]. Only inflammatory form of tinea capitis can lead to scarring hair loss [10].

Cutaneous tuberculosis is an invasion of the skin by *Mycobacterium tuberculosis* characterized by the presence of caseating epithelioid granulomas. The disease presents in various clinical manifestations. There can be inflammatory papules, ulcers, nodules, pustules, verrucous plaques, or any other type of lesions. Mucous membranes can also be affected [11].

Based on clinical picture, trichoscopy and histopathological examination, the diagnosis of sarcoidosis was established. Due to a long history and progressive character of the cutaneous lesion as well as the lung involvement, the patient was administered prednisone at a starting dose of 40 mg/day and methotrexate subcutaneously at a dose of 10 mg/week with good results.

Key Points
- Specific skin involvement is observed in 9–15% of patients with sarcoidosis.
- Skin sarcoidosis presents as brown-reddish papules, nodules, and plaques most frequently located on the face, scalp, back, and extensor surfaces of the extremities.
- Scalp sarcoidosis can lead to scarring alopecia.

References

1. Valeyre D, Prasse A, Nunes H, Uzunhan Y, Brillet PY, Muller-Quernheim J. Sarcoidosis. Lancet. 2014;383(9923):1155–67.
2. Bennett D, Bargagli E, Refini RM, Rottoli P. New concepts in the pathogenesis of sarcoidosis. Expert Rev Respir Med. 2019;13(10):981–91.
3. Arkema EV, Cozier YC. Epidemiology of sarcoidosis: current findings and future directions. Ther Adv Chronic Dis. 2018;9(11):227–40.
4. Haimovic A, Sanchez M, Judson MA, Prystowsky S. Sarcoidosis: a comprehensive review and update for the dermatologist: Part I. Cutaneous disease. J Am Acad Dermatol. 2012;66(5):699 e1–18. quiz 717-8
5. Errichetti E, Stinco G. Dermatoscopy of granulomatous disorders. Dermatol Clin. 2018;36(4):369–75.
6. Koyama T, Ueda H, Togashi K, Umeoka S, Kataoka M, Nagai S. Radiologic manifestations of sarcoidosis in various organs. Radiographics. 2004;24(1):87–104.
7. Haimovic A, Sanchez M, Judson MA, Prystowsky S. Sarcoidosis: a comprehensive review and update for the dermatologist: part II. Extracutaneous disease. J Am Acad Dermatol. 2012;66(5):719 e1–10. quiz 29-30
8. Blakely K, Gooderham M. Management of scalp psoriasis: current perspectives. Psoriasis (Auckl). 2016;6:33–40.
9. Adesiji YO, Omolade FB, Aderibigbe IA, Ogungbe O, Adefioye OA, Adedokun SA, et al. Prevalence of tinea capitis among children in Osogbo, Nigeria, and the associated risk factors. Diseases. 2019;7(1):13.
10. Stein LL, Adams EG, Holcomb KZ. Inflammatory tinea capitis mimicking dissecting cellulitis in a postpubertal male: a case report and review of the literature. Mycoses. 2013;56(5):596–600.
11. Lyon SM, Rossman MD. Pulmonary tuberculosis. Microbiol Spectr. 2017;5(1)

Chapter 15
A 43-Year-Old Woman with a Solitary, Asymptomatic Nodule on the Scalp

Alina Graczyk, Anna Waśkiel-Burnat, and Marta Sar-Pomian

A 43-year-old woman presented with a two-year history of a slowly growing solitary nodule on the scalp. The patient did not complain of any symptoms. No history of dermatological or oncological diseases were reported.

A physical examination revealed a pink nodule (1 cm × 1 cm) on the vertex area of the scalp with coexisted hair loss (Fig. 15.1).

Based on the case description and the photographs, what is your diagnosis?

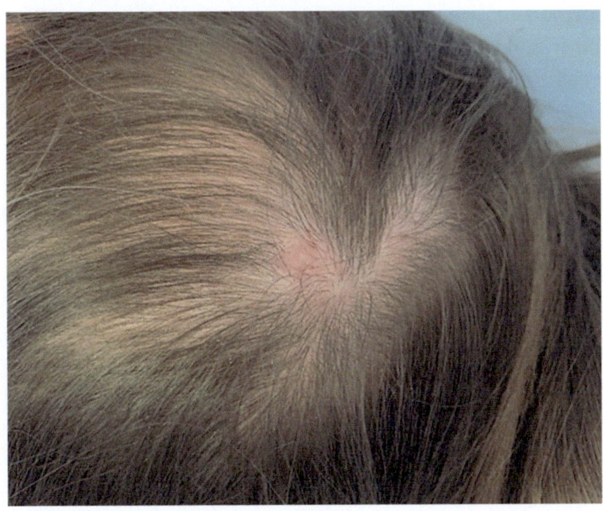

Fig. 15.1 A 43-year-old woman with a pink nodule with coexisted hair loss on the vertex area

A. Graczyk (✉) · A. Waśkiel-Burnat · M. Sar-Pomian
Department of Dermatology, Medical University of Warsaw, Warsaw, Poland
e-mail: anna.waskiel@wum.edu.pl

A. Waśkiel-Burnat et al. (eds.), *Clinical Cases in Scalp Disorders*, Clinical Cases in Dermatology, https://doi.org/10.1007/978-3-030-93426-2_15

Differential Diagnoses
1. Furuncle.
2. Pilar cyst.
3. Lipoma.
4. Skin metastasis.

Diagnosis
Pilar cyst.

Discussion

Pilar cyst, also known as trichilemmal cyst, is a common form of dermal cyst. It arises from the epithelium located between the sebaceous gland and the arrector pili muscle [1]. Pilar cyst is lined by stratified squamous epithelium without a granular cell layer and is filled with keratin. It is most commonly observed in young women. Family history may be present since the disease follows autosomal dominant inheritance in some cases. Clinically, pilar cyst presents as a flesh-colored, smooth, movable, firm, and well-circumscribed nodule. In case of long duration, hair loss on the skin surface immediately above the cyst may be presented. Most commonly, they are multiple lesions, but sometimes, single lesion might be presented. Pilar cyst usually occurs in areas with dense hair follicle especially the scalp, but they may also be found on the face, head, and neck. It is usually asymptomatic. Calcification or eruption lead to inflammatory process and cause pain in the affected area. Diagnosis of pilar cysts is mainly based on the clinical picture. Radiological studies sometimes are needed to exclude other differentials and determine the extent of the lesion. A histopathological examination is characterized by the presence of epithelial lined cyst filled with brightly eosinophilic keratinaceous debris. In case of focal rupture of the cyst, giant cell reaction may be presented. The treatment is a radical surgical excision of the lesion including the wall of the cysts [1].

Pilar cyst should be differentiated from furuncle, lipoma and skin metastasis.

Furuncle is a common bacterial infection of the hair follicle with purulent extension into the adjacent subcutaneous tissue leading to abscess formation [2]. The most common infectious agent is *Staphylococcus aureus*, but other bacteria may also be causative. Furuncle presents as a red, swollen, and tender nodule. Fever and enlarged lymph nodes are rarely observed [3]. Furuncle may occur on any hair-bearing area. However, it most frequently appears on the extremities. The lesion may lead to scarring upon healing [3].

Lipoma is the most common subcutaneous soft-tissue tumor composed of adipocytes. It presents as a solitary, slow-growing nodule with a firm, rubbery consistency. Lipomas are usually asymptomatic. The lesions typically occur on the trunk, shoulders, posterior neck, and axillae [4].

Scalp involvement is observed in 4% to 7% of patients with skin metastases. Clinically, they present as a single or multiple non-tender nodules which are characterized by rapid growth. Disfigurement, pain, bleeding, and drainage may occur. The lesions may develop a long-time after the initial diagnosis or be the first sign of an internal malignancy [5].

In the presented patient based on the clinical manifestation the initial diagnosis of pilar cyst was established. A radical surgical excision of the lesion was performed. A histopathological examination confirmed the initial diagnosis.

Key Points
- In case of nodular lesion of the scalp pilar cyst should be included into differential diagnosis.
- Pilar cyst presents as a slow-growing, flesh-colored, smooth, movable, firm, and well-circumscribed nodule.

References

1. Al Aboud DM, Yarrarapu SNS, Patel BC. Pilar cyst. Treasure Island (FL): StatPearls; 2020.
2. Clebak KT, Malone MA. Skin infections. Prim Care. 2018;45(3):433–54.
3. Ibler KS, Kromann CB. Recurrent furunculosis – challenges and management: a review. Clin Cosmet Investig Dermatol. 2014;7:59–64.
4. Luba MC, Bangs SA, Mohler AM, Stulberg DL. Common benign skin tumors. Am Fam Physician. 2003;67(4):729–38.
5. Strickley JD, Jenson AB, Jung JY. Cutaneous metastasis. Hematol Oncol Clin North Am. 2019;33(1):173–97.

Chapter 16
A 49-Year-Old Woman with a Temporary Bleeding, Solitary Lesion on the Left Temporal Area

Anna Waśkiel-Burnat, Marta Sar-Pomian, Małgorzata Olszewska, and Lidia Rudnicka

A 49-year-old woman presented with a one-year history of a solitary, brown lesion on the left temporal area. The patient complained of sporadic bleeding from the lesion after hair brushing.

On physical examination, a sharply demarcated, verrucous, brown-pinkish lesion on the left temporal area was presented (Fig. 16.1). Dermoscopy showed a lesion with a sharply demarked border with brown and black hyperkeratotic areas on the left side and pink hyperkeratotic areas with harpin vessels on the right side (Fig. 16.2). On dermoscopy with immersion fluid, comedo-like openings were detected.

Based on the case description and the photographs, what is your diagnosis?

Differential Diagnoses
1. Seborrheic keratosis.
2. Melanoma.
3. Pigmented basal cell carcinoma.
4. Melanotic nevus.

Diagnosis
Serborrheic keratosis.

A. Waśkiel-Burnat (✉) · M. Sar-Pomian · M. Olszewska · L. Rudnicka
Department of Dermatology, Medical University of Warsaw, Warsaw, Poland
e-mail: anna.waskiel@wum.edu.pl; malgorzata.olszewska@wum.edu.pl; lidia.rudnicka@wum.edu.pl

A. Waśkiel-Burnat et al. (eds.), *Clinical Cases in Scalp Disorders*, Clinical Cases in Dermatology, https://doi.org/10.1007/978-3-030-93426-2_16

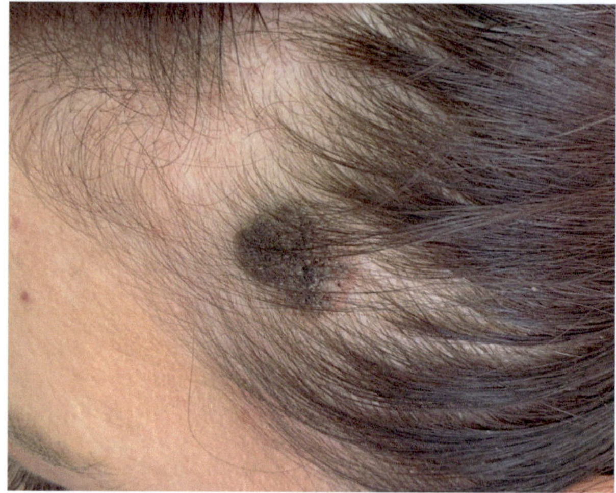

Fig. 16.1 A 49-year-old woman with a sharply demarcated, verrucous, brown-pinkish lesion on the left temporal area

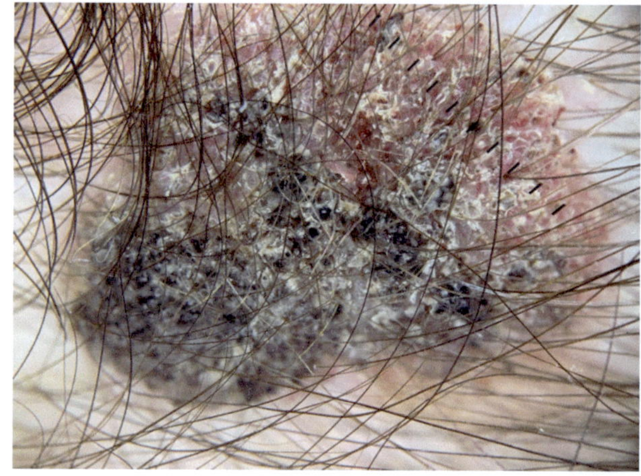

Fig. 16.2 Dermoscopy shows a lesion with a sharply demarked border with brown and black hyperkeratotic areas on the left side and pink hyperkeratotic areas with harpin vessels on the right side (×10)

Discussion

Seborrheic keratosis, also known as verruca seborrhoica and seborrheic wart, is one of the most common benign skin tumor that results from benign clonal expansion of epidermal keratinocytes [1]. The etiology and pathogenesis of seborrheic keratosis are still not well understood. However the role of genetic predisposition, older age and ultraviolet light has been suggested [1]. Seborrheic keratosis is most commonly observed in the middle-aged and elderly, however it may also present in young adults. No gender predisposition is observed. Seborrheic keratosis is mostly presented in individuals with low Fitzgerald's skin phototypes [2]. Typical lesion is sharply demarcated, round or oval-shaped, elevated and stuck on the skin with a verrucous, dull, uneven, or punched-out surface. Flat seborrheic keratosis often has a smooth, velvety surface and is barely elevated above the surface of the skin [1]. The color of the lesions varies from skin color, yellowish, light to dark brown, grey, and black. Seborrheic keratosis may present as an isolated or multiple lesions. The lesions appear anywhere on the body with the exception of the palms, soles and mucous membranes. The chest, back, scalp (mainly the temporal areas) and neck are most commonly affected. Seborrheic keratosis is generally slow-growing and asymptomatic condition. Irritation or trauma may cause itching, pain and bleeding with erythema or crusting [1]. Rarely spontaneous resolution may occur [1, 2]. The diagnosis of seborrheic keratosis is mainly established based on clinical manifestation. Dermoscopy may be helpful to differentiate benign features from dysplastic or malignant tumors. Dermoscopic findings of seborrheic keratosis are milia cysts, comedo-like openings, fissures and ridges, hairpin blood vessels, sharp demarcation, and moth-eaten borders [3]. In case of ambiguity or features of malignancy such as ulcerated or large lesion and rapid change in size, a skin biopsy with histopathological examination may be recommended [2]. In histopathological examination, a proliferation of keratinocytes with keratin-filled cysts are typically observed [2]. In inflamed or irritated lesions lymphocytic infiltration may be present. There are numerous histopathological subtypes of seborrheic keratosis that vary in degrees of hyperkeratosis, acanthosis, pseudocysts, hyperpigmentation, inflammation, and dyskeratosis [1, 2]. Seborrheic keratosis is benign and typically does not require any treatment. However, lesions are frequently removed because of esthetic reason. The therapeutic options include cryotherapy (liquid nitrogen or CO_2), shave excision or topical agents (tazarotene, imiquimod cream, alpha-hydroxy acids, and urea ointment) [2].

Differential diagnoses for the presented patient were melanoma, pigmented basal carcinoma and melanotic nevus.

Melanoma is the most fatal form of skin cancer which most commonly affects the adult population. The typical cutaneous melanoma occurs as an asymmetric macule or nodule with irregular borders, frequently with variations in color within the lesion. Pink or red lesion may be also presented [4].

Basal cell carcinoma is the most common type of skin malignancy. The incidence rate of the disease increases with age. Basal cell carcinoma presents as a tiny, hardly visible papule, growing into a nodule or a plaque that is sometimes ulcerated [5]. The face, scalp or neck are most commonly affected.

The scalp is an anatomical location for nevi with site-related atypia, a subset of melanocytic nevi that share histologic features with melanoma but that are benign. The clinical patterns of the scalp melanotic nevi are solid brown, solid pink, eclipse and cockade. The lesions are mostly presented on the vertex and the parietal area [6].

Based on the clinical presentation and dermoscopic features, the diagnosis of seborrheic keratosis was established. Cryotherapy with liquid nitrogen was performed with resolution of the skin lesion.

Key Points
- Seborrheic keratosis is a benign skin tumor which may affect the scalp area.
- It presents as a sharply demarcated, round or oval-shaped, elevated and stuck on the skin lesion with a verrucous, dull, uneven, or punched-out surface.
- The color of the seborrheic keratosis varies from skin color, yellowish, light to dark brown, grey, and black.

References

1. Hafner C, Vogt T. Seborrheic keratosis. J Dtsch Dermatol Ges. 2008;6(8):664–77.
2. Greco MJ, Bhutta BS. Seborrheic keratosis. Treasure Island (FL): StatPearls; 2020.
3. Braun RP, Rabinovitz HS, Krischer J, Kreusch J, Oliviero M, Naldi L, et al. Dermoscopy of pigmented seborrheic keratosis: a morphological study. Arch Dermatol. 2002;138(12):1556–60.
4. Kibbi N, Kluger H, Choi JN. Melanoma: clinical presentations. Cancer Treat Res. 2016;167:107–29.
5. Marzuka AG, Book SE. Basal cell carcinoma: pathogenesis, epidemiology, clinical features, diagnosis, histopathology, and management. Yale J Biol Med. 2015;88(2):167–79.
6. Tcheung WJ, Bellet JS, Prose NS, Cyr DD, Nelson KC. Clinical and dermoscopic features of 88 scalp naevi in 39 children. Br J Dermatol. 2011;165(1):137–43.

Chapter 17
A 50-Year-Old Man with Itchy, Polymorphic Lesions on the Scalp

Joanna Golińska and Anna Waśkiel-Burnat

A 50-year-old man was admitted to the Department of Dermatology with a one-month history of widespread skin lesions with coexisting itch. The lesions started on his buttocks and then spread into the scalp, elbows, knees and forearms. No other family member was affected. The patient denied having any gastroenterological symptoms.

A physical examination revealed erosions with crusts and single vesicles on the occipital area of the scalp (Fig. 17.1). Moreover, erythematous areas with vesicles and numerous erosions with crusts were present on the elbows, forearms, buttocks and knees.

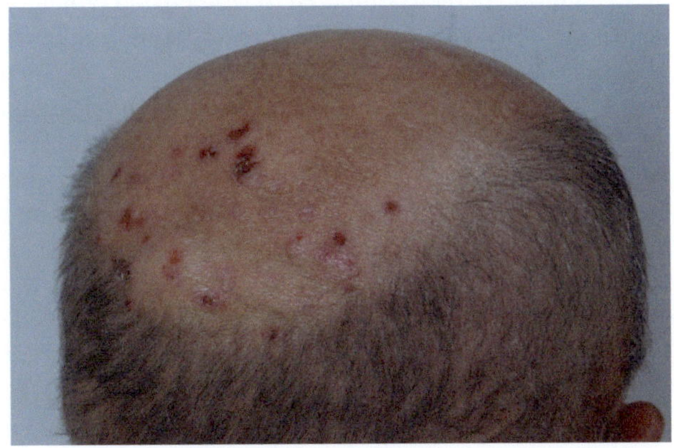

Fig. 17.1 A 50-year-old man with erosions covered by crusts and single vesicles on the occipital area

J. Golińska (✉) · A. Waśkiel-Burnat
Department of Dermatology, Medical University of Warsaw, Warsaw, Poland
e-mail: joanna.golinska@wum.edu.pl; anna.waskiel@wum.edu.pl

© The Author(s), under exclusive license to Springer Nature Switzerland AG 2022
A. Waśkiel-Burnat et al. (eds.), *Clinical Cases in Scalp Disorders*, Clinical Cases in Dermatology, https://doi.org/10.1007/978-3-030-93426-2_17

Laboratory tests were normal. A direct immunofluorescence test from the perilesional skin of the buttock revealed granular IgA (++) and IgM (+) deposits in the dermal papillae. An indirect immunofluorescence showed the presence of IgA anti-endomysial antibodies (IgA-EMA).

Based on the case description and the photographs, what is your diagnosis?

Differential Diagnoses
1. Pemphigus foliaceus.
2. Dermatitis herpetiformis.
3. Bullous pemphigoid.
4. Linear IgA dermatosis.

Diagnosis
Dermatitis herpetiformis.

Discussion

Dermatitis herpetiformis is a cutaneous manifestation of coeliac disease, in which gluten induces development of skin lesions in genetically susceptible individuals with the human leucocyte antigen (HLA) DQ2 or DQ8 haplotypes [1]. In both, celiac disease and dermatitis herpetiformis, the development of IgA autoantibodies against transglutaminases is observed. In the case of dermatitis herpetiformis, IgA autoantibodies are deposited in the superficial papillary dermis [2]. The disease is more common in men compared to women and typically occurs in the fourth decade of life [3]. In dermatitis herpetiformis, polymorphic skin lesions with the presence of vesicles, papules and macules with coexisted itch are observed. However, because of scratching, only erosions and crusts may be detected. The predilection sites for the dermatitis herpetiformis rash are the elbows, knees and buttocks [1]. Scalp involvement is observed in 30% of cases. Hair loss is rarely observed [2, 4]. 20% of patients with dermatitis herpetiformis exhibit gastrointestinal symptoms at time of initial diagnosis [3]. The diagnosis of dermatitis herpetiformis is based on typical clinical picture and direct immunofluorescence test. In direct immunofluorescence test, granular IgA in the papillary dermis are observed. Moreover, the presence of circulating anti-transglutaminase 2 antibodies supports the diagnosis, but their absence does not exclude dermatitis herpetiformis [1]. Therapy of dermatitis herpetiformis consists of a strict life-long gluten-free diet and sulphonamide drugs (dapsone). Moreover, short term use of potent topical corticosteroids may be helpful to decrease the itch [3].

Differential diagnoses for the presented patient included pemphigus foliaceous, bullous pemphigoid and linear IgA dermatosis.

Pemphigus foliaceus is a form of an autoimmune bullous disease affecting the skin. The disease most commonly affects women between 50 and 60 years of age [2]. Skin involvement is characterized by flaccid blisters and erosions localized mainly on the face, scalp, trunk and proximal extremities [5].

Bullous pemphigoid is the most frequent autoimmune bullous disease that mainly affects elderly individuals, usually above 70 years [6]. It presents as itchy, tense blisters over normal skin or over erythematous and edematous background [6]. Mucosal involvement is rarely reported (10–30% of the cases) [6].

Linear IgA bullous dermatosis is a subepidermal vesiculobullous disease that occurs in both adults and children. In children it presents as annular or polycyclic plaques and papules with blistering around the edges, primarily around the mouth and eyes, lower abdomen, thighs, buttocks, genitals, wrists and ankles. In contrast, the adult-onset is characterized by the lesions on the trunk, head and extremities [7].

Based on clinical features and immunofluorescence tests, the patient was diagnosed with dermatitis herpetiformis. Dapsone (100 mg daily) was initiated. Gluten-free diet and gastroenterological consultation was recommended.

Key Points
- Dermatitis herpetiformis presents as itchy, polymorphic skin lesions mainly localized on the elbows, knees and buttocks areas.
- Scalp involvement is observed in 30% of patients with dermatitis herpetiformis; hair loss is rarely observed.

References

1. Salmi TT. Dermatitis herpetiformis. Clin Exp Dermatol. 2019;44(7):728–31.
2. Salmi TT, Hervonen K, Kautiainen H, Collin P, Reunala T. Prevalence and incidence of dermatitis herpetiformis: a 40-year prospective study from Finland. Br J Dermatol. 2011;165(2):354–9.
3. Mirza HA, Gharbi A, Bhutta BS. Dermatitis herpetiformis. Treasure Island (FL): StatPearls; 2020.
4. Gul U, Soylu S, Heper A. An unusual case of dermatitis herpetiformis presenting with initial scalp localization. Indian J Dermatol Venereol Leprol. 2009;75(6):620–2.
5. Kridin K. Pemphigus group: overview, epidemiology, mortality, and comorbidities. Immunol Res. 2018;66(2):255–70.
6. Miyamoto D, Santi CG, Aoki V, Maruta CW. Bullous pemphigoid. An Bras Dermatol. 2019;94(2):133–46.
7. Lammer J, Hein R, Roenneberg S, Biedermann T, Volz T. Drug-induced linear IgA bullous dermatosis: a case report and review of the literature. Acta Derm Venereol. 2019;99(6):508–15.

Chapter 18
A 57-Year-Old Woman with Crusted Erosions on the Scalp

Joanna Golińska and Anna Waśkiel-Burnat

A 57-year-old woman was admitted to the Department of Dermatology with a four-month history of skin and mucosal lesions. Initially, erythematous lesions on the scalp were present. Based on clinical features, the diagnosis of psoriasis was established and treatment with topical corticosteroids was initiated. One month later, a small erosion appeared on the nose. Because of the suspicion of basal cell carcinoma, the lesion was surgically removed. A histopathological examination revealed features of syringiocystadenoma papilliferum. Subsequently, erosions on the erythematous background appeared on the other body areas such as the face, chest and back. Moreover, painful erosions on oral and genital mucosa appeared.

A physical examination revealed erosions covered with thick crusts on the scalp with coexisted hair loss (Fig. 18.1). Moreover, widespread erosions with crusts and single bullae on erythematous background on the face, chest and the upper part of the back were observed. Multiple erosions on oral and genital mucosa were detected. Trichoscopy showed extravasations and yellow hemorrhagic crusts (Fig. 18.2).

In laboratory tests, elevated C-reactive protein was observed. Other laboratory tests including complete blood count, electrolytes, liver enzymes and creatinine were within normal limits. A direct immunofluorescence test revealed intercellular substance deposition of immunoglobulin G (IgG). In indirect immunofluorescence test, intercellular deposits of IgG and C3 were observed.

Based on the case description and the photographs, what is your diagnosis?

Differential Diagnoses
1. Pemphigus foliaceus.
2. Pemphigus vulgaris.

J. Golińska (✉) · A. Waśkiel-Burnat
Department of Dermatology, Medical University of Warsaw, Warsaw, Poland
e-mail: joanna.golinska@wum.edu.pl; anna.waskiel@wum.edu.pl

A. Waśkiel-Burnat et al. (eds.), *Clinical Cases in Scalp Disorders*, Clinical Cases in Dermatology, https://doi.org/10.1007/978-3-030-93426-2_18

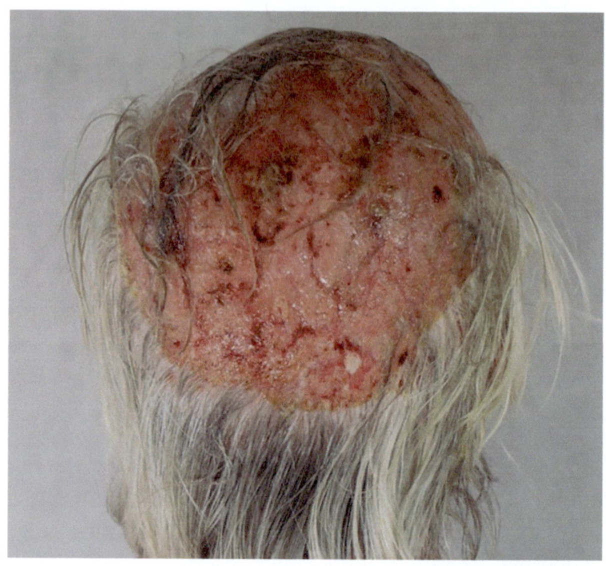

Fig. 18.1 A 57-year-old woman with hair loss and crusted erosions on the erythematous background on the scalp

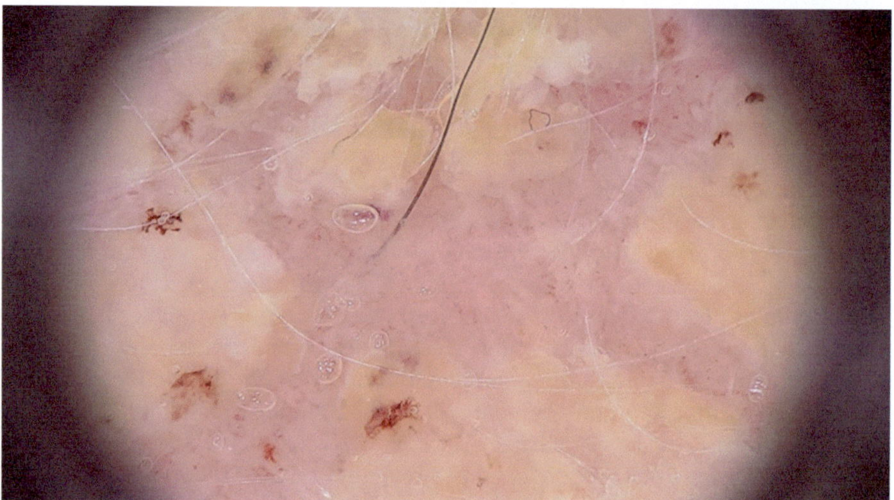

Fig. 18.2 Trichoscopy with the presence of extravasations and yellow hemorrhagic crusts (×20)

3. Bullous pemphigoid.
4. Linear IgA dermatosis.

Diagnosis

Pemphigus vulgaris.

Discussion

Pemphigus vulgaris is a form of an autoimmune bullous disease affecting the skin and mucous membranes. It is the most prevalent type of pemphigus, comprising up to 70% of all cases of pemphigus [1]. The etiopathogenesis of the disease is characterized by acantholysis and intraepidermal blisters formation, resulting from IgG autoantibodies directed against transmembrane desmosomal glycoprotein desmoglein 3, and in some cases desmoglein 1 [1, 2]. Pemphigus vulgaris predominantly affects women between 50 and 60 years of age [3]. The initial clinical presentation usually includes erosions on the mucous membranes. The oral mucosa is most frequently affected, leading to dysphagia and weight loss. The other mucosal surfaces, including the pharyngo-laryngeal, esophageal, conjunctival mucosae, genital, and, anal may be also involved [3]. Skin involvement is characterized by flaccid blisters and erosions localized mainly on the face, scalp, trunk and proximal extremities [1]. The scalp is affected in 16–65% of patients with pemphigus vulgaris. In 9–15% of cases the scalp is the first location [4]. Clinically, pemphigus vulgaris on the scalp presents as crusted erosions on erythematous background. Hair loss, observed in 5.4% of cases, is usually non-scarring, except single cases of prolonged course with staphylococcal suprainfection [4]. The diagnosis of pemphigus vulgaris is mainly established based on clinical features and immunofluorescence tests. In direct immunofluorescence test, IgG or C3 binding to the intercellular cement substance in the mid-lower or entire epidermis is observed. An indirect immunofluorescence reveals the presence of serum autoantibodies against desmosomal antigens. Trichoscopy can be a useful supplementary diagnostic method. Trichoscopic features of pemphigus vulgaris include extravasations, yellow hemorrhagic crusts, and yellow dots with whitish halo [5]. In histopathologic examination, suprabasalar acantholysis and infiltration with predominantly neutrophils and eosinophils are detected [3]. Treatment of pemphigus vulgaris include systemic corticosteroids with/or without immunosuppressive agent (azathioprine, mycophenolate mofetil, mycophenolic acid or dapsone) or rituximab. Topical antiseptic agents and topical corticosteroids can be also useful [6].

Differential diagnoses for the presented patient included pemphigus foliaceous, bullous pemphigoid and linear IgA dermatosis.

Pemphigus foliaceous is the second most prevalent variant of pemphigus. Similarly to the pemphigus vulgaris, it presents as erosions surrounded by erythema that heal with crusting and scaling. On the contrary to pemphigus vulgaris, mucous membranes are spared [1].

Bullous pemphigoid is the most frequent autoimmune bullous disease that mainly affects elderly individuals, usually above 70 years [7]. It presents as itchy, tense blisters on normal skin or on erythematous and edematous background. Mucosal involvement is rarely reported (10–30% of the cases) [7].

Linear IgA bullous dermatosis is a relatively rare subepidermal vesiculobullous disease that occurs in both adults and children [6]. In children the disease is characterized by the presence of annular or polycyclic plaques and papules with blistering around the edges, primarily around the mouth and eyes, lower abdomen, thighs, buttocks, genitals, wrists and ankles. In contrast, the adult-onset form presents as lesions on the trunk, head and extremities. In both children and adults, the mucous membranes can be affected [8].

In the presented patient, based on clinical presentation and immunofluorescence tests, the diagnosis of pemphigus vulgaris was established. The patient was treated with rituximab (two infusions of 1 g 2 weeks apart). Four weeks after the treatment initiation resolution of skin lesions with hair regrowth were observed.

Key Points

- The scalp is involved in 16–65% of patients with pemphigus vulgaris, while in 9–15% of cases it is the first affected location.
- Pemphigus vulgaris on the scalp presents as crusted erosions on erythematous background leading to hair loss in 5.4% of cases.
- The hair loss in the course of pemphigus vulgaris is non-scarring, except the prolonged course with staphylococcal suprainfection.

References

1. Kridin K. Pemphigus group: overview, epidemiology, mortality, and comorbidities. Immunol Res. 2018;66(2):255–70.
2. Venugopal SS, Murrell DF. Diagnosis and clinical features of pemphigus vulgaris. Dermatol Clin. 2011;29(3):373–80.
3. Kasperkiewicz M, Ellebrecht CT, Takahashi H, Yamagami J, Zillikens D, Payne AS, et al. Pemphigus. Nat Rev Dis Primers. 2017;3:17026.
4. Sar-Pomian M, Konop M, Gala K, Rudnicka L, Olszewska M. Scalp involvement in pemphigus: a prognostic marker. Adv Dermatol Allergol Postępy Dermatologii i Alergologii. 2018;35(3):293–8.
5. Sar-Pomian M, Kurzeja M, Rudnicka L, Olszewska M. The value of trichoscopy in the differential diagnosis of scalp lesions in pemphigus vulgaris and pemphigus foliaceus. An Bras Dermatol. 2014;89(6):1007–12.
6. Schmidt E, Sticherling M, Sárdy M, Eming R, Goebeler M, Hertl M, et al. S2k guidelines for the treatment of pemphigus vulgaris/foliaceus and bullous pemphigoid: 2019 update. J Dtsch Dermatol Ges. 2020;18(5):516–26.
7. Miyamoto D, Santi CG, Aoki V, Maruta CW. Bullous pemphigoid. An Bras Dermatol. 2019;94(2):133–46.
8. Lammer J, Hein R, Roenneberg S, Biedermann T, Volz T. Drug-induced linear IgA bullous dermatosis: a case report and review of the literature. Acta Derm Venereol. 2019;99(6):508–15.

Chapter 19
A 65-Year-Old Man with Erosions and Leafy Scaling on the Scalp

Aleksandra Wielgoś

A 65-year-old man presented with a three-month history of disseminated erosions located on the scalp, face, trunk, and upper extremities. He reported the presence of similar skin lesions 13 years ago, when he was successfully treated with systemic prednisone at a maximum dose of 100 mg per day and chloroquine at a maximum dose of 500 mg per day. The patient had hypertension, type 2 diabetes mellitus, obesity, polyneuropathy and vitiligo.

On physical examination, erosions, yellowish crusts and leafy scaling on the frontoparietal and vertex areas were observed (Fig. 19.1). Moreover, erosions on the face, trunk and upper extremities were detected. No mucosal lesions were present.

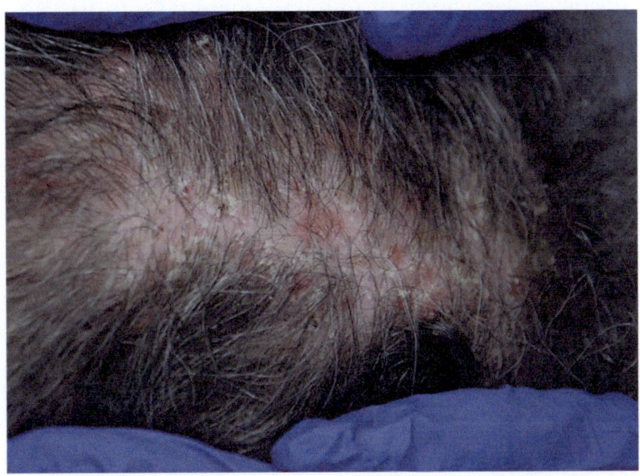

Fig. 19.1 A 65-year-old man with erosions, yellowish crusts and leafy scaling on the scalp

A. Wielgoś (✉)
Department of Dermatology, Medical University of Warsaw, Warsaw, Poland

© The Author(s), under exclusive license to Springer Nature Switzerland AG 2022
A. Waśkiel-Burnat et al. (eds.), *Clinical Cases in Scalp Disorders*, Clinical Cases in Dermatology, https://doi.org/10.1007/978-3-030-93426-2_19

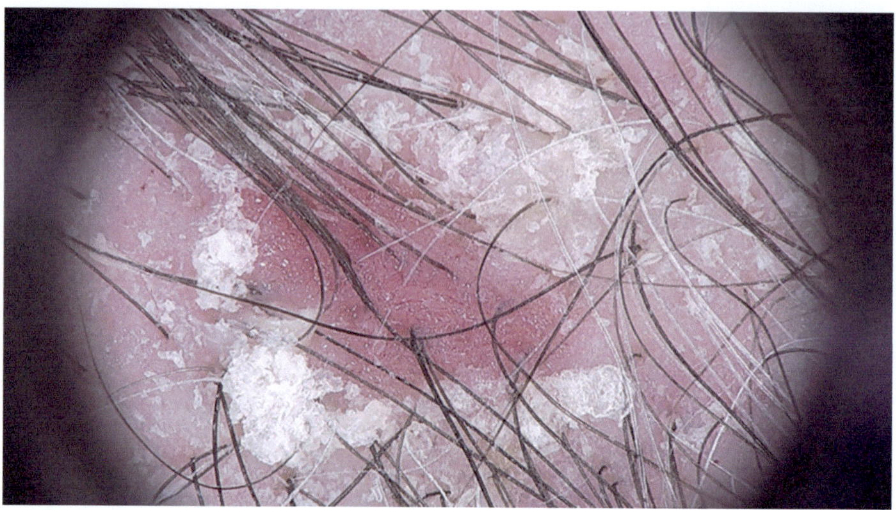

Fig. 19.2 Trichoscopy shows a red area with polymorphic vessels surrounded by whitish scaling (×20)

Trichoscopy showed yellowish and whitish scaling, extravasations and red areas with polymorphic vessels (Fig. 19.2).

Laboratory tests revealed hyperglycemia and an elevated activity of gammaglutamyltranspeptidase. In chest X-ray and abdominal ultrasound no significant abnormalities were observed. Direct immunofluorescence test revealed intercellular substance deposition of immunoglobulin G. In ELISA, anti-desmoglein 1 antibodies were found to be positive.

Based on the case description and the photographs, what is your diagnosis?

Differential Diagnoses
1. Bullous pemphigoid.
2. Pemphigus foliaceus.
3. Pemphigus vulgaris.
4. Linear IgA dermatosis.

Diagnosis
Pemphigus foliaceus.

Discussion

Pemphigus foliaceus is an intraepidermal autoimmune blistering disease affecting the skin. It is the second most prevalent variant of pemphigus [1]. The etiopathogenesis of the disease is characterized by acantholysis and intraepidermal blisters formation, resulting from IgG autoantibodies directed against transmembrane desmosomal glycoprotein desmoglein 1 [1, 2]. Pemphigus foliaceus usually presents between fourth and sixth decade of life and its prevalence is comparable in both sexes. Clinically, it presents as skin erosions surrounded by erythema that heal with crusting and scaling, with sparing of the mucosal surfaces. The vesicles are superficial and fragile, thus only the resultant erosions are observed in most cases [1]. The lesions are most commonly presented on the seborrheic regions (the central face, neck, chest, and upper back). The scalp is affected in 16–65% of patients with pemphigus. In 9–15% of cases the scalp is the first location [3]. Hair loss, observed in 5.4% of cases, is usually non-scarring, except single cases of prolonged course with staphylococcal suprainfection [3]. The diagnosis of pemphigus foliaceus is mainly established based on clinical features and immunofluorescence tests. On direct immunofluorescence, IgG or C3 binding to the intercellular cement substance in the upper epidermis is observed. A indirect immunofluorescence microcopy reveals the presence of pemphigus autoantibodies. In ELISA, autoantibodies against desmoglein-1 are observed. Trichoscopy can be a useful supplementary diagnostic method. Trichoscopic features of pemphigus foliaceus include extravasations, yellow hemorrhagic crusts, yellow dots with whitish halo and white polygonal structures [4]. In histopathologic examination, acantholysis within the stratum granulosum and infiltration with predominantly neutrophils and eosinophils are detected [5]. Treatment of pemphigus foliaceus includes systemic corticosteroids with/ or without an immunosuppressive agent (azathioprine, mycophenolate mofetil, mycophenolic acid or dapsone) or rituximab. Topical antiseptic agents and topical corticosteroids can also be useful [6].

The differential diagnoses for the presented patient were bullous pemphigoid, pemphigus vulgaris and linear IgA dermatosis.

Bullous pemphigoid is the most frequent autoimmune bullous disease that mainly affects elderly individuals, usually above 70 years of age [7]. It presents as itchy, tense blisters over normal skin or over erythematous and edematous background [7].

Pemphigus vulgaris is a form of an autoimmune bullous disease affecting the skin and the mucous membranes. It is the most prevalent type of pemphigus [1]. Pemphigus vulgaris predominantly affects women between 50 and 60 years of age [3]. It initially presents as erosions on the mucous membranes. Skin involvement is characterized by flaccid blisters and erosions localized mainly on the face, scalp, trunk and proximal extremities [1].

Linear IgA bullous dermatosis is a relatively rare subepidermal vesiculobullous disease that occurs in both adults and children [6]. In children the disease is characterized by the presence of annular or polycyclic plaques and papules with blistering around the edges, primarily around the mouth and eyes, lower abdomen, thighs, buttocks, genitals, wrists and ankles. In contrast, the adult-onset form presents as lesions on the trunk, head and extremities. In both children and adults, the mucous membranes can be affected [8].

Based on the patient's clinical presentation and immunofluorescence tests, the diagnosis of pemphigus foliaceus was established. The patient was treated with rituximab (two infusions of 1 g 2 weeks apart) with good tolerance and partial clinical response. A complete resolution of scalp lesions was achieved after intralesional treatment with triamcinolone acetonide (10 mg/ml) every four-six weeks.

Key Points
- Pemphigus foliaceus is characterized by the presence of skin erosions surrounded by erythema that heal with crusting and scaling.
- The scalp is affected in 16–65% of patients with pemphigus, while in 9–15% of cases the scalp is the first location.
- Pemphigus on the scalp presents as crusted erosions on erythematous background leading to hair loss in 5.4% of cases.
- The hair loss in the course of pemphigus is non-scarring, except the prolonged course with staphylococcal suprainfection.

References

1. Kridin K. Pemphigus group: overview, epidemiology, mortality, and comorbidities. Immunol Res. 2018;66(2):255–70.
2. Venugopal SS, Murrell DF. Diagnosis and clinical features of pemphigus vulgaris. Dermatol Clin. 2011;29(3):373–80. vii
3. Sar-Pomian M, Konop M, Gala K, Rudnicka L, Olszewska M. Scalp involvement in pemphigus: a prognostic marker. Postepy Dermatol i Alergol. 2018;35(3):293–8.
4. Sar-Pomian M, Kurzeja M, Rudnicka L, Olszewska M. The value of trichoscopy in the differential diagnosis of scalp lesions in pemphigus vulgaris and pemphigus foliaceus. An Bras Dermatol. 2014;89(6):1007–12.
5. Kasperkiewicz M, Ellebrecht CT, Takahashi H, Yamagami J, Zillikens D, Payne AS, et al. Pemphigus. Nat Rev Dis Prim. 2017;3:17026.
6. Schmidt E, Sticherling M, Sárdy M, Eming R, Goebeler M, Hertl M, et al. S2k guidelines for the treatment of pemphigus vulgaris/foliaceus and bullous pemphigoid: 2019 update. J Dtsch Dermatol Ges. 2020;18(5):516–26.
7. Miyamoto D, Santi CG, Aoki V, Maruta CW. Bullous pemphigoid. An Bras Dermatol. 2019;94(2):133–46.
8. Lammer J, Hein R, Roenneberg S, Biedermann T, Volz T. Drug-induced linear IgA bullous dermatosis: a case report and review of the literature. Acta Derm Venereol. 2019;99(6):508–15.

Chapter 20
A 67-Year-Old Man with an Ulcerated Nodule on the Scalp

Agnieszka Kaczorowska, Paulina Chmielińska, Marta Sar-Pomian, and Joanna Czuwara

A 67-year-old man presented with a five-month history of an enlarging nodule of the scalp. The lesion started as a small erythematous and scaly plaque and had been rapidly growing with occasional bleeding and crusting. He complained of a pain in this area. The patient had been working outdoors as a farmer and he denied using proper sunlight protection. He was a heavy smoker (40 pack-year smoking history). There was no personal or family history of skin cancers.

A physical examination revealed an ulcerated nodule, measuring 3.5 cm × 3 cm, on the vertex area of the scalp (Fig. 20.1). Local lymph nodes were not palpable. On dermoscopy, central mass of keratin, ulceration and linear-irregular vessels arranged radially were observed (Fig. 20.2).

A histopathological examination showed atypical hyperplastic epidermis without maturation and columns of parakeratosis. An early invasion into the dermis was associated with tongues of atypical keratinocytes with inflammatory response at the bottom of the lesion (Fig. 20.3).

Based on the case description and the photographs, what is your diagnosis?

Differential Diagnoses
1. Basal cell carcinoma.
2. Squamous cell carcinoma.
3. Merkel cell carcinoma.
4. Cutaneous metastasis.

Diagnosis
Squamous cell carcinoma.

A. Kaczorowska (✉) · P. Chmielińska · M. Sar-Pomian · J. Czuwara
Department of Dermatology, Medical University of Warsaw, Warsaw, Poland
e-mail: agnieszka.kaczorowska@wum.edu.pl

A. Waśkiel-Burnat et al. (eds.), *Clinical Cases in Scalp Disorders*, Clinical Cases in Dermatology, https://doi.org/10.1007/978-3-030-93426-2_20

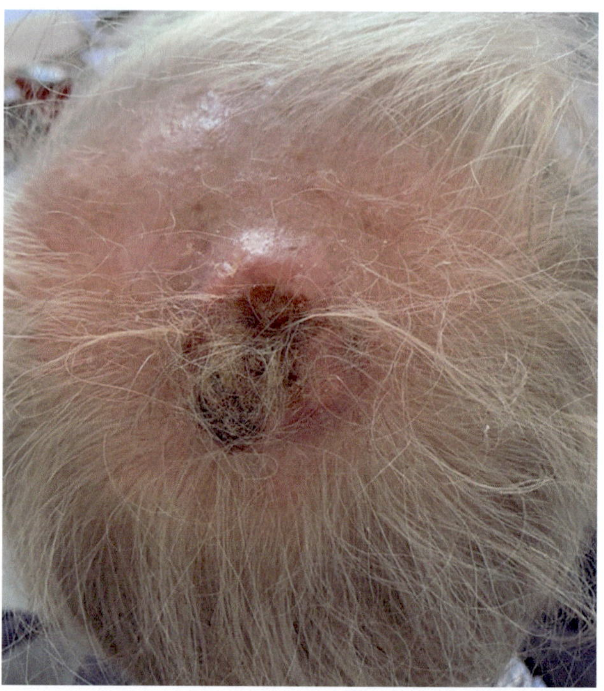

Fig. 20.1 A 67-year-old man with an ulcerated nodule on the vertex area

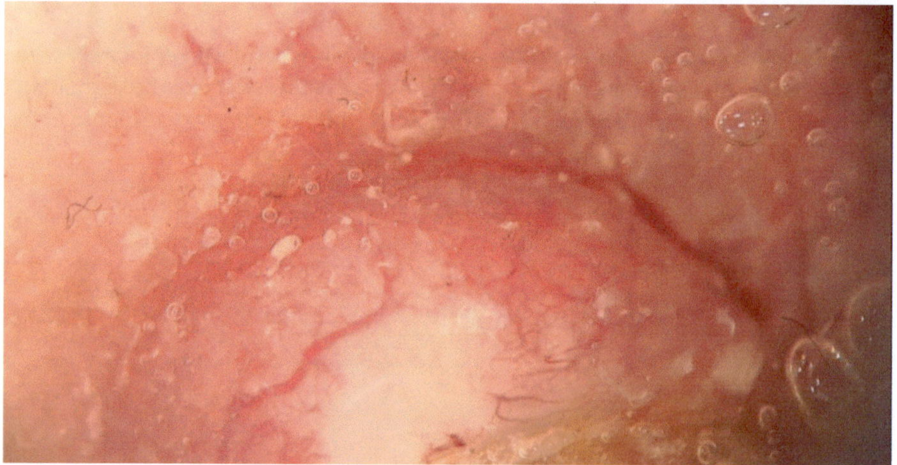

Fig. 20.2 Dermoscopy shows linear-irregular vessels (×20)

Discussion

Squamous cell carcinoma is the second most common non-melanoma skin cancer. It accounts for 20–50% of skin cancers, with an increasing incidence worldwide [1]. Cumulative sun exposure (primarily ultraviolet b) is the greatest risk factor [2].

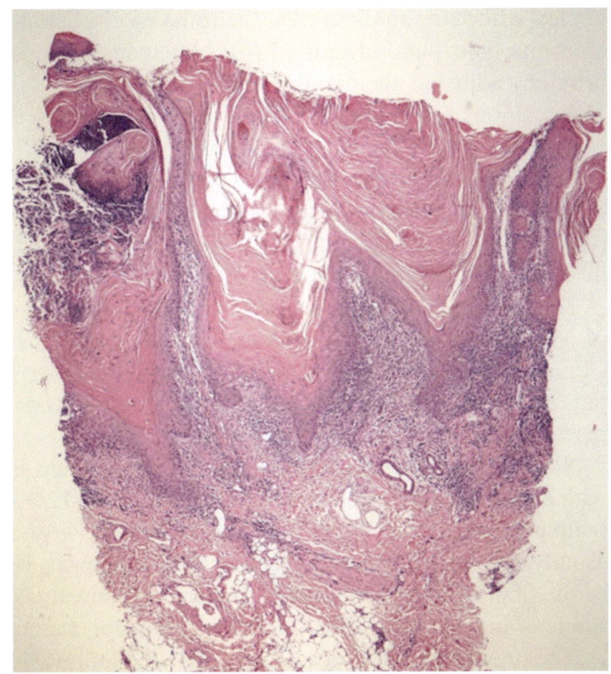

Fig. 20.3 Histopathology shows atypical hyperplastic epidermis without maturation and columns of parakeratosis. An early invasion into the dermis is associated with tongues of atypical keratinocytes with inflammatory response at the bottom of the lesion

Other risk factors include fair skin (Fitzpatrick skin types I-II), older age, immunosuppression, outdoor occupation, smoking, human papillomavirus infection (types 16, 18, and 31), exposure to arsenic and ionizing radiation, chronic skin conditions (burn scars, discoid lupus erythematosus, lichen sclerosus) and treatment with BRAF inhibitors [3–5]. Familial syndromes (xeroderma pigmentosum, epidermolysis bullosa, epidermolysis verruciformis, albinism) predispose to multiple squamous cell carcinoma [2]. Squamous cell carcinoma originates from epidermal keratinocytes or adnexal structures [3]. It can arise within precursor lesions (actinic keratosis, Bowen's disease) or occur de novo [4]. The incidence of squamous cell carcinoma increases with age, with an average age of onset in the mid-60s. It is more common in men than women (3:1). Clinically, squamous cell carcinoma presents as a papule, plaque, or indurated nodule with a smooth, scaly, verrucous, or ulcerative surface. Lesions are typically solitary, but sometimes multiple "in transit" metastases may be present [2]. Squamous cell carcinoma may be asymptomatic or may cause pruritus, pain or even local neuropathic symptoms if associated with perineural invasion [3, 4]. In fair-skinned individuals, it typically develops in the areas of photo-damaged skin, mainly on the head and neck (55%), the extensor surfaces of hands and forearms (18%), and lower extremities (13%). Non-sun-exposed areas are the most common location among dark-skinned individuals [3]. Histopathology is a gold standard diagnostic method in squamous cell carcinoma. Dermoscopy may be helpful to establish the initial diagnosis. Characteristic dermoscopic features of squamous cell carcinoma include scales, blood spots, white circles, white structureless areas, hairpin vessels, linear-irregular vessels, perivascular white halos, and ulceration [6]. Management is primarily surgical, rarely followed by adjuvant chemoradiation.

Squamous cell carcinoma needs to be differentiated from basal cell carcinoma, Merkel cell carcinoma and skin metastasis.

Basal cell carcinoma is the most common skin malignancy. The incidence rate of the disease increases with age. Basal cell carcinoma presents as a tiny, hardly visible papule, growing into a nodule or a plaque that is sometimes ulcerated [7]. Areas of the face, scalp and neck are most commonly affected.

Merkel cell carcinoma is a rare but highly aggressive skin cancer. The incidence of Merkel cell carcinoma increases with age and is higher in men than women. Clinically, it presents as a rapidly growing tumour or solid infiltration of the skin, red to violet in colour. The head and neck are most commonly affected. Ulceration in Merkel cell carcinoma is rarely observed [8].

Skin metastases from primary visceral malignancy are uncommon clinical entity, with a reported incidence ranging from 0.22% to 12% of all malignancies [9]. The scalp involvement is observed in approximately 5% of cases. Cutaneous metastases usually develop a long-time after the initial diagnosis. However, sometimes they can be the first sign of an internal malignancy. Clinically, skin metastasis presents as a single or multiple non-tender nodules which are characterized by rapid growth.

The presented patient was diagnosed with an invasive squamous cell carcinoma and treated with complete surgical excision—T2N0M0. His lymph nodes and abdomen ultrasound as well as chest radiograph results were normal. He had follow-up visits every three months and showed no signs of local recurrence or metastases.

Key Points
- Squamous cell carcinoma is the second most common non-melanoma skin cancer, which is frequently located on the scalp.
- It presents as a papule, plaque, or indurated nodule with a smooth, scaly, verrucous, or ulcerative surface.

References

1. Que SKT, Zwald FO, Schmults CD. Cutaneous squamous cell carcinoma: incidence, risk factors, diagnosis, and staging. J Am Acad Dermatol. 2018;78(2):237–47.
2. Waldman A, Schmults C. Cutaneous squamous cell carcinoma. Hematol Oncol Clin North Am. 2019;33(1):1–12.
3. Kallini JR, Hamed N, Khachemoune A. Squamous cell carcinoma of the skin: epidemiology, classification, management, and novel trends. Int J Dermatol. 2015;54(2):130–40.
4. Parekh V, Seykora JT. Cutaneous squamous cell carcinoma. Clin Lab Med. 2017;37(3):503–25.
5. Dusingize JC, Olsen CM, Pandeya NP, Subramaniam P, Thompson BS, Neale RE, et al. Cigarette smoking and the risks of basal cell carcinoma and squamous cell carcinoma. J Invest Dermatol. 2017;137(8):1700–8.
6. Kato J, Horimoto K, Sato S, Minowa T, Uhara H. Dermoscopy of melanoma and non-melanoma skin cancers. Front Med (Lausanne). 2019;6:180.

7. Marzuka AG, Book SE. Basal cell carcinoma: pathogenesis, epidemiology, clinical features, diagnosis, histopathology, and management. Yale J Biol Med. 2015;88(2):167–79.
8. Dudzisz-Śledź M, Zdzienicki M, Rutkowski P. Merkel cell carcinoma (MCC) – neuroendocrine skin cancer. Nowotwory J Oncol. 2019;69(3–4):111–6.
9. Yu Q, Subedi S, Tong Y, Wei Q, Xu H, Wang Y, Gong Y, Shi Y. Scalp metastases as first presentation of pulmonary adenocarcinomas: a case report. Onco Targets Ther. 2018;11:6147–51.

Chapter 21
A 67-Year-Old Man with Erosions and Scarring on the Scalp

Marta Muszel and Mariusz Sikora

A 67-year-old man was admitted to the Department of Dermatology due to erosive and scarring lesions presented on the scalp for two years. The patient was treated with oral and topical antibiotics without any improvement. The patient complained of a pain and tenderness at touch. He denied history of the scalp trauma or an extensive sun exposure.

On physical examination, erosions partially covered with hemorrhagic and yellowish crusts and surrounded by scarring areas on the frontoparietal region were observed. Moreover, non-scarring hair loss on the vertex area was presented (Fig. 21.1). No other skin or mucosal lesions were observed.

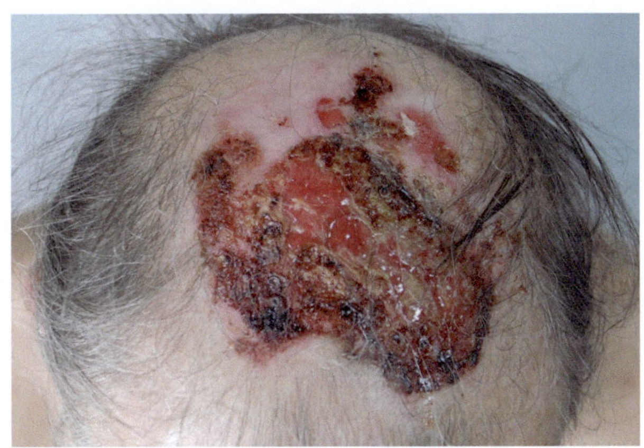

Fig. 21.1 A 67-year-old man with erosions partially covered with hemorrhagic and yellowish crusts surrounded by scarring areas on the frontoparietal region. Moreover, non-scarring hair loss on the vertex area is presented

M. Muszel (✉)
Department of Dermatology, Medical University of Warsaw, Warsaw, Poland

M. Sikora
National Institute of Geriatrics, Rheumatology and Rehabilitation, Warsaw, Poland
e-mail: mariusz.sikora@spartanska.pl

A. Waśkiel-Burnat et al. (eds.), *Clinical Cases in Scalp Disorders*, Clinical Cases in Dermatology, https://doi.org/10.1007/978-3-030-93426-2_21

Laboratory tests were within normal range. Direct immunofluorescence test of perilesional skin showed linear depositions of IgG and C3 at the basement membrane zone. An indirect immunofluorescence test was negative. In histopathological examination, erosion and inflammatory infiltrate composed of lymphocytes, plasmacytes and neutrophils in the dermis were observed.

Based on the case description and the photographs, what is your diagnosis?

Differential Diagnoses
1.   Erosive pustular dermatosis of the scalp.
2.   Discoid lupus erythematosus.
3.   Basal cell carcinoma.
4.   Brunsting-Perry pemphigoid.

Diagnosis
Brunsting-Perry pemphigoid.

Discussion

Brunsting-Perry pemphigoid is a form of mucous membrane pemphigoid [1, 2]. To date, the pathogenesis of Brunsting-Perry pemphigoid remains to be elucidated [3]. The role of BP180, type VII collagen, laminin 332, BP230, and LAD-1 as autoantigens has been suggested [3]. The disease is mostly observed in elderly patients. Men are more commonly affected [1]. Clinically, Brunsting-Perry pemphigoid is characterized by the bullous and erosive lesions limited to the head, neck, scalp, and upper trunk with mild or no mucosal involvement. In the case of the scalp lesions, scarring alopecia may occur [1]. The condition is generally slowly progressing, however possible severe variants have been reported [4]. The diagnosis of Brunsting-Perry pemphigoid is based on clinical presentation and immunopathological and histopathological examinations. A direct immunofluorescence test of perilesional skin shows linear deposition of IgG and complement along the dermal-epidermal junction. Indirect immunofluorescence studies are usually negative. In histopathological examination, subepidermal blisters with mixed inflammatory cell infiltration are detected [4]. Treatment of Brunsting-Perry pemphigoid is similar to the therapy of other forms of pemphigoid. Potent topical corticosteroids are usually the first-line therapeutic option. Low-dose methotrexate, tetracyclines or dapsone are recommended for more severe or refractory cases [5].

Differential diagnoses for the presented patient included erosive pustular dermatosis of the scalp, discoid lupus erythematosus and basal cell carcinoma.

Erosive pustular dermatosis of the scalp is a rare, inflammatory disorder that occurs mostly in elderly patients. Clinically, it is characterized by recurrent pustules, inflamed erosions and grey, yellow or yellow-brown crusts that lead to scarring alopecia [6].

Discoid lupus erythematosus is a form of lymphocytic primary cicatricial alopecia. Typically, it occurs in women between 20 and 40 years of age. The disease is characterized by well-circumscribed erythematous indurated plaques with coexisted scaling. When the adherent scale is removed, follicular plugging may be observed (carpet tack sign). Telangiectasias, atrophy, depigmentation, and hyperpigmentation may be detected. Erosions are not typically presented [2].

Basal cell carcinoma is the most common skin malignancy. The incidence rate of the disease increases with age. Basal cell carcinoma presents as a tiny, hardly visible papule, growing into a nodule or a plaque that is sometimes ulcerated. The face, scalp or neck area are most commonly affected [6].

In the presented patient, based on clinical features, immunofluorescence and histopathological examinations, the diagnosis of Brunsting-Perry pemphigoid was established. The patient was treated with oral methotrexate (7.5 mg once a week) and clobetasol propionate 0.05% cream. A significant improvement was observed three months after the treatment initiation.

Key Points
- Brunsting-Perry pemphigoid is a rare, bullous disease which may lead to scarring alopecia.
- It presents as bullous and erosive lesions limited to the head, neck, scalp, and upper trunk with mild or no mucosal involvement.

References

1. Brunsting LA, Perry HO. Benign pemphigoid; a report of seven cases with chronic, scarring, herpetiform plaques about the head and neck. AMA Arch Derm. 1957;75(4):489.
2. Jedlickova H, Niedermeier A, Zgažarová S, Hertl M. Brunsting-Perry pemphigoid of the scalp with antibodies against laminin 332. Dermatology. 2011;222(3):193–5.
3. Zhou S, Zou Y, Pan M. Brunsting-Perry pemphigoid transitioning from previous bullous pemphigoid. JAAD Case Rep. 2020;6(3):192–4.
4. Leenutaphong V, von Kries R, Plewig G. Localized cicatricial pemphigoid (Brunsting-Perry): electron microscopic study. J Am Acad Dermatol. 1989;21(5 Pt 2):1089–93.
5. Martín JM, Pinazo I, Molina I, Monteagudo C, Villalón G, Reig I, Jordá E. Cicatricial pemphigoid of the Brunsting-Perry type. Int J Dermatol. 2009 Mar;48(3):293–4.
6. Karanfilian KM, Wassef C. Erosive pustular dermatosis of the scalp: causes and treatments. Int J Dermatol. 2021;60(1):25–32.

Chapter 22
A 67-Year-Old Woman with an Acute Scalp Erythema

Anna Waśkiel-Burnat, Monika Łukiewicz, Małgorzata Olszewska, and Lidia Rudnicka

A 67-year-old woman with a history of androgenetic alopecia presented with an erythema and scaling of the scalp since one week. The patient was treated with topical minoxidil solution for one month. She complained of severe itching of the scalp.

A physical examination revealed erythematous lesions extending onto the forehead with erosions and whitish scaling (Figs. 22.1 and 22.2). On trichoscopy, yellowish and white scaling as well as dotted vessels arranged in clusters were observed (Fig. 22.3).

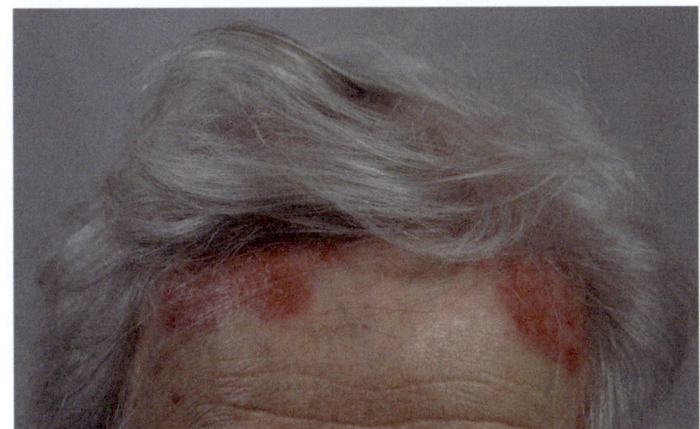

Fig. 22.1 A 67-year-old woman with erythematous lesions extending onto the forehead

A. Waśkiel-Burnat (✉) · M. Łukiewicz · M. Olszewska · L. Rudnicka
Department of Dermatology, Medical University of Warsaw, Warsaw, Poland
e-mail: anna.waskiel@wum.edu.pl; malgorzata.olszewska@wum.edu.pl;
lidia.rudnicka@wum.edu.pl

© The Author(s), under exclusive license to Springer Nature Switzerland AG 2022
A. Waśkiel-Burnat et al. (eds.), *Clinical Cases in Scalp Disorders*, Clinical Cases in Dermatology, https://doi.org/10.1007/978-3-030-93426-2_22

Fig. 22.2 An erythema, whitish scaling and erosions on the scalp

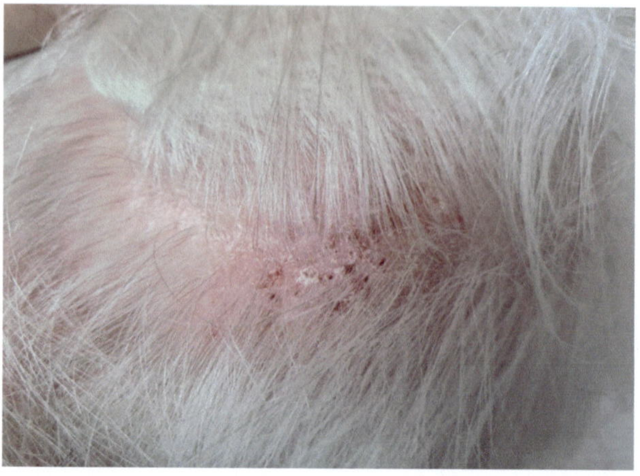

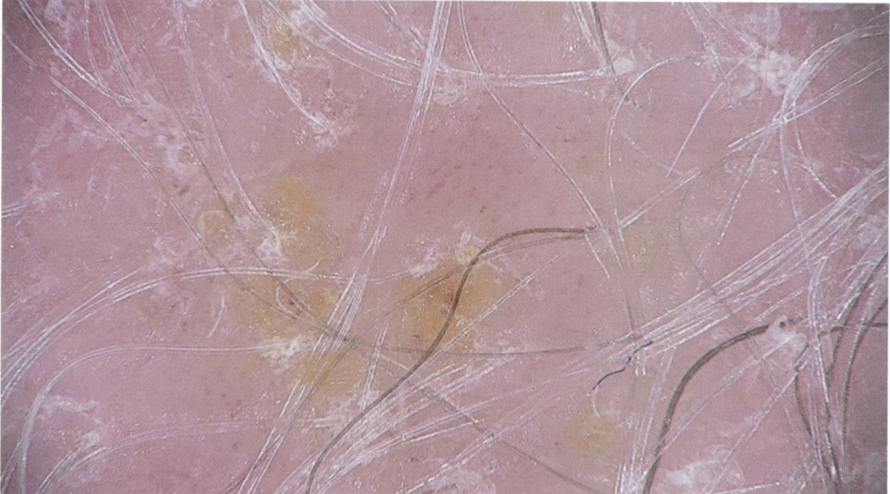

Fig. 22.3 Trichoscopy shows whitish and yellowish scaling as well as dotted vessels arranged in clusters (×40)

The patient was patch tested to a series of allergens and demonstrated a positive reaction to propylene glycol.

Based on the case description and the photographs, what is your diagnosis?

Differential Diagnoses
1. Psoriasis.
2. Seborrheic dermatitis.
3. Allergic contact dermatitis.
4. Diffuse lichen planopilaris.

Diagnosis
Allergic contact dermatitis.

Discussion

Contact dermatitis (eczema) is an inflammatory condition of the skin induced by external agents [1]. There are two types of contact dermatitis: irritant and allergic. Irritant contact dermatitis occurs as a result of direct damage to the stratum corneum by chemicals or physical agents with an inflammatory nonimmunologic cutaneous reaction. The likelihood of developing irritant contact dermatitis depends on individuals susceptibility as well as the duration, intensity, and concentration of the substance [2]. Prior sensitization is not required. The lesions may present after a single episode of exposure to a strong irritant or repeated exposure to weak irritants [1]. Women, infants, elderly, and individuals with atopic history are more commonly affected [2]. Allergic contact dermatitis is a delayed type IV hypersensitivity reaction to external chemicals (allergens) that only occurs in susceptible individuals who have previously been sensitized. The sensitization phase of allergic dermatitis typically lasts 10–14 days. The re-exposure of the skin to the allergen after sensitization results in dermatitis [1]. Risk factors for allergic contact dermatitis include age, occupation, and history of atopic dermatitis [1]. Contact dermatitis is characterized by the presence of erythema, papules, scaling, vesiculation, and bullae during the acute phase as well as lichenification and fissuring in chronic disease. In most cases, the lesions are limited to the site of contact [1]. Itching, burning, stinging, or pain may be reported. The scalp is particularly resistant to contact dermatitis. An allergens applied to this area often produce dermatitis of the eyelids, ears and neck. Nevertheless, potent allergens may also cause severe reactions of the scalp. The most important allergens eliciting contact allergy of the scalp are found in bleaches and dyes, shampoos and conditioners, products for perm waves and straighteners as well as topical drugs [3]. Diagnosis of contact dermatitis is mainly established clinically. Dermoscopy and histopathological examination are useful. Dermoscopy of contact dermatitis is characterized by dotted vessels distributed in clusters or randomly, yellow scales and serocrusts [4]. Histopathology of contact irritant dermatitis presents with mild spongiosis, epidermal cell necrosis, and neutrophilic infiltration of the epidermis. In allergic contact dermatitis dermal inflammatory infiltrate predominately contains lymphocytes and other mononuclear cells [2]. Patch testing is the gold standard in diagnosing contact allergic dermatitis and is used to determine the exact cause. Identification and avoidance of the underlying cause is the most important in contact dermatitis treatment. Friction should be also avoided as well as the use of soaps, perfumes, and dyes [2]. The regular use of emollients is recommended [1]. High-potent and potent topical corticosteroids are usually the first-line therapeutic option. Topical tacrolimus ointment and pimecrolimus may be also helpful. Antihistamines such as hydroxyzine and cetirizine are recommended to control pruritus. Systemic steroids are advised in severe cases. Psoralen and ultraviolet A therapy, narrow-band ultraviolet B, systemic treatment with immunomodulators (methotrexate, cyclosporine) and targeted biologics may be considered in patients with chronic dermatitis that is unresponsive to other measures [1]. Topical minoxidil solution (consisting of minoxidil, alcohol, propylene glycol, and purified water) is a hypertrichotic agent commonly used in androgenetic alopecia. Some patients treated with topical minoxidil complain of pruritus and scaling of the scalp. The most common causes of these symptoms are irritant contact dermatitis, allergic contact dermatitis, or an exacerbation of seborrheic dermatitis. Propylene glycol is found to be the agent most frequently responsible for allergic contact dermatitis to minoxidil solution [5].

Differential diagnoses for the presented patient included psoriasis, seborrheic dermatitis and tinea capitis.

Scalp psoriasis is characterized by the presence of red, thickened plaques with a silver-white scale, either contained within the hairline, or extending onto the forehead, ears, and posterior neck. Other body areas such as knees, elbows and lumbosacral region are commonly affected [6].

Tinea capitis, a fungal infection of the scalp that affects mainly children. The disease is characterized by the presence of hair loss areas with coexisted scaling, inflammation or pustules [7].

Seborrheic dermatitis is a chronic inflammatory dermatologic condition. It presents as well-delimited erythematous plaques with greasy-looking, yellowish scales [8]. The scalp is most commonly affected, however the disease can appear also on the other body areas such as the face, chest, back, axilla, and groin [8, 9]. Seborrheic dermatitis is characterized by a seasonal pattern, presenting more frequently during winter, and improving usually during summer [8].

Based on the clinical picture, trichoscopic examination and patch tests, the presented patient was diagnosed with allergic contact dermatitis. Mometasone furoate 0.1% solution once a day was initiated with resolution of the skin lesions. A propylene glycol–free topical minoxidil solution was recommended.

Key Points
- Contact dermatitis, both irritant and allergic, rarely affects the scalp area.
- The disease is characterized by the presence of an erythema, papules, scaling and vesiculation.
- Topical minoxidil may cause irritant contact dermatitis, allergic contact dermatitis, or an exacerbation of seborrheic dermatitis.
- Propylene glycol is most frequently responsible for allergic contact dermatitis to minoxidil solution.

References

1. Tan CH, Rasool S, Johnston GA. Contact dermatitis: allergic and irritant. Clin Dermatol. 2014;32(1):116–24.

2. Litchman G, Nair PA, Atwater AR, Bhutta BS. Contact dermatitis. Treasure Island (FL): StatPearls; 2020.
3. Koch L, Aberer W. [Allergic contact dermatitis of the scalp]. Der Hautarzt. Zeitschrift fur Dermatologie, Venerologie, und verwandte Gebiete. 2017;68(6):466–71.
4. Errichetti E. Dermoscopy of inflammatory dermatoses (inflammoscopy): an up-to-date overview. Dermatol Pract Concept. 2019;9(3):169–80.
5. Friedman ES, Friedman PM, Cohen DE, Washenik K. Allergic contact dermatitis to topical minoxidil solution: etiology and treatment. J Am Acad Dermatol. 2002;46(2):309–12.
6. Blakely K, Gooderham M. Management of scalp psoriasis: current perspectives. Psoriasis (Auckl). 2016;6:33–40.
7. Adesiji YO, Omolade FB, Aderibigbe IA, Ogungbe O, Adefioye OA, Adedokun SA, et al. Prevalence of tinea capitis among children in Osogbo, Nigeria, and the associated risk factors. Diseases. 2019;7(1):13.
8. Clark GW, Pope SM, Jaboori KA. Diagnosis and treatment of seborrheic dermatitis. Am Fam Physician. 2015;91(3):185–90.
9. Borda LJ, Wikramanayake TC. Seborrheic dermatitis and dandruff: a comprehensive review. J Clin Investig Dermatol. 2015;3(2) https://doi.org/10.13188/2373-1044.1000019.

Chapter 23
A 70-Year-Old Woman with a Brown Nodule on the Scalp

Marta Sar-Pomian and Joanna Czuwara

A 70-year old woman was presented with a history of asymptomatic scalp lesion of unknown duration.

On physical examination, a brown-pinkish nodule in a size of 10 × 13 mm, localized on the parietal scalp was observed (Fig. 23.1). On dermoscopy of the right side of the lesion, brown and grey confluent blotches were presented, whereas on the left

Fig. 23.1 A 70-year-old woman with a brown-pinkish nodule on the parietal area

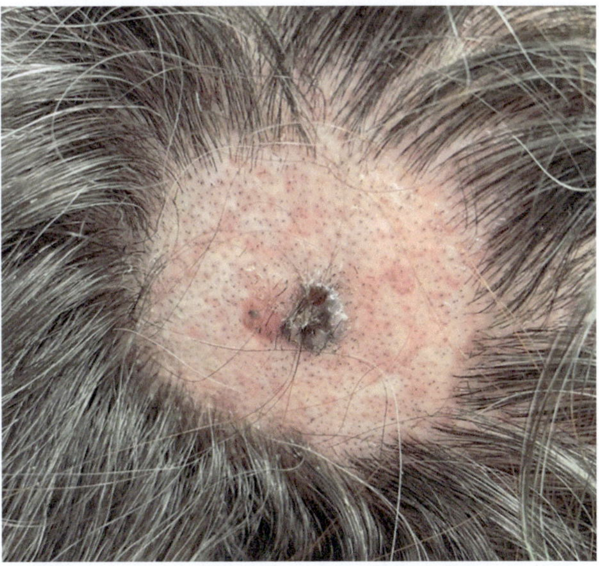

M. Sar-Pomian (✉) · J. Czuwara
Department of Dermatology, Medical University of Warsaw, Warsaw, Poland
e-mail: joanna.czuwara@wum.edu.pl

A. Waśkiel-Burnat et al. (eds.), *Clinical Cases in Scalp Disorders*, Clinical Cases in Dermatology, https://doi.org/10.1007/978-3-030-93426-2_23

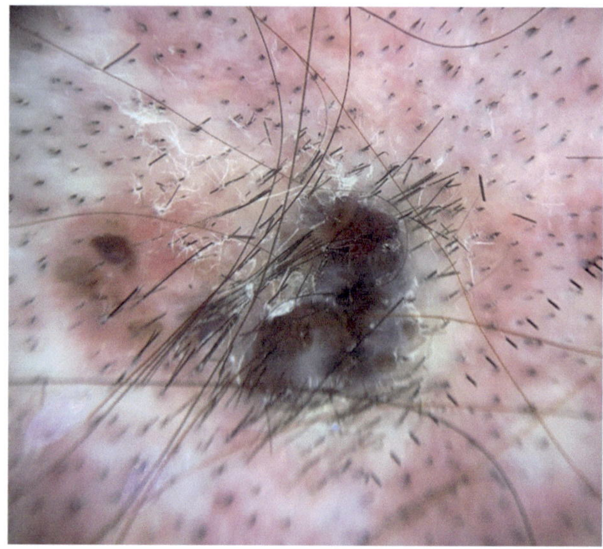

Fig. 23.2 Dermoscopy shows brown and grey confluent blotches on the right side of the lesion, whereas on the left side of the lesion brown globules on the erythematous background are presented (×10)

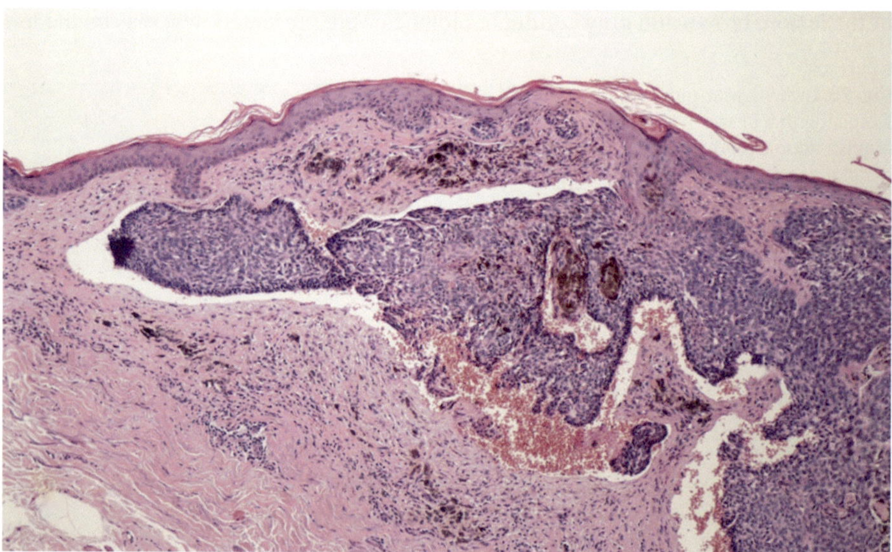

Fig. 23.3 A histopathological examination shows the nodules with a peripheral palisade of basaloid cells and slit-like retraction with a surrounding stroma due to mucin deposition. Melanin is present in tumor nodules and in melanophages mixed with inflammatory infiltrate around the tumor mass

side of the lesion brown globules on the erythematous background were observed (Fig. 23.2). The patient was referred for surgical removal of the lesion.

A histopathological examination revealed the nodules with a peripheral palisade of basaloid cells and slit-like retraction with a surrounding stroma due to mucin deposition. Melanin was observed in tumor nodules and in melanophages mixed with inflammatory infiltrate around the tumor mass (Fig. 23.3).

Based on the case description and the photographs, what is your diagnosis?

Differential Diagnoses
1. Melanoma.
2. Seborrheic keratosis.
3. Melanocytic nevus.
4. Basal cell carcinoma.

Diagnosis
Basal cell carcinoma.

Discussion

Basal cell carcinoma is a skin carcinoma derived from epidermal cells [1]. It is the most common malignant tumor in white populations which accounts for 75% of all skin cancers [1]. In pathogenesis of basal cell carcinoma the role of constitutive activation of patched/hedgehog intracellular signaling pathway is described. The malignancy is more common in individuals with Fitzpatrick skin types I and II. Ultraviolet radiation exposure is the most important environmental risk factor. Other risk factors include older age, childhood sunburns, tanning bed use, chronic immunosuppression, photosensitizing drugs, ionizing radiation, exposure to carcinogenic chemicals, especially arsenic and personal or family history of skin cancer [2]. Basal cell carcinoma is most frequently observed in adults, especially in the elderly population. It is more common in men than in women [1]. It presents as a tiny, hardly visible papule, growing usually for years into a nodule or a plaque, sometimes ulcerated [1]. More than 26 different clinicopathological subtypes of basal cell carcinoma have been described in the literature. A few forms of common basal cell carcinoma, such as superficial, nodular, morphoeic, ulcerated and pigmented are clinically recognized [1, 3]. However, basal cell carcinomas are usually highly polymorphic and sometimes difficult to classify into one of the standard subtypes. Destructive growth and invasion of surrounding tissues usually occur while the rate of metastasis is very low [1]. The malignancy is mainly localized on the body areas exposed to the sun and is the most common on the head and neck (80% of cases) followed by the trunk (15% of cases), arms and lower extremities [1]. The gold standard for diagnosis of basal cell carcinolma is histopathological examination. However, dermoscopy is a useful additional tool [4]. Characteristic dermoscopic features of basal cell carcinoma include arborizing vessels, superficial (short) fine telangiectasias, blue–grey ovoid nests, multiple blue–grey globules, infocus dots, maple leaf-like areas, spoke-wheel areas, concentric structures, ulceration, multiple small erosions, shiny white-red structureless areas and white streaks [4]. The key histopathological feature of the basal cell carcinoma is the presence of a basaloid epithelial tumor arising from the epidermis. Histopathological subtypes of basal cell carcinomas stratified by the risk of recurrence described in the current WHO classification are as follows: (1) lower risk: nodular, superficial, pigmented, infundibulocystic (a variant of basal cell carcinoma with adnexal differentiation), fibroepithelial; (2) higher risk: basosquamous carcinoma, sclerosing/morphoeic, infiltrating [1].

Scalp basal cell carcinoma constitutes for 2.7% of all basal cell carcinomas. Risk factors for the development of scalp basal cell carcinoma are scalp irradiation, ultraviolet exposure and immunosuppression. The tumor may also evolve from pre-existing Jadassohn's sebaceous nevus. It is more commonly observed in men what may be explained by higher prevalence of androgenetic alopecia or shorter hair as compared to women. This may lead to insufficient sun protection [5]. The mean age for the development of scalp basal cell carcinoma is 66.9 ± 15.1 years [5]. Scalp basal cell carcinomas are larger than in other sites, which may be explained by the abundant blood supply and the presence of hair masking growth of the nodule [6]. Rarely, giant basal cell carcinoma on the scalp, characterized by aggressive biological behaviors with intracranial invasion, may occur [7]. Basal cell carcinomas on the scalp tend to present more pigmented compared to other body sites. At least one melanocytic pattern is observed in 63% of patients with scalp basal cell carcinoma. In histopathological examination, nodular and mixed types of basal cell carcinoma are most commonly described [5].

The first-line treatment of basal cell carcinoma is a complete surgery. Topical therapies (5% imiquimod, 5% fluorouracil) and destructive approaches (curettage, electrocautery, cryotherapy, laser ablation, photodynamic therapy) should be considered in patients with a low-risk superficial malignancy. Hedgehog inhibitors, vismodegib or sonidegib, may be offered to patients with a locally advanced and metastatic basal cell carcinoma [1].

In the presented patient, differential diagnoses included melanoma, seborrheic keratosis and melanocytic nevus.

Melanoma is the most fatal form of skin cancer [8]. It most commonly affects the elderly. However, it may also occur in young adults and children. The typical cutaneous melanoma occurs as an asymmetric macule or nodule with irregular borders, frequently with variations in color within the lesion. Pink or red lesion may be also presented [8].

Seborrheic keratosis is one of the most common benign skin tumor that results from benign clonal expansion of epidermal keratinocytes. It is more common in the middle-aged and elderly. Seborrheic keratosis is more commonly presented in individuals with low Fitzpatrick skin phototypes. Typical lesions are sharply demarcated, round or oval-shaped, elevated and stuck on the skin with a verrucous, uneven, dull, or punched-out surface. Flat seborrheic keratoses often have a smooth, velvety surface and are barely elevated above the surface of the skin The color of the lesions varies from skin color, yellowish, light to dark brown, grey, and black. Seborrheic keratosis may present as an isolated lesion to tens or even hundreds of the lesions [9].

The scalp is an anatomical location for nevi with site-related atypia, a subset of melanocytic nevi that share histologic features with melanoma but that are benign. The clinical pattern of scalp melanotic nevi include solid brown, solid pink, eclipse and cockade. Melanotic nevi are most commonly presented on the vertex and parietal areas [10].

In the presented patient, diagnosis of basal cell carcinoma was established. A surgical excision was performed.

Key Points
- Scalp basal cell carcinoma constitutes for 2.7% of all basal cell carcinomas.
- It presents as a tiny, hardly visible papule, growing usually for years into a nodule or a plaque, sometimes ulcerated.

References

1. Peris K, Fargnoli MC, Garbe C, Kaufmann R, Bastholt L, Seguin NB, et al. Diagnosis and treatment of basal cell carcinoma: European consensus-based interdisciplinary guidelines. Eur J Cancer (Oxford, England: 1990). 2019;118:10–34.
2. Kim DP, Kus KJB, Ruiz E. Basal cell carcinoma review. Hematol Oncol Clin North Am. 2019;33(1):13–24.
3. Dourmishev LA, Rusinova D, Botev I. Clinical variants, stages, and management of basal cell carcinoma. Indian Dermatol Online J. 2013;4(1):12–7.
4. Wozniak-Rito A, Zalaudek I, Rudnicka L. Dermoscopy of basal cell carcinoma. Clin Exp Dermatol. 2018;43(3):241–7.
5. Cho M, Lee J, James CL, Marshman G, Huilgol SC. Scalp basal cell carcinoma: review of 2,202 cases. Dermatol Surg. 2016;42(7):834–41.
6. Castanheira A, Soares P, Boaventura P. Scalp basal cell carcinoma: a different entity? Dermatol Ther. 2019;32(2):e12828.
7. Kwon CS, Awar OA, Ripa V, Said G, Rocka S. Basal cell carcinoma of the scalp with destruction and invasion into the calvarium and dura mater: report of 7 cases and review of literature. J Clin Neurosci. 2018;47:190–7.
8. Kibbi N, Kluger H, Choi JN. Melanoma: clinical presentations. Cancer Treat Res. 2016;167:107–29.
9. Hafner C, Vogt T. Seborrheic keratosis. J Dtsch Dermatol Ges. 2008;6(8):664–77.
10. Tcheung WJ, Bellet JS, Prose NS, Cyr DD, Nelson KC. Clinical and dermoscopic features of 88 scalp naevi in 39 children. Br J Dermatol. 2011;165(1):137–43.

Chapter 24
A 71-Year-Old Woman with Erosions on the Scalp

Anna Waśkiel-Burnat, Marta Muszel, Małgorzata Olszewska, and Lidia Rudnicka

A 71-year-old woman was admitted to the Department of Dermatology with erosions on the scalp presented since two days. The patient was diagnosed with seborrheic keratosis which was treated with liquid nitrogen cryotherapy. The day after the procedure, blistering on the forehead and frontoparietal area of the scalp occurred. She applied topical gentian violet on the lesions. The patient had hypertension and diabetes mellitus type 2.

On physical examination erosions surrounded by an erythema on the forehead and frontoparietal area were observed (Fig. 24.1). Palpation caused some tenderness. Her temperature was 98.8 °F, pulse was 85 beats per minute, and blood pressure was 130/80 mmHg.

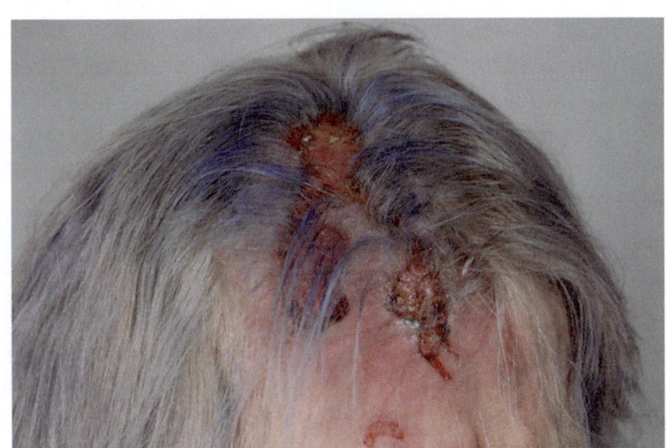

Fig. 24.1 A 71-year-old woman with erosions surrounded by an erythema on the forehead and frontoparietal area

A. Waśkiel-Burnat (✉) · M. Muszel · M. Olszewska · L. Rudnicka
Department of Dermatology, Medical University of Warsaw, Warsaw, Poland
e-mail: anna.waskiel@wum.edu.pl; malgorzata.olszewska@wum.edu.pl;
lidia.rudnicka@wum.edu.pl

A. Waśkiel-Burnat et al. (eds.), *Clinical Cases in Scalp Disorders*, Clinical Cases in Dermatology, https://doi.org/10.1007/978-3-030-93426-2_24

In laboratory tests, an increased number of white blood cell count (12.5 × 10⁹/L_ and C-reactive protein (25 mg/dl) were detected.

Based on the case description and the photographs, what is your diagnosis?

Differential Diagnoses
1. Herpes zoster.
2. Erysipelas.
3. Erosive pustular dermatosis of the scalp.
4. Liquid nitrogen cryotherapy induced cellulitis.

Diagnosis
Liquid nitrogen cryotherapy cellulitis.

Discussion

Cryotherapy is a commonly used technique to treat a variety of dermatologic conditions such as seborrheic dermatitis and actinic keratosis [1]. It is performed using a cyrogen, typically liquid nitrogen, to cool the targeted tissue to subzero temperatures. This effect induces tissue damage in two mechanisms. The first mechanism is induction of tissue ischemia by damaging blood vessels and capillaries. The second mechanism damages the cells by forming ice crystals and inducing osmotic cell injury and cellular membrane disruption [2]. There are several different techniques for the administration of liquid nitrogen. The most common cryosurgical technique is the open technique in which liquid nitrogen is sprayed onto the target lesion. In the semi-open technique, a cone or plate covers or directs liquid nitrogen to the target area what allows for a more targeted treatment area. The closed/contact technique uses a probe cooled with liquid nitrogen applied directly to the skin [2]. Cryotherapy is commonly well-tolerated [1]. Freezing of the skin's surface causes a pain, erythema, and edema. Blistering, crusting, and hypopigmentation may be also presented. These side effects are mild for the majority of cases and resolve within one or two weeks. On the scalp or other hair-bearing areas, alopecia can result from cold-induced destruction of hair bulge cells and lead to permanent alopecia [1].

Cellulitis is an acute, inflammatory infection of the dermis and subcutaneous tissues. It is a rare but important complication of cryotherapy as it may lead to significant patient morbidity [1]. Cellulitis is caused by beta-hemolytic streptococci, generally group A streptococci (i.e., *Streptococcus pyogenes*), followed by the methicillin-sensitive *Staphylococcus aureus* [3]. Risk factors for cellulitis include any breakdown in the skin barrier such as a wound or ulcer. Low temperature of liquid nitrogen initiates apoptosis of all skin cells in the treatment region, leaving the area vulnerable to infection [1]. Cellulitis typically presents as a poorly demarcated, warm, erythematous area with associated edema and tenderness to palpation. Malaise, fatigue, and fever may occur. The diagnosis of cellulitis is mainly established clinically. The treatment includes systemic antibiotic such as penicillin, cephalosporin, clindamycin, sulfamethoxazole/trimethoprim, doxycycline and vancomycin [3].

Differential diagnoses for the presented patient included herpes zoster, erysipelas and erosive pustular dermatosis of the scalp.

Herpes zoster is a result of reactivation of latent varicella zoster virus. The disease most frequently occurs in older adults. It presents as painful, unilateral dermatomal, vesicular lesions on the erythematous background that do not cross the midline. Crusts can be also presented. The most common locations are the thoracic nerves and the ophthalmic division of the trigeminal nerve [4].

Erosive pustular dermatosis of the scalp is a rare, inflammatory disorder that occurs mostly in elderly patients. Clinically, it is characterized by recurrent pustules, inflamed erosions and grey, yellow or yellow-brown crusts that lead to scarring alopecia. No fever is observed [5].

Erysipelas is considered as a form of cellulitis. However, it is a more superficial infection affecting the upper dermis and superficial lymphatic system. It caused by group A streptococci (*Streptococcus pyogenes*). On the contrary to cellulitis, which tends to be more mildly erythematous (pink) and flat with less distinct boundaries, erysipelas is characterized by a bright red erythema, elevation of the affected skin, and well-demarcated borders [3].

In the presented patient diagnosis of liquid nitrogen cryotherapy cellulitis was established. She was treated with intravenous cefuroxime (1.5 g three times a day) for 14 days. Complete resolution of skin lesions with hair regrowth was observed.

Key Points
- Cellulitis is an acute inflammatory infection of the dermis and subcutaneous tissues that may affect the scalp area.
- It typically presents as a poorly demarcated, warm, erythematous area with associated edema and tenderness to palpation.
- Cellulitis may be induced by liquid nitrogen cryotherapy.

References

1. Huang CM, Lu EY, Kirchhof MG. Cellulitis secondary to liquid nitrogen cryotherapy: case report and literature review. J Cutan Med Surg. 2017;21(4):334–8.
2. Prohaska J, Jan AH. Cryotherapy. Treasure Island (FL): StatPearls; 2020.
3. Brown BD, Hood Watson KL. Cellulitis. Treasure Island (FL): StatPearls; 2020.
4. Schmader K. Herpes zoster. Ann Int Med. 2018;169(3):Itc19–itc31.
5. Starace M, Alessandrini A, Baraldi C, Piraccini BM. Erosive pustular dermatosis of the scalp: challenges and solutions. Clin Cosmet Investig Dermatol. 2019;12:691–8.

Chapter 25
A 71-Year-Old Woman with Progressing Multiple Vesicles on the Scalp

Anna Pasierb, Joanna Misiewicz-Wroniak, and Joanna Czuwara

A 71-year-old woman presented with a 13-year history of asymptomatic multiple vesicles and bullae on the scalp area. The patient did not complain of any symptoms. Pemphigus vulgaris was initially suspected, however the diagnosis was excluded based on histopathological and immunofluorescence examination. Due to suspicion of malignancy, a numerous punch biopsies and surgical excisions with skin graft were performed. Each surgical trauma induced formation of new vesicles and disease progression. Histopathological examinations showed features of syringoma, trichoepithelioma, hidradenoma, basal cell carcinoma, and hemangioma.

On physical examination, area of scarring hair loss on the frontoparietal and vertex areas was observed. On the periphery, multiple vesicles with a tendency to coalescence into bullae were presented (Fig. 25.1). Moreover, on the right side of the frontal area, an erythematous plague with an erosion and arborizing blood vessels was detected (Fig. 25.2). Trichoscopy revealed multiple yellowish well-circumscribed lacunas separated by whitish septa at the periphery of the hair loss area (Fig. 25.3). Moreover, on the frontal region an erosion and arborizing vessels were observed.

A histopathological examination of vesicular lesions showed the upper part of the dermis densely packed with thin walled irregular vascular channels with a single layer of endothelial cells. Channels were separated by collagen bundles and were either empty or contain a lymphatic fluid (Fig. 25.4). Histopathology of an erythematous plaque showed wide irregular vascular channels separated by clusters of basophilic cells with cysts formation.

A. Pasierb · J. Misiewicz-Wroniak · J. Czuwara (✉)
Department of Dermatology, Medical University of Warsaw, Warsaw, Poland
e-mail: anna.pasierb@wum.edu.pl; joanna.czuwara@wum.edu.pl

A. Waśkiel-Burnat et al. (eds.), *Clinical Cases in Scalp Disorders*, Clinical Cases in Dermatology, https://doi.org/10.1007/978-3-030-93426-2_25

Fig. 25.1 A 71-year old woman with an area of scarring hair loss on the frontoparietal and vertex areas. On the periphery, multiple vesicles with a tendency to coalescence into bullae are presented

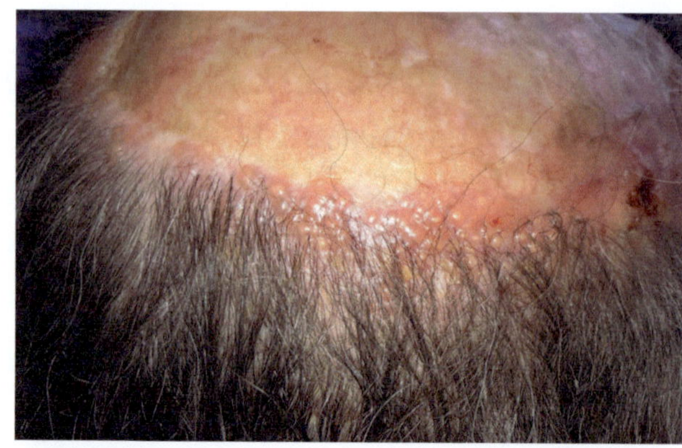

Fig. 25.2 An erythematous plague with an erosion and arborizing blood vessels

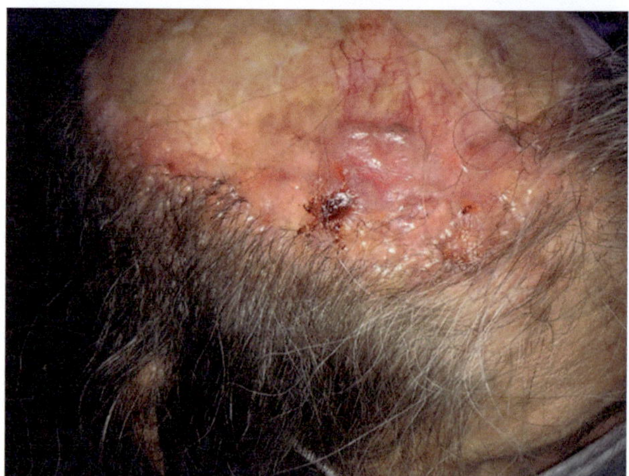

Fig. 25.3 Trichoscopy shows multiple yellowish lacunas separated by whitish septa (×20)

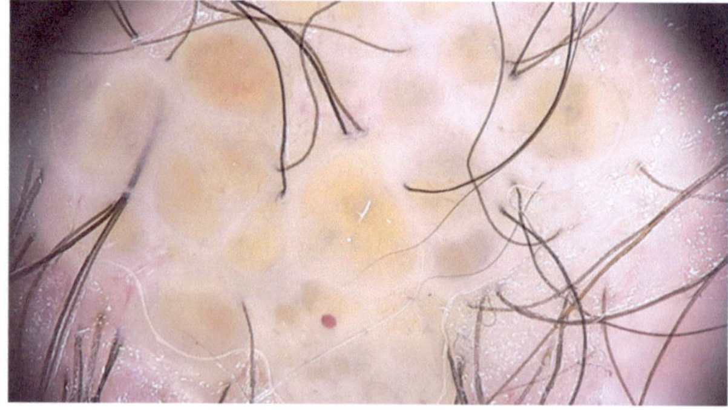

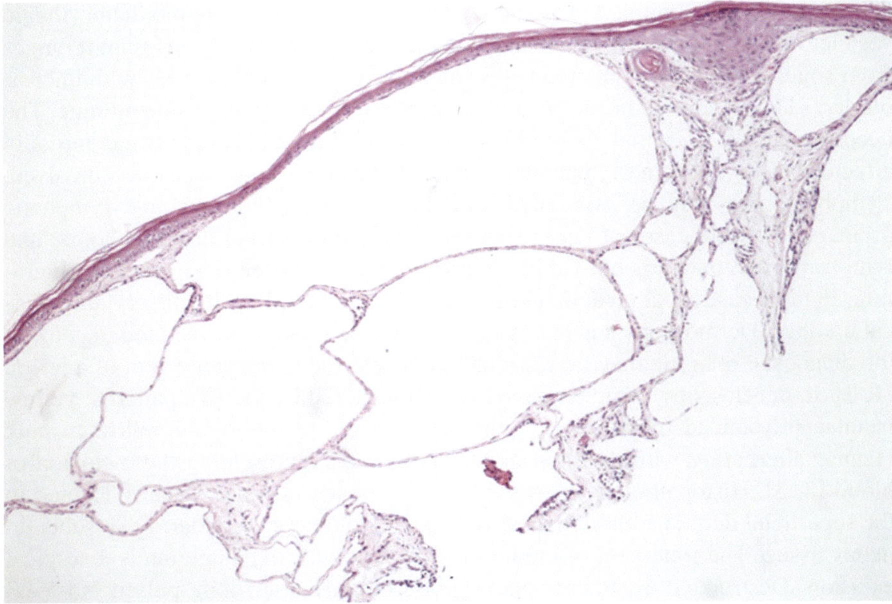

Fig. 25.4 A histopathological examination of a vesicular lesion with the presence of epidermis and dermis filled up with thin walled, jagged, irregular and devoid of erythrocytes vascular spaces distributed between collagen bundles

Based on the case description and the photographs, what is your diagnosis?

Differential Diagnoses
1. Basal Cell Carcinoma.
2. Lymphangioma.
3. Bullous pemphigoid.
4. Linear IgA dermatosis.

Diagnosis
Lymphangioma associated with basal cell carcinoma.

Discussion

Lymphangioma is a hamartomatous, congenital or acquired malformation of the lymphatic vessels that may involve the skin and subcutaneous tissues [1]. Congenital lymphangiomas form due to the blockage of the lymphatic system during fetal development, though the cause remains unknown. The lesions typically appear before the age of five years. Acquired lymphangiomas occur in association with chronic lymphedema that leads to disruption of previously normal lymphatic channels [1, 2]. They usually appear in adults after surgery, trauma, infection, malignancy, or radiation therapy [2]. A spontaneous occurrence has been also described.

Clinically, lymphangioma is characterized by clusters of translucent or hemorrhagic vesicles resembling frog spawn located on the dull pink to violaceous skin. It ranges from small and well-demarcated malformations to large, diffuse ones with unclear borders [1]. The lesions occur on any cutaneous surface or mucous membrane. The head and neck, proximal extremities, buttocks, and trunk are most commonly affected. The intestines, pancreas, and mesentery may also be involved. Lymphangioma may be associated with pruritus, pain, burning, and lymphatic drainage [3]. Rare cases of squamous cell carcinoma, verruciform xanthoma, and lymphangiosarcoma arising within lymphangioma have been reported in the literature. In most cases, a clinical diagnosis can be made based on the history and clinical findings. Dermoscopy and histopathological examination can be used to confirm the diagnosis. Imaging may be warranted to assess the depth and extent of a lesion [1, 2]. In dermoscopy, lymphangioma is characterized by the two patterns: yellow lacunae surrounded by pale septa without inclusion of blood and yellow to pink lacunae alternating with dark-red or bluish lacunae, representing the inclusion of blood [2, 3]. Histopathology shows dilated lymphatic channels usually located in the superficial dermis, although they may extend to the reticular dermis or subcutaneous tissue. The treatment of choice for any type of lymphangioma is a surgical excision. Destructive treatments with carbon dioxide laser, long-pulsed Nd-YAG laser, and electrosurgery have been reported to be effective. Other therapeutic options include cryotherapy, superficial radiotherapy, and sclerotherapy [1–3].

Differential diagnoses for the presented patient were basal cell carcinoma, bullous pemphigoid and linear IgA dermatosis.

Basal cell carcinoma is the most common skin malignancy. The incidence rate of the disease increases with age. Basal cell carcinoma presents as a tiny, hardly visible papule, growing into a nodule or a plaque that is sometimes ulcerated. The lesion is most commonly observed on the face, scalp or neck [4].

Bullous pemphigoid is an autoimmune bullous disease that mainly affects elderly individuals, usually above 70 years. It presents as itchy, tense blisters over normal skin or over erythematous and edematous background [5].

Linear IgA bullous dermatosis is a relatively rare subepidermal vesiculobullous disease that occurs in both adults and children. In children, annular or polycyclic plaques and papules with blistering around the edges, primarily around the mouth and eyes, on the lower abdomen, thighs, buttocks, genitals, wrists and ankles are observed. In contrast, the adult-onset form presents as lesions on the trunk, head and extremities [6].

Based on the patient's presentation, dermoscopic and histopathological examination, the diagnosis of acquired lymphangioma with coexisted basal cell carcinoma was established. A surgical excision was recommended for basal cell carcinoma. A superficial radiotherapy for lymphangioma treatment was planned after the surgery.

Key Points
- Lymphangioma is an uncommon, benign malformation of the lymphatic system that may affect the scalp area.
- It presents as clusters of translucent or hemorrhagic vesicles resembling frog spawn located on the dull pink to violaceous skin.

- Basal cell carcinoma, squamous cell carcinoma, verruciform xanthoma, and lymphangiosarcoma may arise within lymphangioma.

References

1. Patel GA, Schwartz RA. Cutaneous lymphangioma circumscriptum: frog spawn on the skin. Int J Dermatol. 2009;48(12):1290–5.
2. Jha AK, Lallas A, Sonthalia S. Dermoscopy of cutaneous lymphangioma circumscriptum. Dermatol Pract Concept. 2017;7(2):37–8.
3. Massa AF, Menezes N, Baptista A, Moreira AI, Ferreira EO. Cutaneous Lymphangioma circumscriptum – dermoscopic features. An Bras Dermatol. 2015;90(2):262–4.
4. Marzuka AG, Book SE. Basal cell carcinoma: pathogenesis, epidemiology, clinical features, diagnosis, histopathology, and management. Yale J Biol Med. 2015;88(2):167–79.
5. Miyamoto D, Santi CG, Aoki V, Maruta CW. Bullous pemphigoid. Anais brasileiros de Dermatol. 2019;94(2):133–46.
6. Lammer J, Hein R, Roenneberg S, Biedermann T, Volz T. Drug-induced linear IgA bullous dermatosis: a case report and review of the literature. Acta Derm Venereol. 2019;99(6):508–15.

Chapter 26
A 72-Year-Old Man with Crusted Erosions on the Scalp

Marta Kurzeja, Marta Sar-Pomian, Małgorzata Olszewka, and Lidia Rudnicka

A 72-year-old-man was admitted to the Dermatology of Department with a six-week history of crusted erosions on the scalp and tense vesicles and bullae on the trunk, upper and lower extremities. The patient had hypertension and hyperlipidemia. He denied having any dermatological disease.

A physical examination revealed multiple erosions covered with hemorrhagic and yellowish crusts on the frontoparietal and vertex areas of the scalp (Fig. 26.1). Additionally, urticarial lesions as well as blisters, bullae and erosions on erythematous background on the trunk and extremities were presented. The patients had no lesions on mucous membranes. On trichoscopy, extravasations and yellow scaling were detected (Fig. 26.2).

Basic laboratory tests did not reveal any abnormalities. Direct immunofluorescence test of the perilesional skin demonstrated linear immunoglobulin G (IgG) and complement C3 deposition at the basal membrane zone. A histopathological examination showed a subepidermal blister containing fibrin and large numbers of eosinophils. Indirect immunofluorescence revealed the presence of IgG circulating autoantibodies against the skin basement membrane component (titer 1:160).

Based on the case description and the photographs, what is your diagnosis?

Differential Diagnoses
1. Pemphigus foliaceous.
2. Linear IgA dermatosis.
3. Erosive pustular dermatosis of the scalp.
4. Bullous pemphigoid.

M. Kurzeja (✉) · M. Sar-Pomian · M. Olszewka · L. Rudnicka
Department of Dermatology, Medical University of Warsaw, Warsaw, Poland
e-mail: marta.kurzeja@wum.edu.pl; malgorzata.olszewska@wum.edu.pl; lidia.rudnicka@wum.edu.pl

A. Waśkiel-Burnat et al. (eds.), *Clinical Cases in Scalp Disorders*, Clinical Cases in Dermatology, https://doi.org/10.1007/978-3-030-93426-2_26

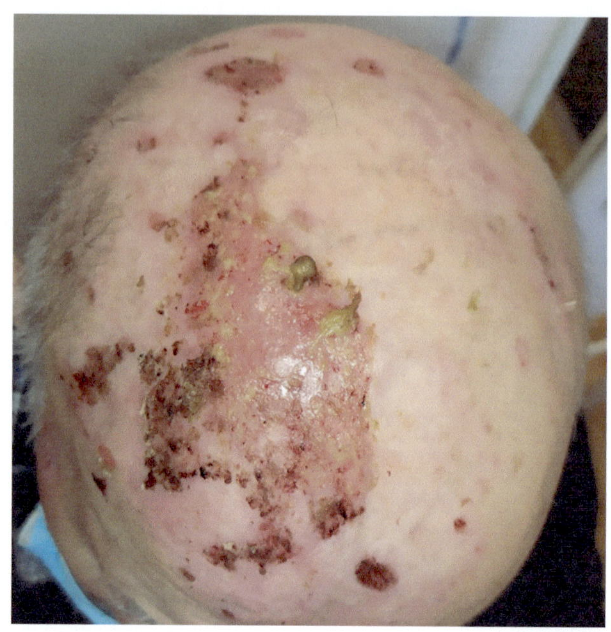

Fig. 26.1 A 72-year-old man with crusted erosions on the scalp. The frontoparietal and vertex area is affected

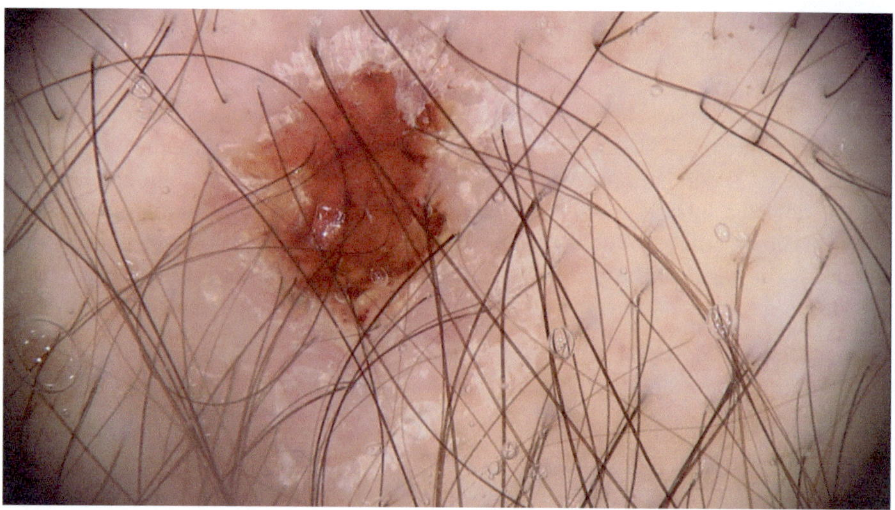

Fig. 26.2 Trichoscopy shows extravasation and yellow scaling (×20)

Diagnosis
Bullous pemphigoid.

Discussion

Bullous pemphigoid is the most frequent autoimmune subepidermal blistering disease. It is characterized by the presence of tissue-bound and circulating autoantibodies against components of the hemidesmosomes: BP230 (BPAg1) and BP180 (BPAg2) [1]. The disease mainly affects elderly individuals, during the eighth decade of life, without gender predilection. The spectrum of clinical presentation is broad. Typically, tense blisters on the apparently normal or erythematosus skin are observed. In non-bullous phase of the disease, signs are extremely polymorphic and include excoriated, eczematous papular or urticarial lesions. The skin lesions are accompanied by an intense pruritus and are most frequently localized on the trunk and extremities. The scalp area is rarely affected [1, 2]. Bullous pemphigoid is commonly associated with various neurological disorders such as Parkinson disease or dementia [1–3]. The association with malignancies has not been clearly confirmed so far. The diagnosis of bullous pemphigoid is established on a basis of immunofluorescence tests. Histopathology may be useful. A direct immunofluorescence test of perilesional skin demonstrates a linear band of immunoglobulin G deposit and/or complement C3 along the dermoepidermal junction. In indirect immunofluorescence test, circulating anti-basement membrane antibodies of the IgG class are detectable in 60%–80% of patients. Autoantibodies classically bind to the epidermal (roof) side of the skin basement membrane. The most characteristic histopathological features of bullous pemphigoid are subepidermal blisters accompanied by composed of eosinophils and mononuclear cells. The first-line therapy of bullous pemphigoid consists of potent topical corticosteroids [4]. The combination of nicotinamide and tetracyclines or doxycycline may be a therapeutic option. In refectory cases oral prednisone with steroid-sparking agents such as azathioprine, mycophenolate mofetil or methotrexate are recommended [4, 5].

For the presented patient, pemphigus foliaceous, erosive pustular dermatosis of the scalp and linear IgA dermatosis were included in differential diagnosis.

Pemphigus foliaceous is the second most prevalent variant of pemphigus. It presents as erosions surrounded by an erythema that heal with crusting and scaling. Flaccid vesicles are rarely observed. Mucous membranes are spared [6].

Erosive pustular dermatosis of the scalp is a rare, inflammatory disorder that occurs mostly in elderly patients. Clinically, it is characterized by recurrent pustules, inflamed erosions and grey, yellow or yellow-brown crusts that lead to scarring alopecia. The lesions are limited to the scalp area [7].

Linear IgA bullous dermatosis is a relatively rare subepidermal vesiculobullous disease that occurs in both adults and children [8]. In children the disease is characterized by the presence of annular or polycyclic plaques and papules with blistering around the edges, primarily around the mouth and eyes, on the lower abdomen, thighs, buttocks, genitals, wrists and ankles. In contrast, the adult-onset form presents as lesions on the trunk, head and extremities [8].

The presented patient, based on the clinical picture, immunofluorescence tests and histopathological examination was diagnosed with bullous pemphigoid. He was treated with doxycycline and nicotinamide along with clobetasol propionate 0.05% cream with resolution of the skin lesions.

Key Points
- Bullous pemhigoid is the most common blistering disease that may affect the scalp area.
- The disease is characterized by the presence of tense blisters on the apparently normal or erythematosus skin and excoriated, eczematous papular or urticarial lesions.

References

1. Bernard P, Antonicelli F. Bullous pemphigoid: a review of its diagnosis, associations and treatment. Am J Clin Dermatol. 2017;18(4):513–28.
2. Miyamoto D, Santi CG, Aoki V, Maruta CW. Bullous pemphigoid. An Bras Dermatol. 2019;94(2):133–46.
3. Bağcı IS, Horváth ON, Ruzicka T, Sárdy M. Bullous pemphigoid. Autoimmun Rev. 2017;16(5):445–55.
4. Fontaine J, Joly P, Roujeau JC. Treatment of bullous pemphigoid. J Dermatol. 2003;30(2):83–90.
5. Feliciani C, Joly P, Jonkman MF, Zambruno G, Zillikens D, Ioannides D, Kowalewski C, Jedlickova H, Kárpáti S, Marinovic B, Mimouni D, Uzun S, Yayli S, Hertl M, Borradori L. Management of bullous pemphigoid: the European Dermatology Forum consensus in collaboration with the European Academy of Dermatology and Venereology. Br J Dermatol. 2015;172(4):867–77.
6. Kridin K. Pemphigus group: overview, epidemiology, mortality, and comorbidities. Immunol Res. 2018;66(2):255–70.
7. Karanfilian KM, Wassef C. Erosive pustular dermatosis of the scalp: causes and treatments. Int J Dermatol. 2021;60(1):25–32.
8. Lammer J, Hein R, Roenneberg S, Biedermann T, Volz T. Drug-induced linear IgA bullous dermatosis: a case report and review of the literature. Acta Derm Venereol. 2019;99(6):508–15.

Chapter 27
A 72-Year-Old Woman with the Scalp Erythema and Weakness of the Muscles of the Arms and Hips

Barbara Borkowska

A 72-year-old woman was admitted to the Department of Dermatology due to a one-year history of erythematous skin lesions and symmetrical weakness of the muscles of the arms and hips. The first skin lesions appeared on the forehead and scalp, then spread to the trunk, upper and lower extremities. She also complained of hypersensitivity to ultraviolet radiation. Previously, she was treated with topical corticosteroids and oral doxycycline without clinical improvement. The patient reported left breast cancer treated with conserving therapy in 2003.

A physical examination revealed a moderate erythema and yellowish scaling on the scalp (Figs. 27.1 and 27.2). Moreover, disseminated erythematous and papular skin lesions on the lateral surfaces of the thighs, hips and over the finger joints were observed. Nail fold erythema and a moderate erythema with swelling of the eyelids

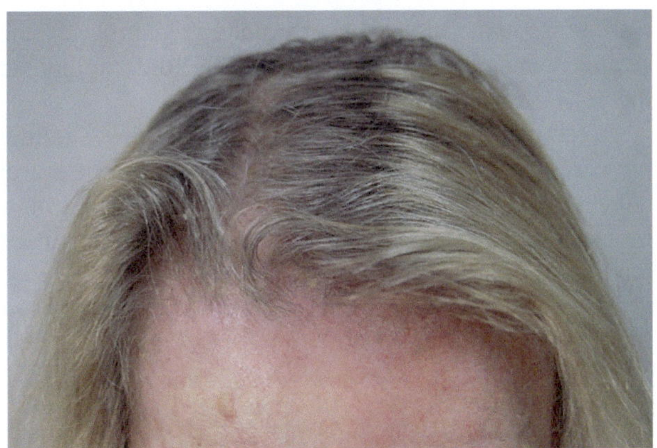

Fig. 27.1 A 72-year-old women with the scalp erythema extending onto the forehead

B. Borkowska (✉)
Department of Dermatology, Medical University of Warsaw, Warsaw, Poland

117

A. Waśkiel-Burnat et al. (eds.), *Clinical Cases in Scalp Disorders*, Clinical Cases in Dermatology, https://doi.org/10.1007/978-3-030-93426-2_27

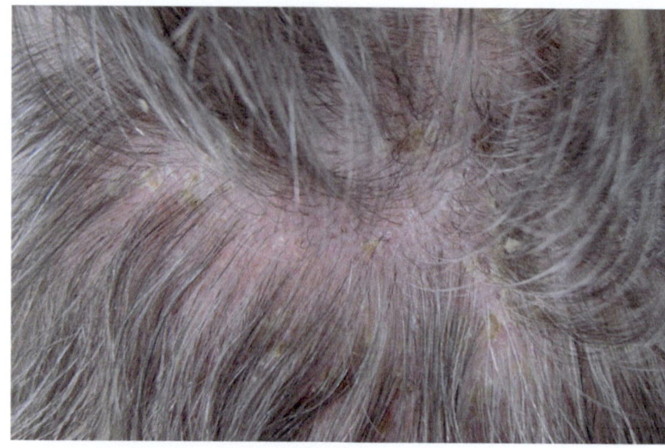

Fig. 27.2 An erythema and yellowish scales of the scalp

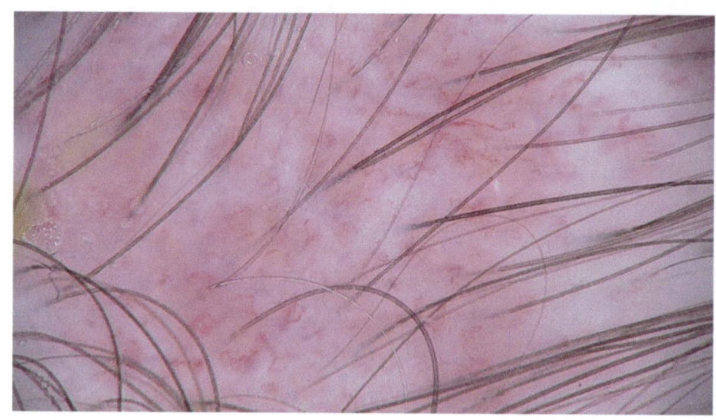

Fig. 27.3 Trichoscopy shows enlarged capillaries (×70)

were presented. On trichoscopy, enlarged capilaries and areas of diffuse yellowish scaling were observed (Fig. 27.3). Nailfold capillaroscopic examination revealed the presence of enlarged capillaries.

In laboratory tests, an accelerated erythrocyte sedimentation rate test as well as increased levels of transaminases, creatine kinase, cardiac isoenzyme phosphocreatine kinase, lactate dehydrogenase and myoglobin were observed. An indirect immunofluorescence test showed ANA antibodies in ratio 1:160. In the immunoblot, TIF1-gamma antibodies were positive.

Based on the case description and the photographs, what is your diagnosis?

Differential Diagnoses
1. Dermatomyositis.
2. Systemic lupus erythematosus.
3. Systemic sclerosis.
4. Trichinellosis.

Diagnosis
Dermatomyositis.

Discussion

Dermatomyositis is an autoimmune disease characterized by the presence of skin changes, skeletal muscles weakness and involvement of different internal organs such as lungs, esophagus, joints and blood vessels [1]. There are a range of factors playing a role in the pathogenesis of dermatomyositis such as genetic, environmental, immune and nonimmune-mediated responses. There is a strong association between the disease and malignancy. The incidence of dermatomyositis is estimated at two to nine in million individuals [2]. The disease affects both, adults and children and is two to three times more common among women compared to men. Skin lesions occur in 30–40% of adults with dermatomyositis and in 95% of juvenile dermatomyositis cases [1]. Characteristic dermatomyositis skin changes include Gothron sign and Gothron papules, heliotrop rash, shawl sing, V-sign, nailfold changes, poikilodema and holster sign. The scalp involvement occurs in up to 82% of adults with dermatomyositis and is more common in women. It presents as psoriasiform dermatitis, non-scarring alopecia, macular violaceous erythema, scale, pigmentary changes, telangiectasias, and background scalp poikiloderma. Pruritus and burning sensation typically occur [2]. Muscle weakness symmetrically affects the proximal muscles and may precede, follow or occur simultaneously with the skin lesions [1]. The evaluation of patients with suspicion of dermatomysositis must include a total body skin examination, objective muscle strength examination, and laboratory tests (phosphocreatine kinase, lactate dehydrogenase, aspartate transaminase, aldolase and auto-antibody testing). Typical autoantibodies are anti—Mi2 and anti—Jo1. Tif1-gamma antibodies are more likely for cancer-associated dermatomyositis. In equivocal cases, skin biopsy, muscle biopsy, or muscle imaging may be helpful to clarify the diagnosis. Nailfold capillaroscopy and trichoscopy show similar findings and are helpful in diagnosing dermatomyositis. Nailfold capillaroscopy reveals enlarged capillaries, hemorrhages and loss of capillaries. On trichoscopy enlarged capillaries, peripilar casts, tufting and interfollicular scales are observed [1, 2]. Treatment of dermatomyositis consists of sun protection, topical therapy with corticosteroids and/or calcineurin inhibitors as well as systemic therapy. Systemic corticosteroids are the first-line treatment for dermatomyositis. Concomitant treatment with steroid-sparing immunosuppressive agents, including methotrexate, azathioprine, cyclosporine mycophenolate mofetil, and cyclophosphamide is usually recommended [2].

Differential diagnoses for the presented patient were systemic lupus erythematosus, systemic sclerosis and trichinellosis.

Systemic lupus erythematous is a chronic autoimmune disease that is characterized by the presence of skin lesions and involvement of internal organs such as kidneys, serosa, nervous system and joints. Additionally, hematological abnormalities are frequently observed. Skin lesions include acute, subacute cutaneous or discoid lupus, oral ulcers and non-scaring alopecia. Muscle weakness is not typical observed. Characteristic antinuclear antibodies for systemic lupus erythematosus are anti-dsDNA, anti-Sm, and anti-phospholipid antibodies [3].

Systemic sclerosis is an immune-mediated disease that is characterized by fibrosis of the skin and internal organs and vasculopathy. Skin lesions in systemic sclerosis include Raynaud's phenomenon, skin thickening of the fingers (puffy finger or sclerodactyly), fingertip ulcers and scars, telangiectasias and abnormal nailfold capillaries [4]. Lungs, kidneys, heart, esophagus, are osteoarticular system can be involved. Systemic sclerosis-related autoantibodies are anti-topoisomerase 1 (Scl-70), anticentromere (ACA), and anti-RNA polymerase III (RNAP-3) [4].

Trichinellosis is a parasitic zoonosis that can be contracted by eating raw or rare meat. Larvae of *Trichinella* migrates through lymphatic and blood vessels of the host to the skeletal muscles and cause severe muscle pain and muscle enzyme elevations. Periorbital and face oedema can be observed. Moreover headaches, fevers, chills, diarrhea, nausea, fatigue or vomiting are reported. An increased white blood cell count with eosinophilia occur [5].

Based on the patient's presentation and laboratory tests, the diagnosis of dermatomyositis was established. The patient was treated with oral prednisone (50 mg daily) with subcutaneous methotrexate (10 mg weekly). The resolution of skin lesions, reduction of muscles weakness and the activity of muscle enzymes were observed. Oncological consultation was recommended.

Key Points
- The scalp involvement occurs in up to 82% of adults with dermatomyositis.
- It presents as psoriasiform dermatitis, non-scarring alopecia, macular violaceous erythema, scale, pigmentary changes, telangiectasias, and background scalp poikiloderma with coexisted itching or burning.

References

1. Bogdanov I, Kazandjieva J, Darlenski R, Tsankov N. Dermatomyositis: current concepts. Clin Dermatol. 2018;36(4):450–8.
2. Jasso-Olivares JC, Tosti A, Miteva M, Domínguez-Cherit J, Díaz-González JM. Clinical and dermoscopic features of the scalp in 31 patients with dermatomyositis. Skin Appendage Disord. 2017;3(3):119–24.
3. Aringer M, Leuchten N, Johnson SR. New criteria for lupus. Curr Rheumatol Rep. 2020;22(6):18.
4. Krasowska D, Rudnicka L, Dańczak-Pazdrowska A, Chodorowska G, Woźniacka A, Lis-Święty A, Czuwara J, Maj J, Majewski S, Sysa-Jędrzejowska A, Wojas-Pelc A. Systemic sclerosis – diagnostic and therapeutic recommendations of the Polish Dermatological Society. Part 1: diagnosis and monitoring. Dermatol Rev. 2017;104:483–98.
5. Shimoni Z, Froom P. Uncertainties in diagnosis, treatment and prevention of trichinellosis. Expert Rev Anti-Infect Ther. 2015;13(10):1279–88.

Chapter 28
A 75-Year-Old Woman with an Unilateral Vesicular Eruption on the Scalp

Sylwia Chrostowska

A 75-year-old woman presented to the emergency room due to a few-day history of clusters of confluent vesicles on the left side of the scalp and forehead. The patient complained of malaise, unilateral facial pain and headache with abnormal skin sensations.

A physical examination revealed unilateral lesions confined to a single dermatome. Vesicles and crusts with a surrounding erythema on the forehead, the frontal and left temporal area of the scalp were presented. Palpation caused some tenderness, with increased itching and burning (Fig. 28.1).

Her temperature was 98.6 °F, pulse was 75 beats per minute, and blood pressure was 115/73 mmHg. An estimated glomerular filtration rate was 60 ml/min/m^2. Other laboratory tests that included complete blood count, erythrocyte sedimentation rate, C-reactive protein, electrolytes, and liver enzymes were normal.

Based on the case description and the photographs, what is your diagnosis?

Differential Diagnoses
1. Herpes gladiatorum.
2. Contact dermatitis.
3. Herpes zoster.
4. Basal cell carcinoma.

Diagnosis
Herpes zoster.

S. Chrostowska (✉)
Department of Dermatology, Medical University of Warsaw, Warsaw, Poland
e-mail: sylwia.chrostowska@wum.edu.pl

A. Waśkiel-Burnat et al. (eds.), *Clinical Cases in Scalp Disorders*, Clinical Cases in Dermatology, https://doi.org/10.1007/978-3-030-93426-2_28

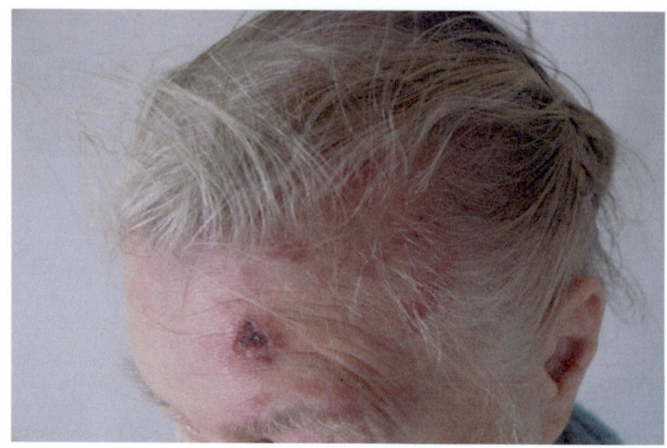

Fig. 28.1 A 75-year-old woman with painful eruption on the left side of the scalp and forehead. Vesicles and crusts with surrounding erythema are observed

Discussion

Chickenpox and herpes zoster are caused by varicella zoster virus (VZV). Varicella is a common childhood illness, characterized by fever, viremia, and scattered vesicular lesions of the skin. After the primary infection, the virus lies dormant in the nerves, including the cranial nerve ganglia, dorsal root ganglia, and autonomic ganglia. Herpes zoster is the result of reactivation of latent VZV. The disease most frequently occurs in older adults. It presents as painful, unilateral dermatomal, vesicular lesions on the erythematous background that do not cross the midline [1]. Crusts can be also presented. The most common locations are the thoracic nerves and the ophthalmic division of the trigeminal nerve with possible eye involvement (keratitis, scarring, and vision loss). The major complication of herpes zoster is an postherpetic neuralgia, defined as a pain persisting for more than 90 days after the resolution of the skin lesions [2]. The diagnosis on herpes zoster is established based on the clinical picture. Polymerase chain reaction, direct fluorescent antigen testing or viral culture are rarely performed [3]. Antiviral drugs (acyclovir, famciclovir, and valacyclovir) should be considered for all patients with herpes zoster and they are especially recommended for patients older than 50 years, those who have a moderate or severe pain or rash, and those with involvement of non-truncal dermatomes [2].

Differential diagnoses for the presented patient included herpes gladiatorum, contact dermatitis and basal cell carcinoma.

Herpes gladiatorum is a skin infection caused by herpes simplex virus type 1. The disease is spread through direct skin-to-skin contact, thus it is more commonly observed in individuals who play sport with the close contact [4]. Clinically, herpes gladiatorum is characterized by the presence of cluster or clusters of clear, fluid-filled vesicles with surrounding erythema. Each body area can be affected. Pain may be reported [4]. The lesions can be multiple and are not limited to one dermatome. Fever and enlarged lymph nodes are rarely reported [4].

Contact dermatitis is an inflammatory eczematous skin disease. The disease is rarely presented on the scalp area, because of the great thickness of the epidermis in this region. In the case of application of irritants or allergens on the scalp symptoms are usually observed on the face or neck. Clinically, contact dermatitis presents as an erythema with scaling and coexisted itch [5]. In acute disease, vesicles or pustules may be presented [5].

Basal cell carcinoma is the most common skin malignancy. The incidence rate of the disease increases with age. Basal cell carcinoma presents as a tiny, hardly visible papule, growing into a nodule or a plaque that is sometimes ulcerated. The face, scalp and neck are most commonly affected [6].

In the presented patient, based on the clinical manifestation the diagnosis of herpes zoster involving ophthalmic branch (V1) of the trigeminal nerve was established. She was treated with 500 mg intravenous acyclovir three times daily per 10 days and oral paracetamol in order to reduce pain. A complete resolution of skin lesions was observed.

Key Points
- Herpes zoster is a viral skin infection that may affect the scalp area.
- It is characterized by the presence of unilateral, dermatomal, painful vesicles and crusts with surrounding erythema.

References

1. Gershon AA, Breuer J, Cohen JI, Cohrs RJ, Gershon MD, Gilden D, et al. Varicella zoster virus infection. Nat Rev Dis Primers. 2015;1:15016.
2. Saguil A, Kane S, Mercado M, Lauters R. Herpes zoster and postherpetic neuralgia: prevention and management. Am Fam Physician. 2017;96(10):656–63.
3. Schmader K. Herpes zoster. Ann Int Med. 2018;169(3):Itc19–itc31.
4. Johnson R. Herpes gladiatorum and other skin diseases. Clin Sports Med. 2004;23(3):473–84. x
5. Rozas-Muñoz E, Gamé D, Serra-Baldrich E. Allergic contact dermatitis by anatomical regions: diagnostic clues. Actas Dermosifiliogr. 2018;109(6):485–507.
6. Marzuka AG, Book SE. Basal cell carcinoma: pathogenesis, epidemiology, clinical features, diagnosis, histopathology, and management. Yale J Biol Med. 2015;88(2):167–79.

Chapter 29
A 79-Year-Old Man with a Pigmented Lesion on the Scalp

Joanna Czuwara and Anna Waśkiel-Burnat

A 79-year-old man presented with an approximately four-year history of a solitary, brown lesion on the back of the scalp. The lesion was first noticed by his family members. The patient observed the lesion to be changing in color and slowly growing, thus he decided for dermatological appointment. No personal or family history of skin cancer was reported.

On physical examination, a 1.2 cm × 1.3 cm greyish-brown lesion on the occipital area was observed (Fig. 29.1). Moreover, non-scarring hair loss on the frontoparietal and vertex areas was presented. Dermoscopy showed hyperpigmented

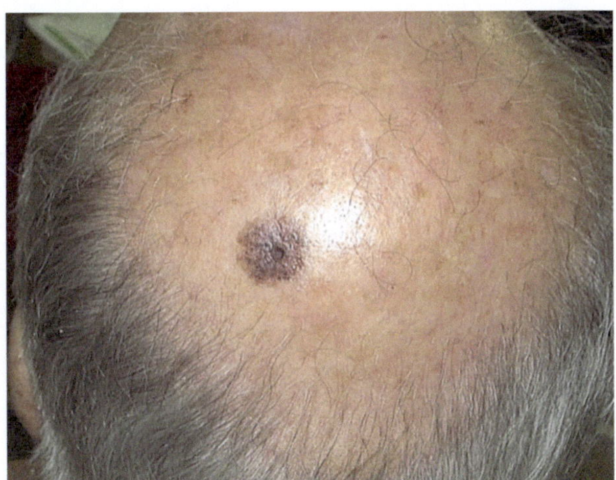

Fig. 29.1 A 79-year-old man with a brown-greyish lesion on the occipital area

J. Czuwara (✉) · A. Waśkiel-Burnat
Department of Dermatology, Medical University of Warsaw, Warsaw, Poland
e-mail: joanna.czuwara@wum.edu.pl; anna.waskiel@wum.edu.pl

A. Waśkiel-Burnat et al. (eds.), *Clinical Cases in Scalp Disorders*, Clinical Cases in Dermatology, https://doi.org/10.1007/978-3-030-93426-2_29

125

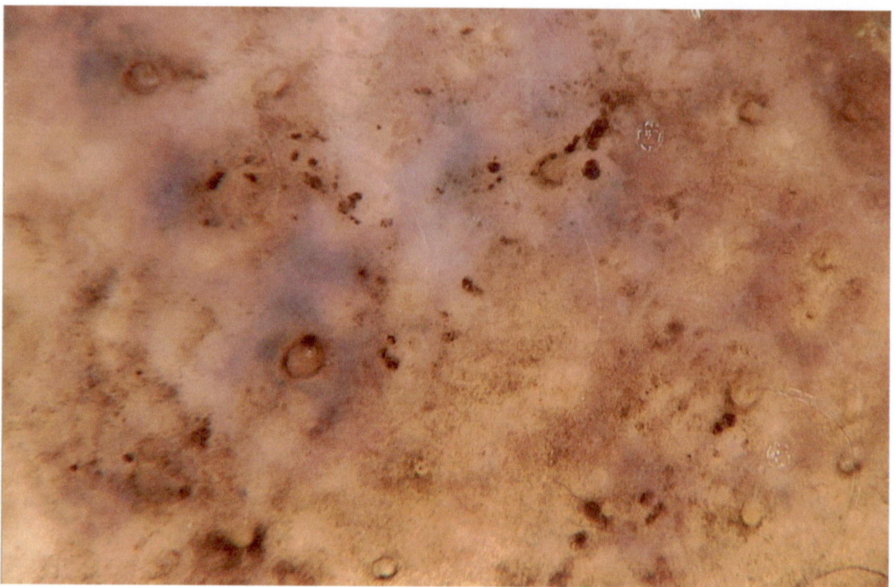

Fig. 29.2 Dermoscopy shows hyperpigmented follicular openings, brown globules and white-bluish structureless areas dispersed between empty hair follicules (×70)

follicular openings, brown globules and white-bluish structureless areas (Fig. 29.2). A diagnostic biopsy was performed from the most suspicious area.

In histopathological examination, a confluent proliferation of basal melanocytes with irregular, hyperchromatic nuclei and uneven melanin production was noticed. There was an early intraepidermal migration of atypical melanocytes, called pagetoid spread. Atypical melanocytes also migrated into hair follicle epithelia tagging their borders. The epidermis was flattened and atrophic. Superficial dermis presented solar elastosis and melanophages (Fig. 29.3).

Based on the case description and the photographs, what is your diagnosis?

Differential Diagnoses
1. Solar lentigo.
2. Lentigo maligna.
3. Seborrheic keratosis.
4. Lichen planus-like keratosis.

Diagnosis
Lentigo maligna.

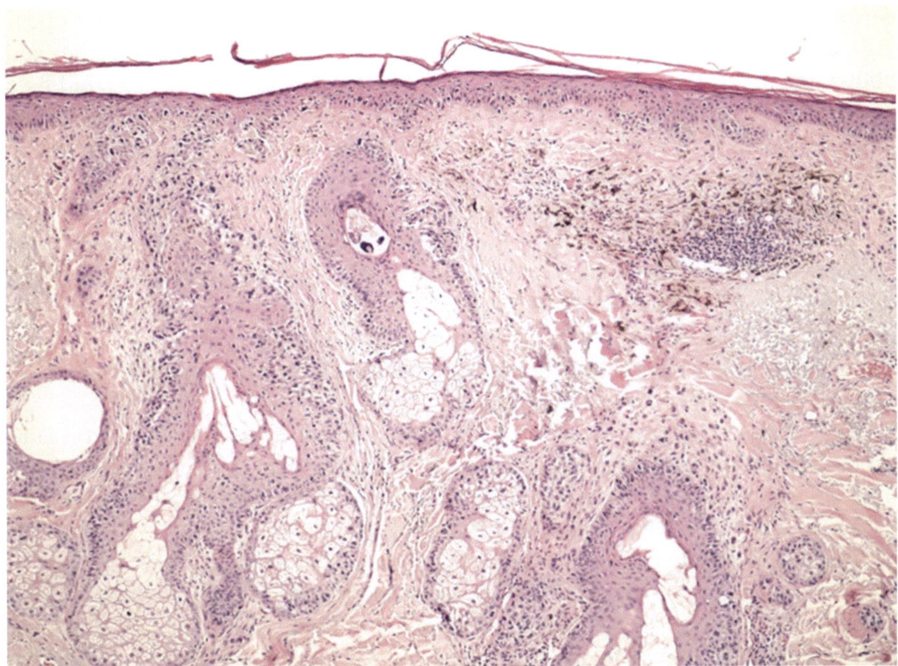

Fig. 29.3 Histopathology of the pigmented lesion on the scalp reveals confluent proliferation of basal melanocytes with irregular, hyperchromatic nuclei and uneven melanin production. There is intraepidermal migration of atypical melanocytes and invasion into hair follicle epithelia. Superficial dermis presents solar elastosis and melanophages (H&E, ×100)

Discussion

Lentigo maligna is classified as a type of melanoma in situ [1]. It accounts for 79%–83% of all cases of melanoma in situ. The lifetime risk of progression from lentigo maligna to lentigo maligna melanoma ranges from 5% to 50% and increases with time. The condition most commonly affects patients aged between 65 and 80 years. However, lentigo maligna has been also reported in patients at the age of 20–30 years. According to the literature, up to 10% of patients with lentigo maligna are younger than 40 years [2]. Men are more commonly affected compared to women [1]. Clinically, lentigo maligna presents as an asymmetric macule, which slowly spreads centrifugally with increasingly irregular borders. The lesion commonly varies in pigmentation, with shades of tan to black. A net-like black pigmentation is often presented [3]. Lentigo maligna affects mainly chronically sun-damaged skin, most commonly on the head and neck [1]. A histopathological examination is the gold standard for diagnosis of lentigo maligna. Dermoscopy may be useful in establishing of initial diagnosis and selection of the biopsy site. Characteristic dermoscopic features of lentigo maligna include hyperpigmented follicular openings, annular-granular pattern, pigmented rhomboidal structures, dark blotches and obliterated hair follicles [4]. A histopathological examination is characterized by a proliferation of predominantly solitary units of melanocytes at the dermoepidermal junction. However, nests of melanocytes may also be displayed. Extension of melanocytes into the superficial portion of hair follicles is commonly observed [1]. A complete surgical removal of lentigo maligna with five to 10 mm clinical margins is the preferred management. Topical imiquimod 5% cream as the second-line treatment for lentigo maligna is recommended when surgery is not possible at the outset (primary setting) or when optimal surgery has been performed (adjuvant setting). Radiotherapy may be also used for nonsurgical candidates [1].

Lentigo maligna should be differentiated from solar lentigo, seborrheic keratosis and lichen planus-like keratosis.

Solar lentigo presents as an irregular brown or tan macule localized on sun-exposed skin such as the face and the back of the hands. Solitary or multiple lesions may be observed. Solar lentigo occurs mainly in elderly, fair-skinned individuals who have had excessive exposure to the sun [5].

Typical seborrheic keratosis is a sharply demarcated, round or oval-shaped, elevated and stuck on the skin lesion with a verrucous, dull, uneven, or punched-out surface. The color of the lesions varies from skin color, yellowish, light to dark brown, grey, and black. Seborrheic keratosis may present as an isolated or multiple lesions. It is most common in the middle-aged and elderly, however it may also present in young adults. The chest, back, scalp (mainly the temporal areas) and neck are most commonly affected [6].

Lichen planus-like keratosis, also known as benign lichenoid keratosis or solitary lichen planus, is a common benign skin lesion. The condition generally develops in fair-skinned patients aged 30–80 years. It is more common in women compared to men. Lichen planus-like keratosis usually appears as a rapidly evolving solitary lesion, ranging from five to 20 mm in diameter. The lesion presents as a papule or plaque with either a smooth or verrucous surface. The colour ranges from pink to violaceous or tan to brown. The upper extremities, face, and chest are most commonly affected [7].

In the presented patient, based on the clinical, dermoscopic and histopathological examination, the diagnosis of lentigo maligna was established. The lesion was surgically removed with a five mm margins with a conformation of the initial diagnosis.

Key Points
- Lentigo maligna is a type of melanoma in situ that is commonly observed on the scalp area.
- The condition presents as an asymmetric macule, which slowly spreads centrifugally with increasingly irregular borders.
- The lesion varies in pigmentation, with shades of tan to black.

References

1. Iznardo H, Garcia-Melendo C, Yélamos O. Lentigo maligna: clinical presentation and appropriate management. Clin Cosmet Investig Dermatol. 2020;13:837–55.
2. Samaniego E, Redondo P. Lentigo maligna. Actas Dermosifiliogr. 2013;104(9):757–75.
3. Kallini JR, Jain SK, Khachemoune A. Lentigo maligna: review of salient characteristics and management. Am J Clin Dermatol. 2013;14(6):473–80.
4. Schiffner R, Schiffner-Rohe J, Vogt T, Landthaler M, Wlotzke U, Cognetta AB, et al. Improvement of early recognition of lentigo maligna using dermatoscopy. J Am Acad Dermatol. 2000;42(1 Pt 1):25–32.
5. Byrom L, Barksdale S, Weedon D, Muir J. Unstable solar lentigo: a defined separate entity. Australas J Dermatol. 2016;57(3):229–34.
6. Hafner C, Vogt T. Seborrheic keratosis. J Dtsch Dermatol Ges. 2008;6(8):664–77.
7. Nagrani N, Jaimes N, Oliviero MC, Rabinovitz HS. Lichen planus-like keratosis: clinical applicability of in vivo reflectance confocal microscopy for an indeterminate cutaneous lesion. Dermatol Pract Concept. 2018;8(3):180–3.

Chapter 30
An 80-Year-Old Man with Erosions on the Scalp

Anna Waśkiel-Burnat, Joanna Golińska, Patrycja Gajda, Adriana Rakowska, Joanna Czuwara, Małgorzata Olszewska, and Lidia Rudnicka

An 80-year-old man presented with a two-year history of progressing erosions on the scalp area. He did not complain of any symptoms associated with the skin lesions. The patient had hypertension, ischemic heart disease and type 2 diabetes mellitus.

A physical examination revealed erosions, yellowish crusts and areas of scarring hair loss on the frontal and parietal areas. Moreover, non-scarring hair loss of the frontal, parietal and vertex regions with multiple areas of actinic keratosis were presented (Fig. 30.1). On trichoscopy, red and milky-red areas with the absence of follicular openings, hemorrhagic and yellowish crusts were detected (Fig. 30.2).

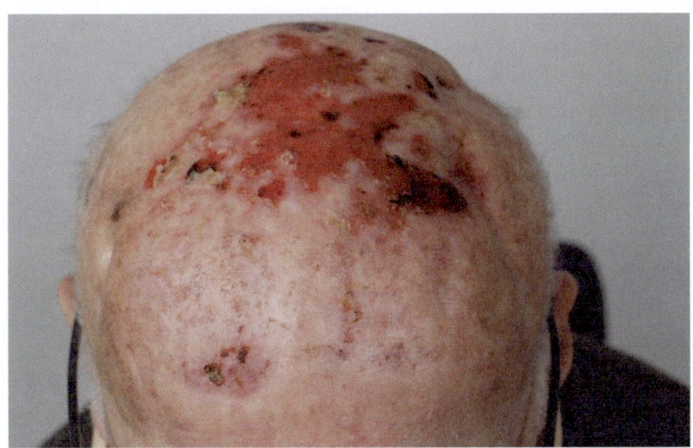

Fig. 30.1 An 80-year-old man with androgenetic alopecia. Erosions on the frontal and parietal areas with yellowish crusts surrounded by areas of scarring alopecia are presented

A. Waśkiel-Burnat (✉) · J. Golińska · P. Gajda · A. Rakowska · J. Czuwara · M. Olszewska
L. Rudnicka
Department of Dermatology, Medical University of Warsaw, Warsaw, Poland
e-mail: anna.waskiel@wum.edu.pl; joanna.golinska@wum.edu.pl;
patrycja.gajda@wum.edu.pl; adriana.rakowska@wum.edu.pl; joanna.czuwara@wum.edu.pl;
malgorzata.olszewska@wum.edu.pl; lidia.rudnicka@wum.edu.pl

A. Waśkiel-Burnat et al. (eds.), *Clinical Cases in Scalp Disorders*, Clinical Cases in Dermatology, https://doi.org/10.1007/978-3-030-93426-2_30

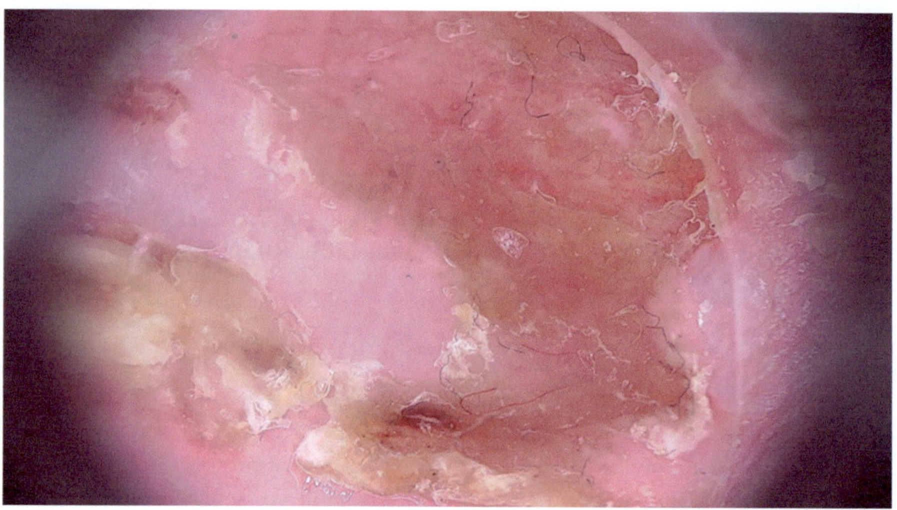

Fig. 30.2 Trichoscopy shows yellowish and hemorrhagic crusts with a surrounding erythema (×20)

Fig. 30.3 Histology shows a zone of epidermal erosion covered with serum, blood and the cornified layer remnants. Moreover, a dense dermal polymorphous inflammation, loss of follicular structures, or in some areas the naked hair shaft surrounded by multinucleated giant cells are visible

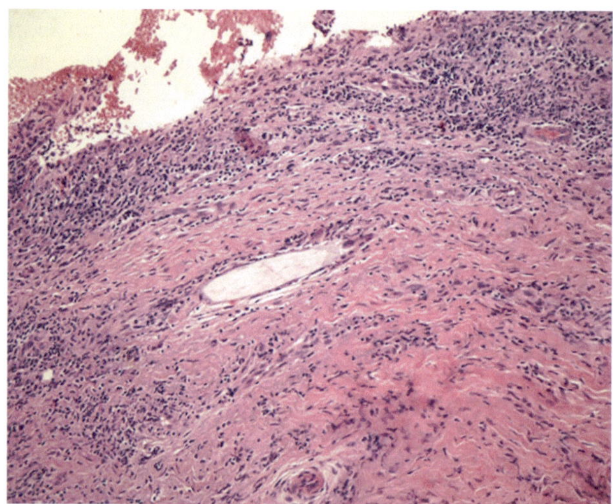

In histopathological examination a zone of epidermal erosion covered with serum, blood and the cornified layer remnants was observed. Moreover, a dense dermal polymorphous inflammation with vascular proliferation suggestive of granulation tissue rich in plasma cells was detected. There was loss of follicular structures, or in some areas the naked hair shaft surrounded by multinucleated giant cells were visible (Fig. 30.3).

Based on the case description and the photographs, what is your diagnosis?

Differential Diagnoses
1. Erosive pustular dermatosis of the scalp.
2. Brunsting-Perry cicatricial pemphigoid.
3. Basal cell carcinoma.
4. Pyoderma gangrenosum.

Diagnosis
Erosive pustular dermatosis of the scalp.

Discussion

Erosive pustular dermatosis of the scalp is a rare inflammatory condition of the scalp [1]. The etiopathology of the disease is not fully described. The possible trigger factors are a prior trauma, radiation, herpes zoster, treatment with topical fluorouracil or imiquimod, cryotherapy, and photodynamic therapy [2]. The lesions typically occurs six months after the triggering event [3]. Erosive pustular dermatosis of the scalp is more common in patients with androgenetic alopecia and actinic damage as well as in individuals with autoimmune disorders such as rheumatoid arthritis, autoimmune hepatitis, Hashimoto thyroiditis, and Takayasu aortitis [3]. It mainly affects elderly with aging of onset at 60–70 years [1, 3]. Clinically, the condition is characterized by recurrent pustules, inflamed erosions and grey, yellow or yellow-brown crusts that lead to the scarring alopecia. Affected areas undergo a continuous cycle of healing and recurrences with a fluctuating course [1]. Pain and pruritus are rarely observed. The vertex is the most common location for erosive pustular dermatosis of the scalp, followed by the frontal and parietal areas [1]. Diagnosis of the disease is based on a combination of history, physical examination, trichoscopy, and histopathology [3]. Trichoscopic features of erosive pustular dermatosis of the scalp include absence of follicular ostia, tufted and broken hair, crusts, serous exudate, dilated vessels, pustules and hyperkeratosis [1]. In histopathological examination, nonspecific changes such as an erosive or hyperplastic epidermis and subcorneal pustules are presented. In the dermis, there are lymphocytic and leukocyte-rich infiltrates, plasma cells and, in some cases, foreign body reactions [2]. The disease management involves a pragmatic multimodal approach. Potent or ultrapotent topical corticosteroids and topical calcineurin inhibitors are usually the first line treatment. Moreover, the improvement after topical calcipotriene (calcipotriol), systemic prednisone, doxycycline, isotretinoin or acitretin, dapsone and zinc has been described [2].

For the presented patient differential diagnoses included Brunsting-Perry cicatricial pemphigoid, basal cell carcinoma and pyoderma gangrenosum.

Brunsting-Perry cicatricial pemphigoid is a chronic inflammatory, autoimmune condition. It is characterized by subepithelial blisters and erosions with following scarring strictly limited to the head and neck. The mucous membranes are spared.

Pyoderma gangrenosum is a rare, noninfectious, neutrophilic dermatosis with an incidence between three and 10 patients per million [4]. It presents as pustules or papules that undergo a central necrosis and extend peripherally to form ulcers. Lower extremities are the most common location, however the scalp involvement has been described in the literature [4]. Classic pyoderma gangrenosum is most common in adults between 20 and 50 years of age. However, the scalp lesions frequently occur in the pediatric and geriatric patient populations [4]. Women are slightly more commonly affected compared to man. Pyoderma gangrenosum is commonly associated with an underlying comorbidity such as inflammatory bowel disease, hematologic disorders (myelodysplastic syndrome, multiple myeloma), or inflammatory arthritis [4].

Basal cell carcinoma is the most common skin malignancy. The incidence rate of the disease increases with age. There are five types of basal cell carcinoma: nodular, pigmented, morpheaform, superficial and premalignant (fibroepithelioma) that vary in clinical presentation. Basal cell carcinoma presents as solitary lesion, most commonly on the face, scalp or neck areas [5].

Based on the clinical manifestation, trichoscopy and histopathological examination, the diagnosis of erosive pustular dermatosis of the scalp was established. Therapy with propionate clobetasol 5% cream was initiated with clinical improvement.

Key Points
- Erosive pustular dermatosis of the scalp is a form of scarring alopecia that is mainly observed in the elderly.
- It presents as recurrent pustules, inflamed erosions and grey, yellow or yellow-brown crusts that lead to scarring alopecia.

References

1. Starace M, Iorizzo M, Trüeb RM, Piccolo V, Argenziano G, Camacho FM, et al. Erosive pustular dermatosis of the scalp: a multicentre study. J Eur Acad Dermatol Venereol. 2020;34(6):1348–54.
2. Kanti V, Rowert-Huber J, Vogt A, Blume-Peytavi U. Cicatricial alopecia. J Dtsch Dermatol Ges. 2018;16(4):435–61.
3. Starace M, Alessandrini A, Baraldi C, Piraccini BM. Erosive pustular dermatosis of the scalp: challenges and solutions. Clin Cosmet Investig Dermatol. 2019;12:691–8.
4. Gupta AS, Nunley JR, Feldman MJ, Ortega-Loayza AG. Pyoderma gangrenosum of the scalp: a rare clinical variant. Wounds Compendium Clin Res Pract. 2018;30(2):e16–20.
5. Marzuka AG, Book SE. Basal cell carcinoma: pathogenesis, epidemiology, clinical features, diagnosis, histopathology, and management. Yale J Biol Med. 2015;88(2):167–79.

Chapter 31
A Boy with Nodular Plaques on the Scalp

Qian Zhang, Hao Guo, and Jiu-Hong Li

A 16-year-old boy presented to the Department of Dermatology with a slowly enlarging scalp lesion. The lesion had been present since birth as a well-defined hairless area. A pink-like nodular plaque was firstly noticed four years ago. No pruritus or pain were reported.

A physical examination revealed a few pink-like, verrucous, and nodular plaques with overlying alopecia on the left parietal area of the scalp (Fig. 31.1a, b).

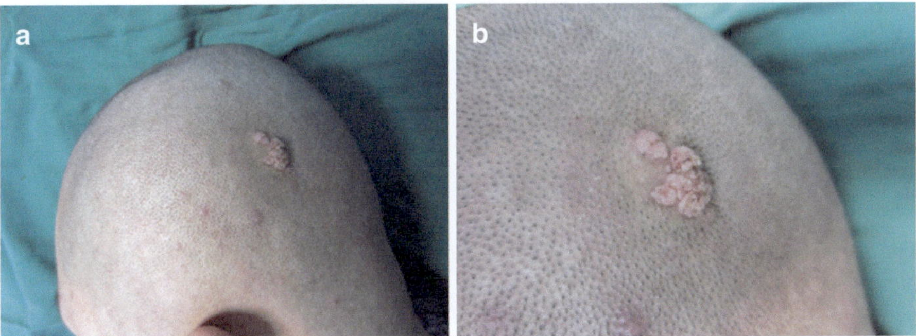

Fig. 31.1 A 16-year-old boy with a few pink-like, verrucous, and nodular plagues with overlying alopecia on the left parietal area of the scalp (**a, b**)

Q. Zhang · H. Guo (✉) · J.-H. Li
Department of Dermatology, The First Hospital of China Medical University,
Shenyang, China

A. Waśkiel-Burnat et al. (eds.), *Clinical Cases in Scalp Disorders*, Clinical
Cases in Dermatology, https://doi.org/10.1007/978-3-030-93426-2_31

Fig. 31.2
Histology shows overlying
papillomatous epidermal
hyperplasia and a large
number of hyperplastic
matured sebaceous glands
without mature hair
follicles (HE × 40)

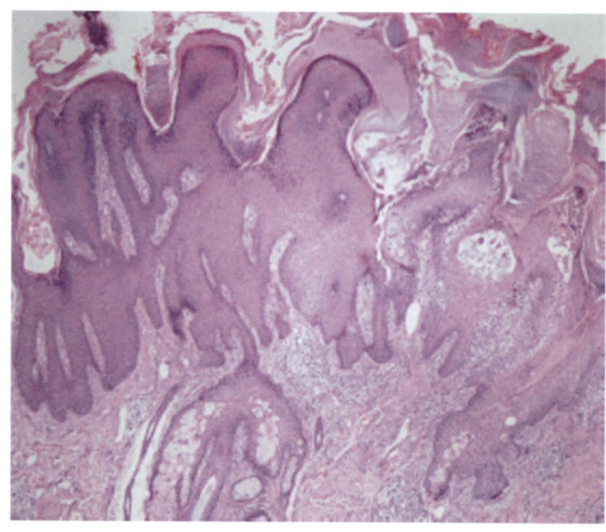

Laboratory tests were within normal limits. A full-thickness surgical excision within local anesthesia was performed. A histopathological examination revealed overlying papillomatous epidermal hyperplasia and a large number of hyperplastic matured sebaceous glands without mature hair follicles (Fig. 31.2).

Based on the case description and the photography, what is your diagnosis?

Differential Diagnoses
1. Nevus sebaceous.
2. Verruca vulgaris.
3. Epidermal nevus.
4. Alpasia cutis congenita.

Diagnosis
Nevus sebaceous.

Discussion

Nevus sebaceous, firstly mentioned by Jadassohn, is also named as an organoid nevus, because it contains any or all components of the skin (mainly sebaceous glands). Nevus sebaceous is a congenital hamartoma that mainly appears as a solitary, well-defined, waxy, pink/yellow/orange color and hairless plaque ranging in size from one to over 10 cm. It is generally located on the face and scalp. Less commonly, oval or round, multiple, and extensive nodular plaques are presented.

Nevus sebaceous often behaves differently depending on the proliferative changes of sebaceous glands, sweat glands, and hair follicles. It usually undergoes three stages. In childhood, nevus sebaceous often shows onset at birth or shortly thereafter, with the prevalence of 0.3% of newborns [1]. The lesion is a smooth or raised, greasy, yellowish, hairless, localized plaque, in a linear arrangement or a round shape. At puberty, with hormonal stmuli on developed sebaceous and apocrine glands, the lesion can undergo rapid growth and become thickened with a nodular, verrucous surface. When the lesion becomes extensive, it may be associated with an extra-cutaneous complex syndrome that includes skeletal, ocular, and neurologic abnormalities. In the third stage, nevus sebaceous can be complicated with epithelial neoplasm. The majority of tumors are benign. The most common benign tumors include trichoblastoma, syringocystadenoma papilliferum (with separately 5%), trichilemmoma, and sebaceoma (with separately 2%–3%). The most common malignant tumors are basal cell carcinoma, apocrine carcinoma, sebaceous carcinoma, and squamous cell carcinoma. The standard treatment of nevus sebaceous is a full-thickness surgical excision. Because of cosmetic reason and potential risk of malignancy, the excision may be recommended before puberty.

The histopathological features of the nevus sebaceous are age-dependent [2]. In childhood, the sebaceous glands are underdeveloped and reduced in size and number, which makes diagnosis difficult. During puberty, the amount of mature or nearly mature sebaceous glands tends to enlarge what induces verrucous, papillomatous hyperplasia of the overlying epidermis. Nevus sebaceous is usually located deeply in the dermis. Ectopic apocrine glands can be seen while terminally differentiated hair follicles are usually lack.

The diagnosis of nevus sebaceous is commonly established based on clinical manifestation. An ultrasound examination and dermoscopy may be useful diagnostic tools. They also help in the early detection of non-melanoma skin cancers, especially basal cell carcinoma [3, 4]. The biopsy is the gold diagnostic standard of nevus sebaceous when the diagnosis remains uncertain.

Nevus sebaceous needs to be differentiated from verruca vulgaris, epidermal nevus and aplasia cutis congenita.

Verruca vulgaris presents as a cauliflower-like papule with a rough, papillomatous and hyperkeratotic surface. It most frequently occurs on the fingers, toes, soles, and the dorsal surface of the hands. It is mostly asymptomatic. A histopathological examination shows hyperkeratosis, spinous hypertrophy, papilloma-like hyperplasia, and koilocytes.

Epidermal nevus presents as enlarging, gray/dark, coarse, hyperkeratotic papules, which are distributed along the lines of Blashko. The head, trunk, and extremities are commonly affected. Sometimes, the lesions can be bilateral, multiple, and extensive. Mucous membranes may be also affected.

Aplasia cutis congenita is characterized by a focal or diffuse defect of the skin present at birth. The typical lesion is pink, oval, or round and has smooth or atrophic surface.

Based on the patient's history, clinical manifestation and histopathological examination, the diagnosis of nevus sebaceous was established.

Key Points
- Nevus sebaceous is a congenital hamartoma characterized by age-dependent clinical and histopathological features.
- A full-thickness surgical excision of nevus sebaceous, because of cosmetic reason and potential risk of malignancy, is usually recommended before puberty.

References

1. Lopez AS, Lam JM. Nevus sebaceous. CMAJ. 2019;191(27):E765.
2. Donati A, Cavelier-Balloy B, Reygagne P. Histologic correlation of dermoscopy findings in a sebaceous nevus. Cutis. 2015;96(6):E8–9.
3. Wortsman X, Ferreira-Wortsman C, Corredoira Y. Ultrasound Imaging of Nevus Sebaceous of Jadassohn. J Ultrasound Med. 2021;40(2):407–15.
4. Micali G, et al. Dermatoscopy of common lesions in pediatric dermatology. Dermatol Clin. 2018;36(4):463–72.

Chapter 32
A Deep Furrowed Forehead

Uwe Wollina

A 66-year-old male patient presented with deep furrows and large longitudinal soft-tissue folds on the forehead and glabella. The lesions were present for decades. He had no subjective symptoms but asked for treatment due to esthetic reasons. His medical history was positive for hyperuricemia and hypertensive heart disease.

On physical examination, convoluted soft-tissue folds and deep furrows on the forehead with a longitudinal direction were observed (Fig. 32.1).

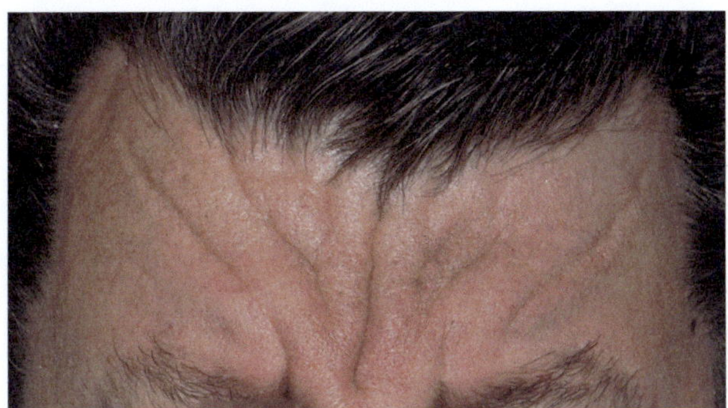

Fig. 32.1 Deep furrows and longitudinal soft-tissue folds on the forehead

U. Wollina (✉)
Department of Dermatology and Allergology, Municipal Hospital of Dresden, Academic Teaching Hospital, Dresden, Germany
e-mail: Uwe.Wollina@klinikum-dresden.de

A. Waśkiel-Burnat et al. (eds.), *Clinical Cases in Scalp Disorders*, Clinical Cases in Dermatology, https://doi.org/10.1007/978-3-030-93426-2_32

Differential Diagnoses
1. Pachydermoperiostosis.
2. Cutis verticis gyrata.
3. Accentuated sleeping folds.
4. Cerebriform intradermal nevus.
5. Cutis laxa.
6. Lymphoma.

Diagnosis
Cutis verticis gyrata.

Discussion

Cutis verticis gyrata is a rare benign cutaneous disorder that is characterized by convoluted folds and deep furrows of the scalp. These lesions mimic cerebral sulci and gyri. The term cutis verticis gyrata was coined by Paul Gerson Unna in 1907 [1], although the first description originates from Jean-Louis Alibert in 1837, who named it cutis sulcata. The clinical appearance is very characteristic.

The disease affects between 0.03 and 1 per 100,000 of the general population [2]. The forehead and glabella are rarely affected compared to the scalp area [2].

The disease is classified into primary and secondary (Table 32.1). The primary cutis verticis gyrata usually occurs in adult men before the age of 30. The secondary form can occur at any age with no gender predilection [3]. Secondary cutis verticis gyrata has been recently seen in patients with melanoma treated with vemurafenib and the whole brain irradiation [4].

The disease can be disfiguring but runs a benign course. Surgical correction needs hair and scalp restoration procedures of plastic and neurosurgery including the use of tissue expansion [5–7].

Table 32.1 Classification of cutis verticis gyrata

Type	Remarks
Primary essential	Absence of associated abnormalities
Primary non-essential	Associated with intellectual disability, neuropsychiatric disorders, seizures, schizophrenia, cerebral palsy, cataracts, strabismus, retinitis pigmentosa, blindness
Secondary	Associated with chronic actinic dermatitis, pachydermoperiostosis, cerebriform intradermal nevus, acromegaly, scleromyxedema, leukemia, lymphoma, syphilis, acanthosis nigricans, neurofibromas, nevus lipomatosus, tuberous sclerosis complex, cylindroma, Ehlers-Danlos syndrome, amyloidosis, diabetes mellitus, cutis laxa, intracerebral aneurysm, cutaneous focal mucinosis, misuse of anabolic steroids, Turner syndrome, Klinefelter syndrome, syndrome, Akesson syndrome, Cohen syndrome, Mcdowall syndrome etc.

Key Points
- Cutis verticis gyrata is a rare cutaneous disease of the scalp.
- It is characterized by the presence of convoluted folds and deep furrows.
- Primary and secondary subtypes of cutis verticis gyrata are described.

References

1. Unna PG. Cutis verticis gyrata. Monatsh Prakt Derm. 1907;45:227–33.
2. Harish V, Clarke F. Isolated cutis verticis gyrata or the glabella and nasal bridge: a case report and review of the literature. J Plast Recontr Aesthet Surg. 2013;66(10):1421–3.
3. Larsen F, Birchall N. Cutis verticis gyrata: three cases with different aetiologies that demonstrate the classification system. Australas J Dermatol. 2007;48(2):91–4.
4. Harding JJ, Barker CA, Carvajal RD, Wolchok JD, Chapman PB, Lacouture ME. Cutis verticis gyrata in association with vemurafenib and whole-brain radiotherapy. J Clin Oncol. 2014;32(14):e54–6.
5. Rallo MS, Nosko M, Agag RL, Xiong Z, Al-Mufti F, Roychowdhury S, Nanda A, Gupta G. Neurosurgical and scalp reconstructive challenges during craniotomy in the setting of cutis verticis gyrata. World Neurosurg. 2019;125:392–7.
6. Eginli A, McMichael A, Cooley J. Combination hair restoration techniques in the treatment of severe cutis verticis gyrata. Dermatol Surg. 2020; https://doi.org/10.1097/DSS.0000000000002833. Epub ahead of Print. PMID: 33165082
7. Zhao D, Li J, Wang K, Guo X, Lang Y, Peng L, Wang Q, Li Y. Treating cutis verticis gyrata using skin expansion method. Cell Biochem Biophys. 2012;62(2):373–6.

Chapter 33
A 4-Month-Old Girl with a Red Ulcerated Nodule on the Temporal Area

Marta Kurzeja, Małgorzata Olszewska, and Lidia Rudnicka

A four-month-old girl was presented with a red ulcerated nodule on the scalp. The lesion appeared as a red macule in the second week of life. Then the lesion began to grow rapidly and developed into a red nodule. An ulceration was presented since two weeks. No personal and family history of dermatological or non-dermatological condition was reported.

A physical examination revealed a 2 cm × 1.8 cm cherry-colored nodule with the central ulceration localized on the left temporal area (Fig. 33.1).

Based on the case description and the photographs, what is your diagnosis?

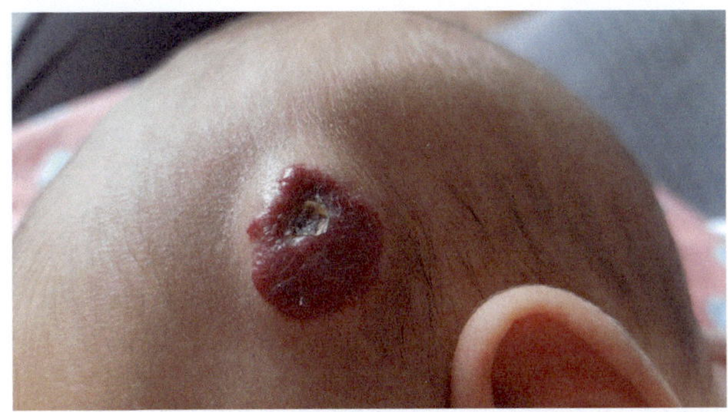

Fig. 33.1 A four-month-old girl with a cherry-colored nodule with the central ulceration localized on the left temporal area

M. Kurzeja (✉) · M. Olszewska · L. Rudnicka
Department of Dermatology, Medical University of Warsaw, Warsaw, Poland
e-mail: marta.kurzeja@wum.edu.pl; malgorzata.olszewska@wum.edu.pl;
lidia.rudnicka@wum.edu.pl

A. Waśkiel-Burnat et al. (eds.), *Clinical Cases in Scalp Disorders*, Clinical Cases in Dermatology, https://doi.org/10.1007/978-3-030-93426-2_33

Differential Diagnoses
1. Nevus flammeus.
2. Pyogenic granuloma.
3. Infantile hemangioma.
4. Kaposiform hemangioendothelioma.

Diagnosis
Infantile hemangioma.

Discussion

Infantile hemangioma is the most common benign tumor of the infancy that affects 4%–5% of newborns [1]. The pathogenesis of infantile hemangiomas has not been fully elucidated. The main hypothesis suggests that circulating endothelial progenitor cells migrate to fields with hypoxia or developmental disturbances and then multiply [1–4]. Infantile hemangiomas are more frequent in Caucasian, premature infants, twins and infants with a low birth weight. There is also a female predominance. Additionally, family history of infantile hemangioma, eclampsia and placental anomalies are also significant risk factors [1, 2]. Infantile hemangiomas are classified as superficial, deep and mixed. Superficial lesions involve the upper part of the dermis and typically appear as elevated red papules, nodules, or plaques. Deep infantile hemangiomas extend to the subcutaneous tissue and are visible as bluish tumors, with blurry borders. There is also a mixed form of infantile hemangiomas with features of both locations [1, 4]. Infantile hemangiomas are characterized by triphasic evolution. Precursor lesion is visible as a pale area of vasoconstriction or a telangiectatic pink spot which appears after birth or in the first weeks of life. In an early proliferative or growth phase, there is a rapid growth during the first three months and a gradual growth in months five to eight of life. A plateau phase is observed between six and 12 months of life. An involution phase occurs after the first year of life and continues for several years. In a regression phase, infantile hemangioma becomes softer and more compressible, and the color changes from bright red to purple or gray. The skin may return to normal, but in 70% of causes there are residual changes (excessive fibrofatty tissue, telangiectasia, skin laxity) [1, 2, 4]. Infantile hemangiomas occur on the skin and mucosal surfaces. They are usually solitary. However, multifocal or segmental lesions may be presented. Five or more infantile hemangiomas on the skin may indicate visceral involvement, most frequently liver or gastrointestinal tract [1]. The head and neck are most commonly affected (60% of cases). This is followed by the lesions on the trunk in 25% of cases, and least commonly, on the extremities, seen in 15% of cases. Infantile hemangiomas localized on the lumbosacral area may associated with an increased risk for tethering of the spinal cord or genitourinary abnormalities (e.g. LUMBAR syndrome). Infantile hemangiomas on the face and neck may be connected with structural anomalies (e.g. PHACES syndrome). They have a high risk of scarring and ulceration and may cause ocular occlusion [4]. Complications occur in 10–15% of infantile hemangiomas. An ulceration is the most frequent and occurs in 10%–25% of patients, commonly between the four and eight months of life [1]. Infantile hemangiomas on the eyelid or close to the eye may lead to visual disturbance, while the lesions involving the lips or oral cavity may cause feeding impairment. Paraglottic or intratracheal infantile haemangiomas may lead to life-threatening obstruction of the airway [1–4]. The diagnosis of infantile hemangioma is established on the basis of clinical picture. Further investigations should be performed when the diagnosis is uncertain, there are five or more cutaneous infantile hemangiomas, or when associated anatomic abnormalities are suspected [1]. Infantile hemangiomas do not usually require treatment. In case of complications therapy is recommended. Oral propranolol is the first-line therapeutic option [5]. Also topical beta-blockers such as timolol may be used off-label for small superficial haemangiomas [4]. Topical, intralesional and systemic corticosteroids may be also helpful [5]. Imiquimod has been reported to be efficient in some cases. The pulse dye laser is recommended in the treatment of residual lesions [1, 4]

Differential diagnoses of infantile hemangioma include nevus flammeus, pyogenic hemangioma and Kaposiform hemangioendothelioma.

Nevus flammeus is the most common vascular malformation, typically presents at birth as pink or red homogenous, variably sized macules and patches and persists throughout life. In 70%–90% of cases, the head and neck are affected. The lesions may be single or multiple, unilateral or bilateral, localized, or widespread [1–4].

Pyogenic granuloma, known as granuloma pyogenicum, is a common, acquired, benign, vascular tumor. The lesion occurs as a solitary, red, pedunculated papule that is very friable. Less commonly, it may present as a sessile plaque. It characterized by a rapid exophytic growth, with a surface that often undergoes ulceration. It is often seen on the cutaneous or mucosal surfaces [1–3].

Kaposiform hemangioendothelioma typically presents as an enlarging, single soft tissue mass with cutaneous findings that range from an erythematous papule, plaque, or nodule to an indurated, purple and firm tumor. The lesions are localized on the trunk, extremities, or retroperitoneum [2, 3].

In the presented patient, based on the clinical manifestation, the diagnosis of infantile hemangioma was established. She was treated with oral propranolol (2 mg/kg/day) with gradual involution of the lesion.

Key Points
- Infantile haemangioma is the most common benign tumor of infancy that is commonly localized on the scalp.
- Infantile hemangioma initially presents as pale area of vasoconstriction or a telangiectatic pink spot which appears after birth or in the first weeks of life. Then a rapid growth is observed followed by a plateau and involution phase.

References

1. Léauté-Labrèze C, Harper JI, Hoeger PH. Infantile haemangioma. Lancet. 2017;390(10089):85–94.
2. Smith CJF, Friedlander SF, Guma M, Kavanaugh A, Chambers CD. Infantile hemangiomas: an updated review on risk factors, pathogenesis, and treatment. Birth Defects Res. 2017;109(11):809–15.
3. De Leye H, Saerens J, Janmohamed SR. News on infantile haemangioma. Part 1: clinical course and pathomechanism. Clin Exp Dermatol. 2020; https://doi.org/10.1111/ced.14502.
4. Krowchuk DP, Frieden IJ, Mancini AJ, Darrow DH, Blei F, Greene AK, Annam A, Baker CN, Frommelt PC, Hodak A, Pate BM, Pelletier JL, Sandrock D, Weinberg ST, Whelan MA. Clinical practice guideline for the management of infantile hemangiomas. Pediatrics. 2019;143(1):e20183475.
5. Darrow DH, Greene AK, Mancini AJ, Nopper AJ. Diagnosis and management of infantile hemangioma: executive summary. Pediatrics. 2015;136(4):786–91.

Chapter 34
A Male Student with a Scalp Nodule

Runping Fang

An 18-year-old male student was presented with a nodule on the top of his scalp for several years. The lesion appeared after scalp injury a few years ago. It was not painful, but the nodule gradually increased. Recently, the nodule burst, and was painfull and bleeding at palpation.

A physical examination showed a red dome-shaped nodule (1 cm × 0.8 cm × 0.3 cm) on the top of the scalp (Fig. 34.1), with a hard texture, smooth surface, and central ulceration. Complete blood count as well as liver and kidney function tests were normal. Syphilis, HIV, and HCV were excluded. A complete surgical excision was performed. A pathological examination showed the tumor cells growing from the epidermis to dermis and forming a wide and interconnected tumor mass. The tumor cells were cubic in shape and uniform in size. The nuclei were round or ovoid. A large number of transparent cells were visible (Fig. 34.2).

Based on the case description and the photographs, what is your diagnosis?

Differential Diagnoses
1. Tricholemmoma.
2. Squamous cell carcinoma.
3. Clear cell hidradenoma.
4. Eccrine poroma.

Diagnosis
Clear cell hidradenoma.

R. Fang (✉)
Department of Dermatology, Shangyou County People's Hospital, Jiangxi Province, Ganzhou, China

© The Author(s), under exclusive license to Springer Nature Switzerland AG 2022

A. Waśkiel-Burnat et al. (eds.), *Clinical Cases in Scalp Disorders*, Clinical Cases in Dermatology, https://doi.org/10.1007/978-3-030-93426-2_34

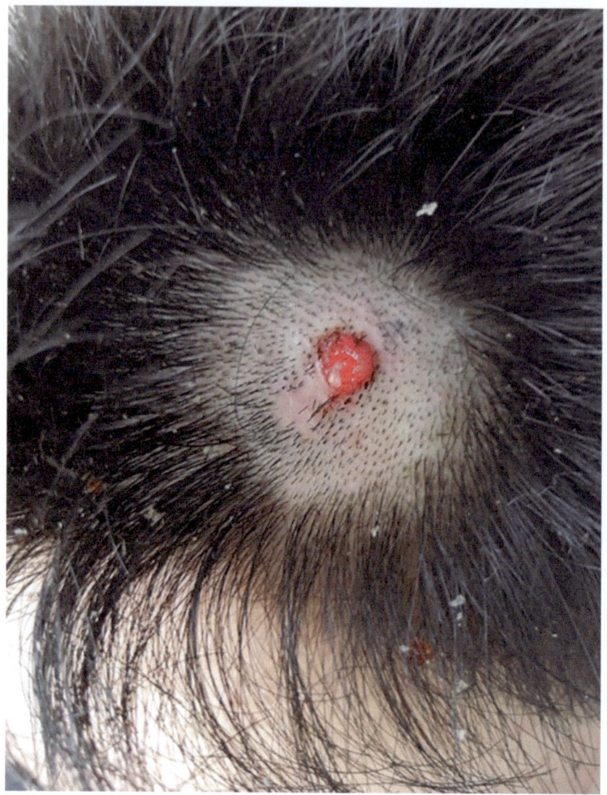

Fig. 34.1 A red solid nodule on the top of the scalp

Discussion

Clear cell hidradenoma is known as nodular hidradenoma, clear cell eccrine adenoma, clear cell myoepithelioma, eccrine acrospiroma or solid cystic hidradenoma, and porosyringoma. On the contrary to other sweat gland tumors, clear cell hidradenoma is dominated by clear cells in histology. The tumor tissue is located in the dermis with clear boundaries and with or without capsule. It may contiguous to the epidermis. The clinical diagnosis of this disease is very difficult. In histology, lobulated or domed structures, findle-shaped or polygonal basophils, and large clear cells are identified. Differential diagnoses for clear cell hidradenoma include tricholemmoma, eccrine poroma, and squamous cell carcinoma [1].

Clear cell hidradenoma may be misdiagnosed as tricholemmoma which contains glycogen-rich clear cells and keratinization. Clear cell hidradenoma often has a large cystic cavity and tubular structure, while tricholemmoma has a gridlike arrangement of cells around the tumor nest [2].

When there is keratosis in the tumor, it should be distinguished from squamous cell carcinoma. Squamous cell carcinoma cells are obviously pleomorphic and lacks the tendency of squamous cell swirls to surround or form lumens in clear cell hidenoma [3].

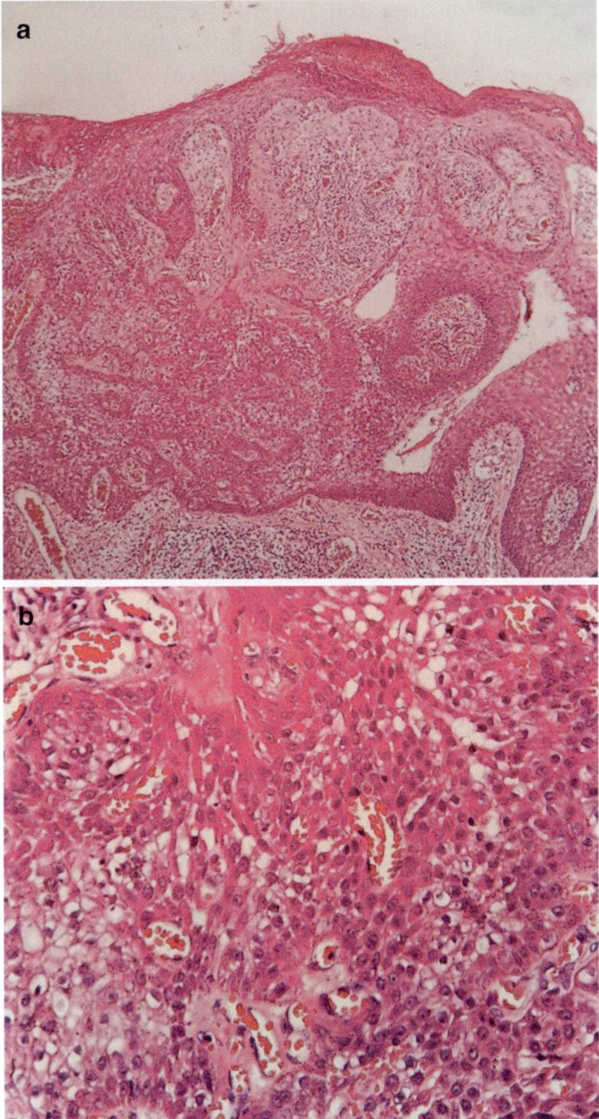

Fig. 34.2 A pathological examination. (**a**) There are masses of neoplastic cells in the dermis, which are associated with the epidermis (HE × 20); (**b**) The tumor is composed of two kinds of cells: 1) with transparent cytoplasm and small nuclei and 2) with eosinophilic cytoplasm, vesicular nuclei and punctate nucleoli. There is no heteromorphism and mitotic activity of the cells. Vascular proliferation and expansion can be seen in the stroma, with inflammatory cell infiltration (HE × 40)

The difference between clear cell hidradenoma and eccrine poroma is that eccrine poroma is mainly located in the lower part of the epidermis. The epidermis of the lesion site is thickened and the skin process is widened and extended. The tumor often extends into the dermis and most of it is in the dry dermis. The boundary between the tumor body and normal epidermis and dermis is clear. The tumor cells are small, cuboidal or fusiform in size, with deep basophilic round nuclei and fine cells. There are intercellular bridges between the cells. They are often closely arranged into broad bands and anastomose with each other. In most tumor cells, narrow lumens or cysts can be seen in the bands, and the gaps are often lined with protective membranes [4].

Based on the patient's medical history, clinical manifestation, and supplementary examination results, the diagnosis is clear cell hidradenoma. The disease is benign and occur in all parts of the body. In most cases, the tumor tissue is connected with the epidermis. In this case, it is located in the dermis and not connected with the epidermis. Malignant transformation is rare in this tumor, but because of its lack of capsule, it is easy to relapse when the surgical resection is incomplete.

Surgical resection is the first choice of treatment, and the tumor is not sensitive to radiotherapy. In this case, conventional prism incision was performed. According to the pathological results, the patients were given extended resection. No recurrence was found in the follow-up.

Key Points
- This disease usually occurs on the scalp, the lesions are simple or lobular solid or cystic nodules.
- Surgical resection needs to be thorough, it is easy to relapse.

Conflict of Interests None

References

1. Shahmoradi Z, Mokhtari F. Clear cell hidradenoma. Adv Biomed Res. 2013;2:40. https://doi.org/10.4103/2277-9175.109742. PMID: 24516840; PMCID: PMC3905631
2. Cao YT, Wang XY, Xuan M, et al. Facial multiple malignant proliferating tricholemmoma: a case report. Hua Xi Kou Qiang Yi Xue Za Zhi. 2009;27(4):466–8. Chinese
3. Nuño-González A, Vicente-Martín FJ, Pinedo-Moraleda F, et al. High-risk cutaneous squamous cell carcinoma. Actas Dermosifiliogr. 2012;103(7):567–78. https://doi.org/10.1016/j.ad.2011.09.005. English, Spanish. Epub 2012 Jan 17
4. Wankhade V, Singh R, Sadhwani V, et al. Eccrine poroma. Indian Dermatol Online J. 2015;6(4):304–5. https://doi.org/10.4103/2229-5178.160296. PMID: 26225348; PMCID: PMC4513423

Chapter 35
A Male with an Erythema, Pustules, and Crusts on the Scalp

Pei-Yu Liao and Lin Dang

A 22-year-old Asian man presented with an eight-year history of recurrent pustules, erosions and crusts on the scalp (Fig. 35.1a). No improvement after topical and oral antimicrobials was observed. Progression of the lesion was reported. The patient had positive family history of androgenic alopecia.

A physical examination revealed small pustules and crusts on the parietal region of the scalp. After crusts removal, superficial erosions with yellowish discharge

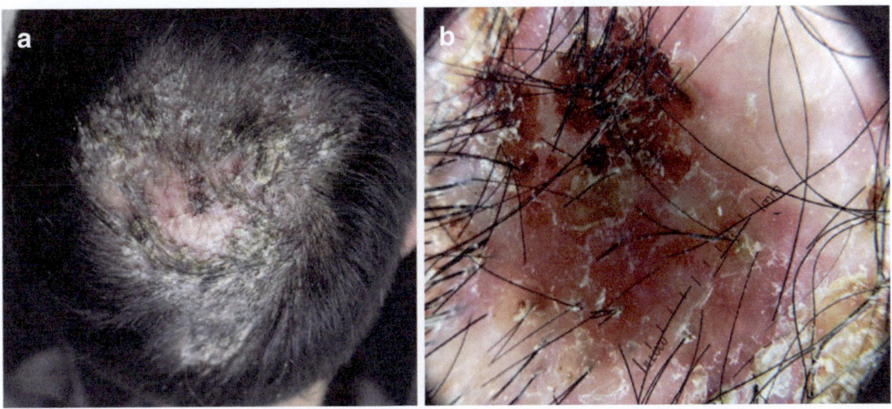

Fig. 35.1 (**a**) A 22-year-old man with superficial erosions and crusted lesions on the atrophic skin. (**b**) Trichoscopy shows erosions, yellowish and hemorrhagic crusts and milky-red areas lacking of follicular openings

P.-Y. Liao · L. Dang (✉)
Department of Dermatology, Shenzhen People's Hospital, The Second Clinical Medical College of Jinan University, The First Affiliated Hospital of Southern University of Science and Technology, Shenzhen, China

151

A. Waśkiel-Burnat et al. (eds.), *Clinical Cases in Scalp Disorders*, Clinical Cases in Dermatology, https://doi.org/10.1007/978-3-030-93426-2_35

were observed. Moreover, a recession of frontal hair line was presented. No other skin lesions were detected.

Dermoscopy showed erosions, yellowish and hemorrhagic crusts as well as milky-read areas lacking of follicular openings (Fig. 35.2b). Routine laboratory tests were normal. A skin biopsy showed acanthosis in the epidermis, the absence of hair follicles and sebaceous glands and an inflammatory infiltrate in the dermis mainly consisting of neutrophils and lymphocytes (Fig. 35.2).

Based on the case description and the photographs, what is your diagnosis?

Differential Diagnoses
1. Pyoderma gangrenosum.
2. Pemphigus.
3. Pustular psoriasis.
4. Bacterial and fungal infections.
5. Erosive pustular dermatosis of the scalp.

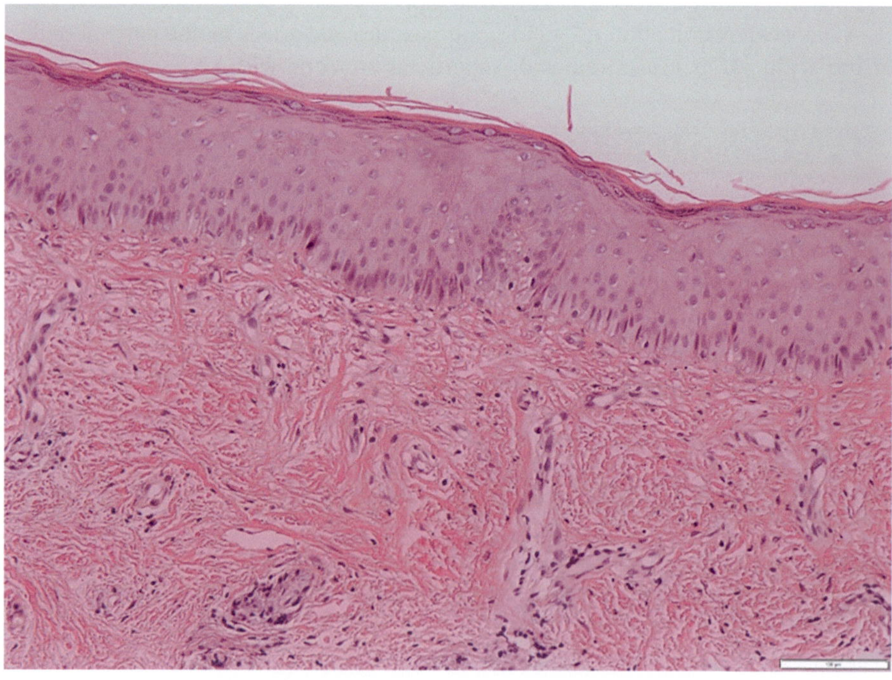

Fig. 35.2 Histopathology shows an epidermal acanthosis, the absence of hair follicles and sebaceous glands and an inflammatory infiltrate in the dermis mainly consisting of neutrophils and lymphocytes (HE × 200)

Diagnosis
Erosive pustular dermatosis of the scalp.

Discussion

Erosive pustular dermatosis of the scalp is a rare entity first described in the late 1970s. A female predominance is observed, with an estimated female to male ratio 3:2 [1]. The etiopathogenesis of the disease remains uncertain. Local trauma, skin grafting, prolonged exposure to sunlight, and the presence of autoimmune diseases have been reported as the predisposing factors [2].

Erosive pustular dermatosis of the scalp predominantly affects elderly individuals at the age of 60–70 years. However, a few cases in children have been reported [3, 4]. Clinically, erosive pustular dermatosis of the scalp is characterized by the presence of multiple pustules, erosions and crusts. With the disease progression, after several months or years, scarring alopecia occurs. The vertex is most commonly affected. No other skin lesions are observed [4].

Erosive pustular dermatosis of the scalp is the diagnosis of exclusion [5]. Histopathological features of usually nonspecific. Histology shows erosions, hyperkeratosis, skin atrophy and occasionally subcorneal pustules. In the dermis, a diffuse or focal inflammatory infiltrate containing lymphocytes and plasma cells is observed. In long-lasting lesions, a loss of hair follicles, fibrosis, and foreign-body giant cells are observed. A direct immunofluorescence test, bacteriologic and mycologic studies are negative [6]. However, secondary colonization with *Staphylococcus aureus* or *Candida albicans* may occur.

Erosive pustular dermatosis of the scalp is a chronic relapsing disease which requires an extended therapy, ranging from weeks to months. Therapeutic options include oral isotretinoin, nimesulide and zinc sulfate, as well as topical corticosteroids, calcipotriol, and tacrolimus [5].

Based on the patient's medical history, clinical feature, and biopsy results, the diagnosis of erosive pustular dermatosis of the scalp was established.

The patient was instructed to avoid the sun exposure, physical trauma and chemical reagents. Tretament with topical tacrolimus and oral isotretinoin 10 mg twice a day was recommended with good results (Fig. 35.3).

Key Points
- Erosive pustular dermatosis of the scalp is characterized by pustular, erosive and crusted lesions on the scalp with progressive scarring alopecia, is a diagnosis of exclusion.
- It responds very well to systemic retinoids and topical tacrolimus, which may be considered as an alternative treatment to corticosteroids.

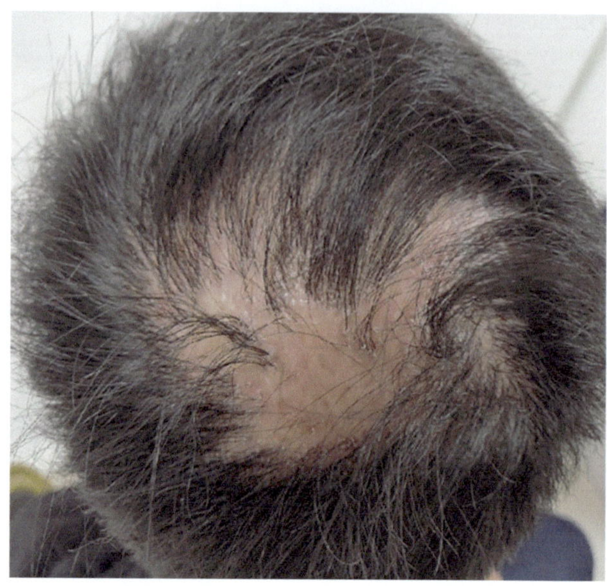

Fig. 35.3 Areas of diffuse scarring alopecia on the scalp with no the disease activity after nine months of treatment

References

1. Ena P, et al. Erosive pustular dermatosis of the scalp in skin grafts: report of three cases. Dermatology. 1997;194(1):80–4.
2. Mastroianni A, et al. Erosive pustular dermatosis of the scalp: a case report and review of the literature. Dermatology. 2005;211(3):273–6.
3. Fertig R, et al. Erosive pustular dermatosis of the scalp after aplasia cutis congenita in a 9-year-old patient: A 5-year follow-up. Pediatr Dermatol. 2017;34(6):695–6.
4. Starace M, et al. Erosive pustular dermatosis of the scalp: challenges and solutions. Clin Cosmet Investig Dermatol. 2019;12:691–8.
5. Allevato M, et al. Erosive pustular dermatosis of the scalp. Int J Dermatol. 2009;48(11):1213–6.
6. Starace M, et al. Erosive pustular dermatosis of the scalp: Clinical, trichoscopic, and histopathologic features of 20 cases. J Am Acad Dermatol. 2017;76(6):1109–14. e2

Chapter 36
A 6-Year-Old Boy with a Generalized Erythema and Scales

Jiahui Hu and Songmei Geng

A six-year-old boy presented to the Department of Dermatology with generalized erythematous scales, lichenification, and dry skin since birth. He complained of an intractable pruritus. The skin lesions progressed extensively but no systemic abnormalities were reported. The patient's mother had allergic rhinitis. There was no family history of similar skin lesions or genetic diseases.

A physical examination revealed a short structure, good general condition and no abnormalites of internal organs. A generalized lichenified erythema and desquamation on the face, trunk, perineum and skin folds was observed. The characteristic double-edged scale was noted at the margin of the erythema on the lower extremities (Fig. 36.1). An edema of external genital organs and sparse hair were prominent. Trichoscopy revealed multiple bamboo hairs and yellow-white scales. Scanning fluorescence microscopy also showed bamboo hairs (Fig. 36.2). A mycological examination was negative.

Laboratory tests showed an elevated level of total immunoglobulin E (1770 IU/mL; normal range: <90 IU/mL) and tumor necrosis factor (25.50 pg/ml; normal range: <8.1 pg/mL). Complete blood count, liver and renal parameters, levels of immunoglobulin A, M and G as well as complements 3 and 4 were within normal limits. Next generation Genetic Screening (NGS) showed two heterozygous mutations in the exon region of SPINK5 gene c.652C > T and c.2423C > T, respectively.

Based on the case description and the photograph, what is your diagnosis?

Differential Diagnoses
1. Omenn syndrome.
2. Wiskott—Aldrich syndrome.
3. Hyper-immunoglobulin E syndrome.
4. Netherton Syndrome.
5. Non-bullous congenital ichthyosiform erythroderma.

J. Hu · S. Geng (✉)
Department of Dermatology, The Second Affiliated Hospital of Xi'an Jiaotong University, Xi'an, China

A. Waśkiel-Burnat et al. (eds.), *Clinical Cases in Scalp Disorders*, Clinical Cases in Dermatology, https://doi.org/10.1007/978-3-030-93426-2_36

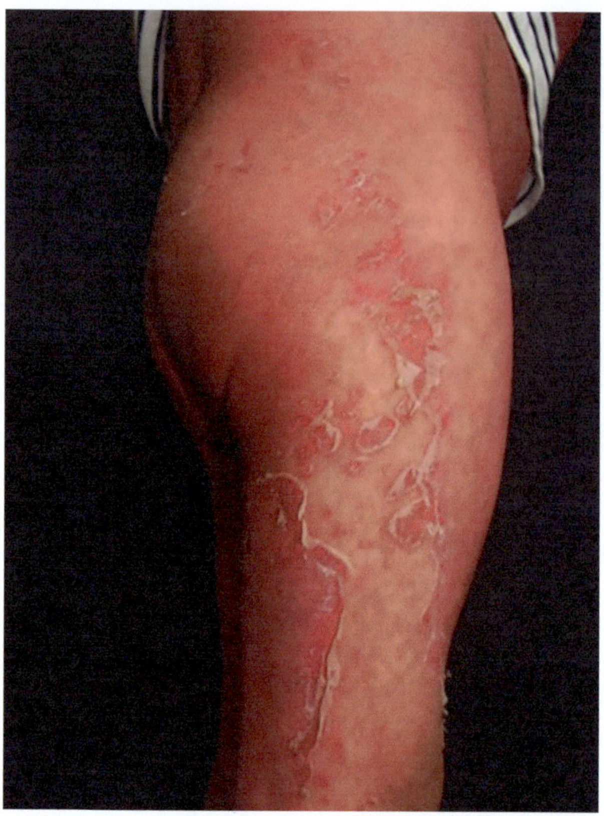

Fig. 36.1 A six-year-old boy with generalized erythematous scales, lichenification, intractable pruritus and dry skin since birth

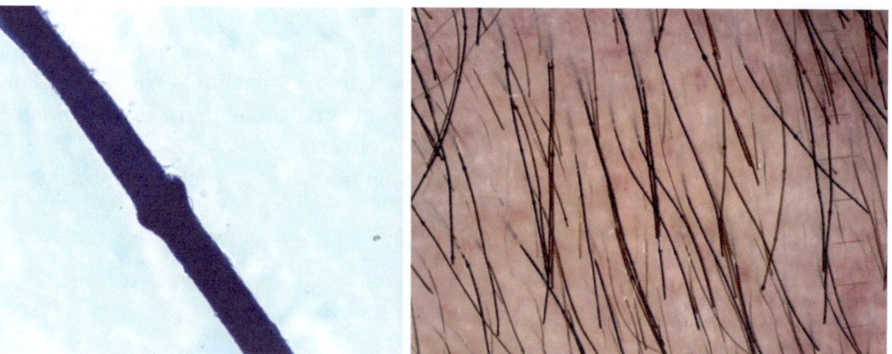

Fig. 36.2 A scanning fluorescence microscopy and dermoscopy show bamboo hairs

Diagnosis
Netherton Syndrome.

Discussion

Netherton Syndrome is a rare autosomal recessive inherited skin disease characterized by a congenital ichthyosis erythroderma, interstitial embrittlement (bamboo hair) and atopic constitution [1]. It is caused by mutations in the SPINK5 gene located on chromosome 5q32 [2].

There are three main clinical characteristics of Netherton syndrome: (1) congenital ichthyosis erythroderma, which appears shortly after birth, with a flaky erythema which is most prominent on the head, upper trunk and skin folds; (2) bamboo-like hairs, also known as intercalated brittle hairs, are dry, rough, easy to fold and short; (3) atopic diseases, such as asthma, allergic rhinitis, urticaria, angioedema, special allergic dermatitis and allergies to various foods or drugs, etc.

Treatment of Netherton syndrome is still challenging. Topical corticosteroids, calmodulin inhibitors, psoralen, ultraviolet irradiation and oral retinoids have been reported as treatment options but with a variable success. Intravenous immunoglobulin, infliximab, omalizumab and secukinumab may be used in critical patients [3, 4].

For the presented patient differential diagnoses included Omenn syndrome, Wiskott-Aldrich syndrome, hyper-immunoglobulin E syndrome, and non-bullous congenital ichthyosiform erythroderma.

Omenn syndrome is an autosomal recessive, severe combined immunodeficiency disease [5]. Clinical manifestations are desquamative erythroderma, which gradually formed a few weeks after birth, hair loss within erythematous areas, accompanied by liver, spleen and lymph nodes enlargement, diarrhea, stunted growth and persistent infection. An immune deficiency is the underlying cause of the disease. Severe infections are the most common cause of death. In laboratory tests, eosinophilia, an increased IgE level, a decreased IgG, IgA, and IgM levels as well as dysfunction of B and T lymphocytes are observed.

Wiskott-Aldrich syndrome is a rare X-linked recessive genetic disease characterized by the presence of persistent eczema, suppurative infections and thrombocytopenia [6].

Hyper-immunoglobulin E syndrome, also called Job's syndrome, is a rare and complex primary immunodeficiency disease characterized by recurrent pulmonary infections, intractable eczematoid dermatitis, skeletal abnormalities and high levels of the serum IgE [7].

Non-bullous congenital ichthyosiform erythroderma belongs to the family of autosomal-recessive ichthyosis. Clinically, it mainly presents as a generalized erythema with fine. Grayish white and semi-adhered scales. In some patients, hyperkeratosis of the palms and soles, eyelid and lip ectropion, scalp involvement, and nail dystrophy are observed [8].

Based on the clinical manifestiation, trichoscopy and genetic tests, the patient was diagnosed with Netherton syndrome. Tacrolimus ointment 0.03% twice a day and moisturizers were recommended. Three months after the treatment initiation, the desquamation, pruritus, and inflammatory lesions improved. No adverse reactions were reported.

Key Points

- Netherton Syndrome is a rare hereditary disease with severe symptoms, refractory course and no satisfactory treatment strategy.
- Bamboo-hair is a characteristic symptom of Netherton syndome.

References

1. Wilkinson RD, Curtis GH, Hawk WA. Netherton's disease: trichorrhexis invaginata (bamboo hair), congenital ichthyosiform erythroderma and the atopic diathesis. A histopathologic study. Arch Dermatol. 1964;89:46–54.
2. Saleem HMK, Shahid MF, Shahbaz A, Sohail A, Shahid MA, Sachmechi I. Netherton syndrome: a case report and review of literature. Cureus. 2018;10(7):e3070.
3. Roda Â, Mendonça-Sanches M, Travassos AR, Soares-de-Almeida L, Metze D. Infliximab therapy for Netherton syndrome: a case report. JAAD Case Rep. 2017;3(6):550–2.
4. Yalcin AD. A case of netherton syndrome: successful treatment with omalizumab and pulse prednisolone and its effects on cytokines and immunoglobulin levels. Immunopharmacol Immunotoxicol. 2016;38(2):162–6.
5. Puzenat E, et al. Congenital erythroderma should be considered as an urgent warning sign of immunodeficiency: a case of Omenn syndrome. Eur J Dermatol. 2017;27(3):313–4.
6. Candotti F. Clinical manifestations and pathophysiological mechanisms of the Wiskott-Aldrich syndrome. J Clin Immunol. 2018;38(1):13–27.
7. Park B, Liu GY. Staphylococcus aureus and hyper-IgE syndrome. Int J Mol Sci. 2020;21(23):9152.
8. Nawaz S, Tariq M, Ahmad I, Malik NA, Baig SM, Dahl N, Klar J. Non-bullous congentital ichthyosiform erythroderma associated with homozygosity for a novel missense mutation in an ATP binding domain of ABCA12. Eur J Dermatol. 2012;22(2):178–81.

Chapter 37
Acne Keloidalis Nuchae

Ghazala Butt and Muhammad Ahmad

A 45-year-old man presented with papulonodular lesions on the nape of the neck (Fig. 37.1) for the last six months. Initially the lesions were erythematous and itchy. The patient was treated with topical medications but his condition didn't improve and aggravated over the course of a few months. He also complained of irritation, dryness and roughness of the lesions along with pain. There was also history of applying lot of over-the-counter drugs and home-made totkas (domestic hacks) but of no use.

Differential Diagnosis
 1. Acne vulgaris.
 2. Acne mechanica.
 3. Molluscum contagiosum.
 4. Tinea capitis.
 5. Bacterial folliculitis.
 6. Folliculitis decalvans.
 7. Dissecting cellulitis.
 8. Lichen planopilaris.
 9. Acne keloidalis nuchae.
10. Follicular cutaneous T-cell lymphoma.
11. Hidradenitis suppurativa.

G. Butt (✉)
King Edward Medical University, Lahore, Pakistan

M. Ahmad
Aesthetic Plastic Surgery & FUE Hair Transplant Institute, Islamabad, Pakistan

A. Waśkiel-Burnat et al. (eds.), *Clinical Cases in Scalp Disorders*, Clinical Cases in Dermatology, https://doi.org/10.1007/978-3-030-93426-2_37

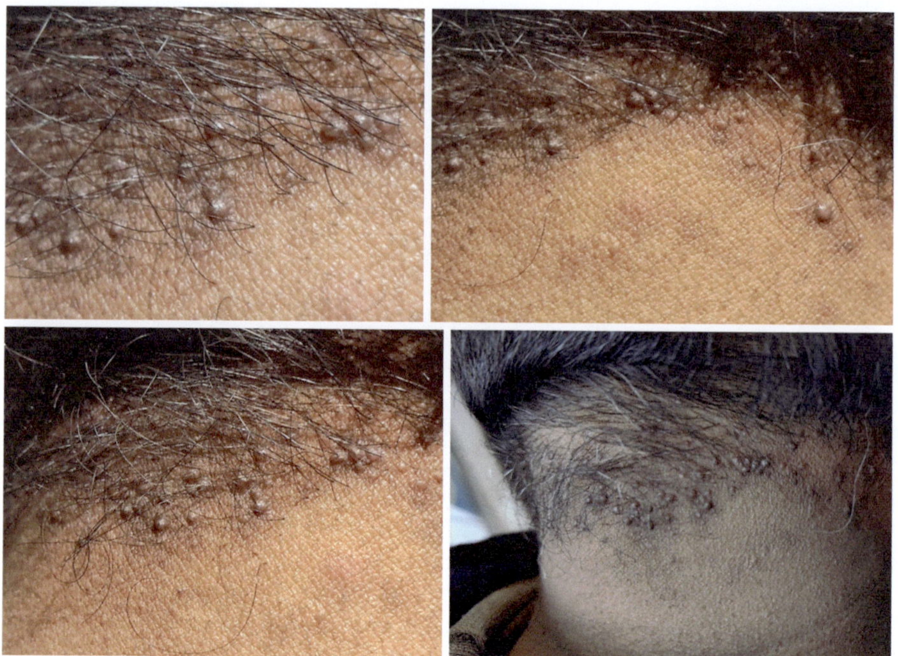

Fig. 37.1 Papulonodular lesions along with some areas of scarring on the nape of the neck

Diagnosis
Acne Keloidalis Nuchae.

Discussion

Acne Keloidalis Nuchae also known as keloidal folliculitis or nuchal keloidal acne is a chronic inflammatory skin condition. The exact pathogenesis of the disease is not known. However, a skin injury and abnormal immunological reaction seem to play an important role. Moreover, chronic irritation, friction, wearing hard wears, and trauma can aggravate the condition [1]. The disease occurs mostly in dark-skinned populations but is also commonly seen in Caucasians. Acne keloidalis nuchae occurs 20 times more frequently in men than in women and it usually starts after adolescence. Initially, erythematous papules are presented. When secondary infection occurs pustules and abscesses are observed. A long term chronic inflammation leads to scarring, and keloids formation. Prevalent sites of involvement are the occipital area of the scalp and the nape of the neck [2, 3]. The prognosis of acne keloidalis nuchae is good if an early treatment is started [4, 5].

Management of acne keloidalis nuchae includes the avoidance of mechanical irritation. Oral and topical antibiotics in combination with oral and topical retinoids can be useful. Intralesional steroids also give good results by decreasing inflammation. Other therapeutic options are catery and cryotherapy. A surgical excision along with skin grafting may be required in some cases. Recently laser therapies including Nd:Yag 1064 nm and diode laser have also been tried with variable results [6]. Clinically, he was diagnosed as a case of Acne Keloidalis Nuchae. He was prescribed azithromycin along with topical clindamycin and retinoid. After a month, his symptoms were much improved but lesions were still there and he is on continuous follow-up (Fig. 37.1).

Key Points
- Acne keloidalis nucahe is characterized by papules and pustules on the occipitial area and the nape of the neck.
- Typically, in patients with acne keloidalis nuchae a history of local iritation is reported.

References

1. Dinehart SM, Herzberg AJ, Kerns BJ, Pollack SV. Acne keloidalis: a review. J Dermatol Surg Oncol. 1989;15(6):642–7. https://doi.org/10.1111/j.1524-4725.1989.tb03603.x.
2. Sperling LC, Homoky C, Pratt L, Sau P. Acne keloidalis is a form of primary scarring alopecia. Arch Dermatol. 2000;136(4):479–84. https://doi.org/10.1001/archderm.136.4.479.
3. Harris H. Acne keloidalis aggravated by football helmets. Cutis. 1992;50(2):154.
4. Alexis A, Heath CR, Halder RM. Folliculitis keloidalis nuchae and pseudofolliculitis barbae: are prevention and effective treatment within reach? Dermatol Clin. 2014;32(2):183–91. https://doi.org/10.1016/j.det.2013.12.001.
5. Sattler ME. Folliculitis keloidis nuchae. WMJ. 2001;100(1):37–8.
6. Dragoni F, Bassi A, Cannarozzo G, Bonan P, Moretti S, Campolmi P. Successful treatment of acne keloidalis nuchae resistant to conventional therapy with 1064-nm ND:YAG laser. G Ital Dermatol Venereol. 2013;148:231–2.

Chapter 38
An Aggressive Skin Tumor in a Patient Treated with Adalimumab for Crohn's Disease

Piotr Brzezinski and Katarzyna Borowska

A 60-year-old man treated with adalimumab for Crohn's disease presented with progressing skin lesions. The first lesions of actinic keratosis (Fig. 38.1a) developed on the forehead five months after adalimumab initation . One month later, a nodular lesion on the forehead occured. With time, the disease progression was reported. Three months later, multiple nodules on the forehead were present (Figs. 38.1b and 38.2). In the meantime, because of the relapse of Crohn's disease, the patient underwent resection of 30 cm of the ileum. Adalimumab was discontinued. This resulted in the progression of tumors in the median forehead region with the presence of numerous satellite nodules (Figs. 38.2b–38.3c). A surgical excision of the lesions was performed (Fig. 38.3).

Based on the case description and the photograph, what is your diagnosis?

Differential Diagnoses
1. Cylindroma.
2. Nodular melanoma.
3. Squamous cell carcinoma.
4. Basal cell carcinoma.
5. Actinic keratosis.

P. Brzezinski (✉)
Department of Physiotherapy and Medical Emergency, Faculty of Health Sciences, Pomeranian Academy, Slupsk, Poland

Department of Dermatology, Provincial Specialist Hospital in Slupsk, Ustka, Poland

K. Borowska
Department of Histology and Embryology with Experimental Cytology Unit, Medical University of Lublin, Lublin, Poland

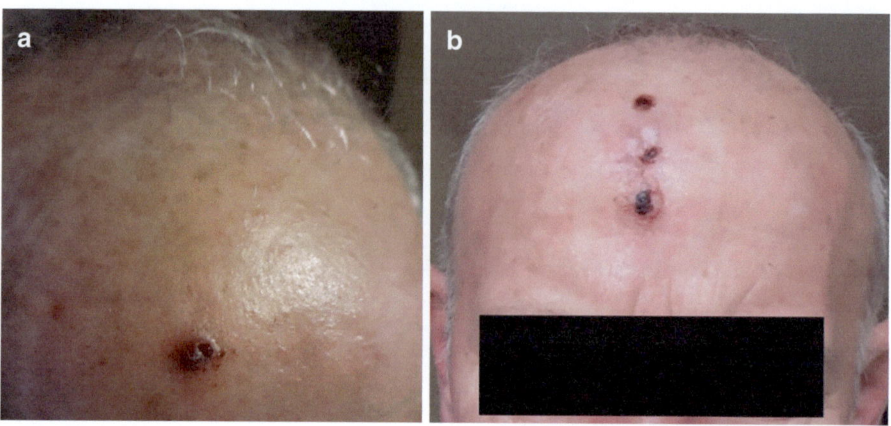

Fig. 38.1 A 60-year-old man with nodular lesions on the forehead

Diagnosis
Squamous cell carcinoma.

Discussion

Tumor necrosis factor (TNF) is a central proinflammatory cytokine which plays an important role in the pathogenesis of many inflammatory diseases. TNF promotes apoptosis of cancer cells by stimulating NK and CD8 + T cells. Adalimumab, a human recombinant immunoglobulin G1 anti-tumor necrosis factor (TNF) mono-clonal antibody, is approved for the treatment of Crohn's disease [1, 2].

Crohn's disease is a progressive inflammation of the digestive tract. The incidence of the disease is increasing worldwide. It has been reported that 15%–25% of inflammatory bowel diseases occur in children and adolescents [3].

The most common side effects of adalimumab in patients with Crohn's disease are: headache (27%), upper respiratory tract infection (22%), nasopharyngitis (21%), diarrhea (19%), and development of squamous cell carcinoma [4–6].

In recent years, an increased risk of skin malignancies in patients treated with TNF inhibitors has been reported [7].

In the meta-analysis, one hundred thirty (0.84%) of 15,418 individuals random-ized to anti-TNF therapy were diagnosed with cancer [8]. A significant risk of non melanoma skin cancer in patients treated with adalimumab or etanercept was described.

In our patient, anti-TNF therapy could increase the risk of squamous cell carci-noma, although the history of sun exposure was also reported.

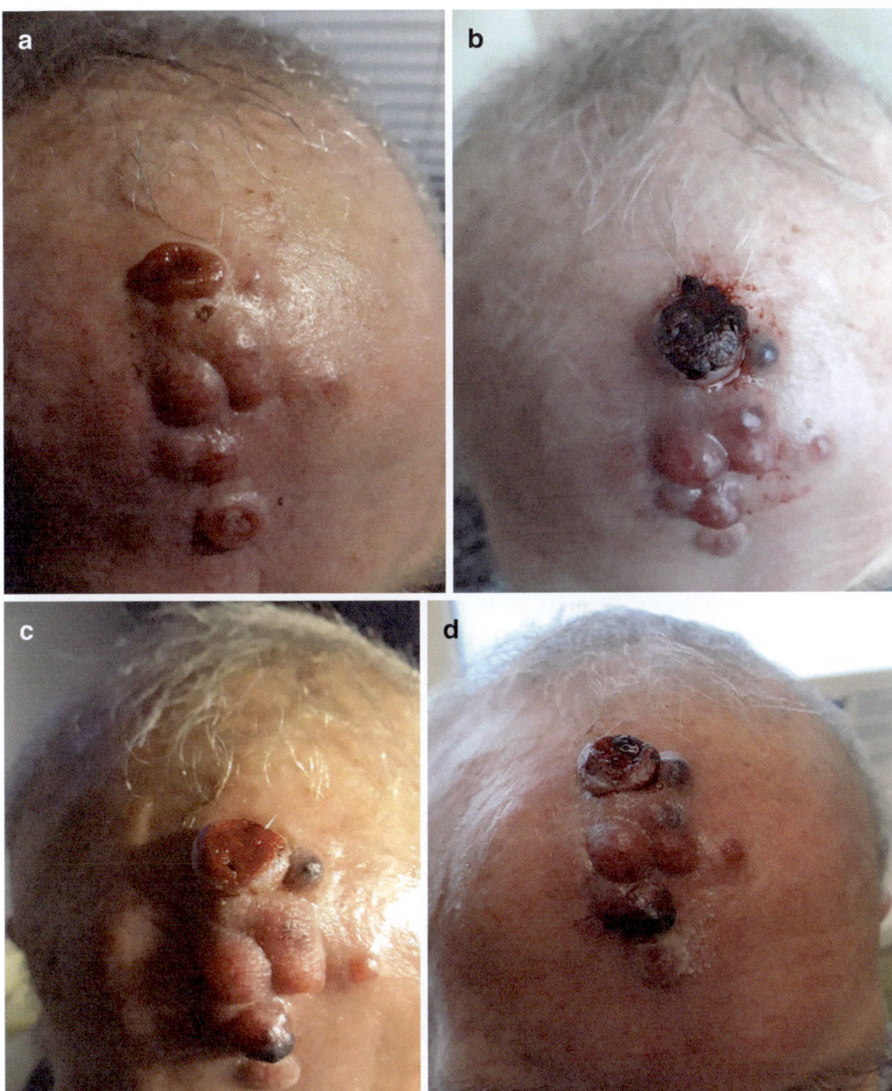

Fig. 38.2 Progression of the nodular lesions on the forehead

Key Points
- Anti-TNF treatment may increase the risk of skin malignancies.
- A regular skin examination in patientes treated with TNF inhibitors should be recommended.

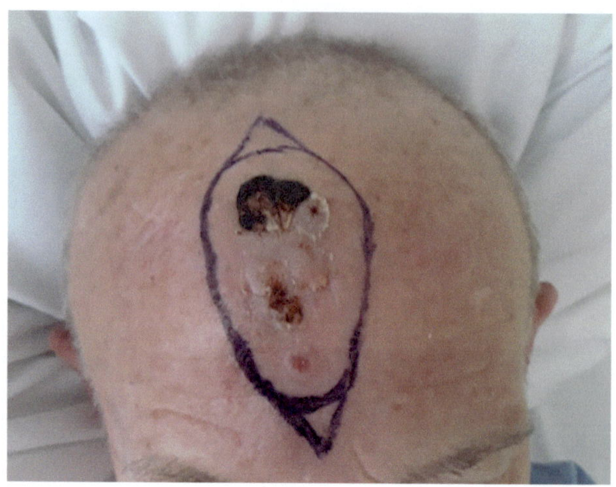

Fig. 38.3 Tumor after a surgical excision

References

1. Matsumoto T, Motoya S, Watanabe K, Hisamatsu T, Nakase H, Yoshimura N, Ishida T, Kato S, Nakagawa T, Esaki M, Nagahori M, Matsui T, Naito Y, Kanai T, Suzuki Y, Nojima M, Watanabe M, Hibi T, DIAMOND Study Group. Adalimumab monotherapy and a combination with azathioprine for Crohn's disease: a prospective, randomized trial. J Crohns Colitis. 2016;10(11):1259–66. https://doi.org/10.1093/ecco-jcc/jjw152. Epub 2016 Aug 26
2. Faubion WA, Dubinsky M, Ruemmele FM, Escher J, Rosh J, Hyams JS, Eichner S, Li Y, Reilly N, Thakkar RB, Robinson AM, Lazar A. Long-term efficacy and safety of adalimumab in pediatric patients with crohn's disease. Inflamm Bowel Dis. 2017;23(3):453–60. https://doi.org/10.1097/MIB.0000000000001021. PMID: 28129288; PMCID: PMC5319394
3. Malik TA. Inflammatory bowel disease: historical perspective, epidemiology, and risk factors. Surg Clin North Am. 2015;95(6):1105–22. https://doi.org/10.1016/j.suc.2015.07.006. Epub 2015 Sep 7
4. Belanouane S, Hali F, Baline K, Chiheb S, Marnissi F, Hliwa W. A rare case of malignant pyoderma associated with ulcerative colitis both treated effectively with adalimumab. Our Dermatol Online. 2020;11(4):393–6. https://doi.org/10.7241/ourd.20204.16.
5. Scheinfeld N. Adalimumab: a review of side effects. Expert Opin Drug Saf. 2005 Jul;4(4):637–41. https://doi.org/10.1517/14740338.4.4.637.
6. Hisamatsu T, Matsumoto T, Watanabe K, Nakase H, Motoya S, Yoshimura N, Ishida T, Kato S, Nakagawa T, Esaki M, Nagahori M, Matsui T, Naito Y, Kanai T, Suzuki Y, Nojima M, Watanabe M, Hibi T, DIAMOND Study Group. Concerns and side effects of azathioprine during adalimumab induction and maintenance therapy for Japanese patients with Crohn's disease: a subanalysis of a prospective randomised clinical trial [DIAMOND Study]. J Crohns Colitis. 2019 Sep 19;13(9):1097–104. https://doi.org/10.1093/ecco-jcc/jjz030.

7. Kouklakis G, Efremidou EI, Pitiakoudis M, Liratzopoulos N, Polychronidis AC. Development of primary malignant melanoma during treatment with a TNF-α antagonist for severe Crohn's disease: a case report and review of the hypothetical association between TNF-α blockers and cancer. Drug Des Devel Ther. 2013;7:195–9. https://doi.org/10.2147/DDDT.S41889. Epub 2013 Mar 27. PMID: 23569358; PMCID: PMC3615922
8. Askling J, Fahrbach K, Nordstrom B, Ross S, Schmid CH, Symmons D. Cancer risk with tumor necrosis factor alpha (TNF) inhibitors: meta-analysis of randomized controlled trials of adalimumab, etanercept, and infliximab using patient level data. Pharmacoepidemiol Drug Saf. 2011 Feb;20(2):119–30. https://doi.org/10.1002/pds.2046.

Chapter 39
An Adolescent with a Peculiar Scar on the Scalp

Alina Suru, Georgiana-Patricia Ogruţan, Răzvan Andrei,
Sabina Andrada Zurac, and Carmen Maria Sălăvăstru

A 16-year-old male was referred to the Dermatology Clinic with an asymptomatic hair loss area presented since two years. The patient was diagnosed with celiac disease and Asperger syndrome.

On physical examination, a well-defined hairless area with coexisted papules on the parietal region was observed (Fig. 39.1). Dermoscopy showed whitish-yellow structureless areas (Figs. 39.2 and 39.3). Laboratory investigations revealed normal serum level of calcium, phosphate, 25-OH-Vitamine D, PTH, TSH, and free T4.

A. Suru (✉)
Dermatology Research Unit, Colentina Clinical Hospital, Bucharest, Romania

"Carol Davila" University of Medicine and Pharmacy, Bucharest, Romania
e-mail: suru.pirvu@drd.umfcd.ro

G.-P. Ogruţan
"Carol Davila" University of Medicine and Pharmacy, Bucharest, Romania

Fundeni Clinical Institute, Bucharest, Romania
e-mail: georgiana-patricia.ogrutan@rez.umfcd.ro

R. Andrei
Pathology Department, Colentina Clinical Hospital, Bucharest, Romania

S. A. Zurac
"Carol Davila" University of Medicine and Pharmacy, Bucharest, Romania

Pathology Department, Colentina Clinical Hospital, Bucharest, Romania
e-mail: sabina.zurac@umfcd.ro

C. M. Sălăvăstru
"Carol Davila" University of Medicine and Pharmacy, Bucharest, Romania

Pediatric Dermatology Department, Colentina Clinical Hospital, Bucharest, Romania
e-mail: carmen.salavastru@umfcd.ro

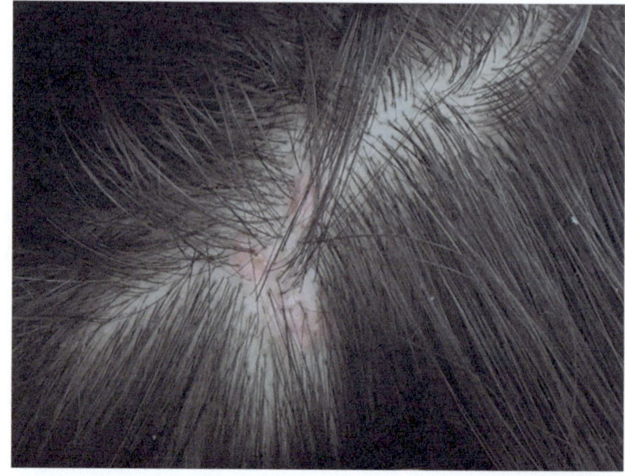

Fig. 39.1 An alopecic plaque with erythematous, well-defined, 5-mm papules on the parietal scalp

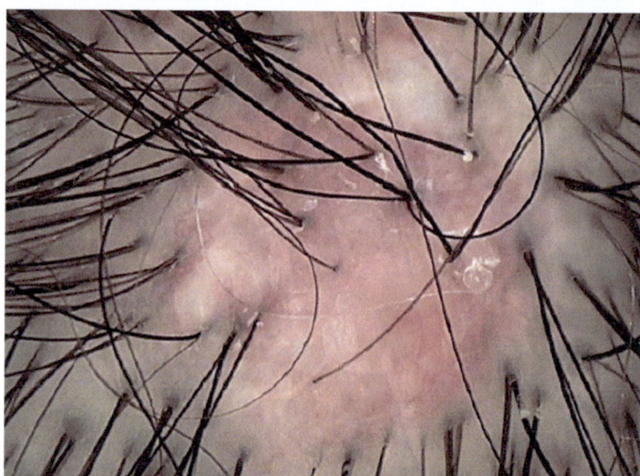

Fig. 39.2 Dermoscopy shows a milky-red and yellowish, structureless area (x30)

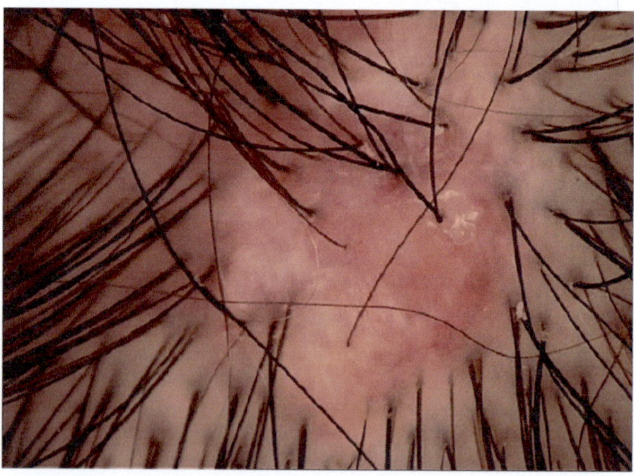

Fig. 39.3 Dermoscopy with the presence of milky-red and yellowish, structureless area (x20)

Hypercalciuria was presented (564 mg/24 h; range 100–300 mg/24 h). X-ray of the skull showed no bone changes.

A punch biopsy was performed under local anesthesia. A histopathological examination showed small spicules to large masses of mature bone present in the superficial and deep dermis (Fig. 39.4). The patient was referred to the Pediatric Nephrology Department. The calcium restriction diet was recommended.

Based on the case description and the photographs, what is your diagnosis?

Differential Diagnoses

1. Osteoma cutis.
2. Calcinosis cutis.
3. Dermoid cyst.
4. Keloid scar.
5. Pilomatrixoma.

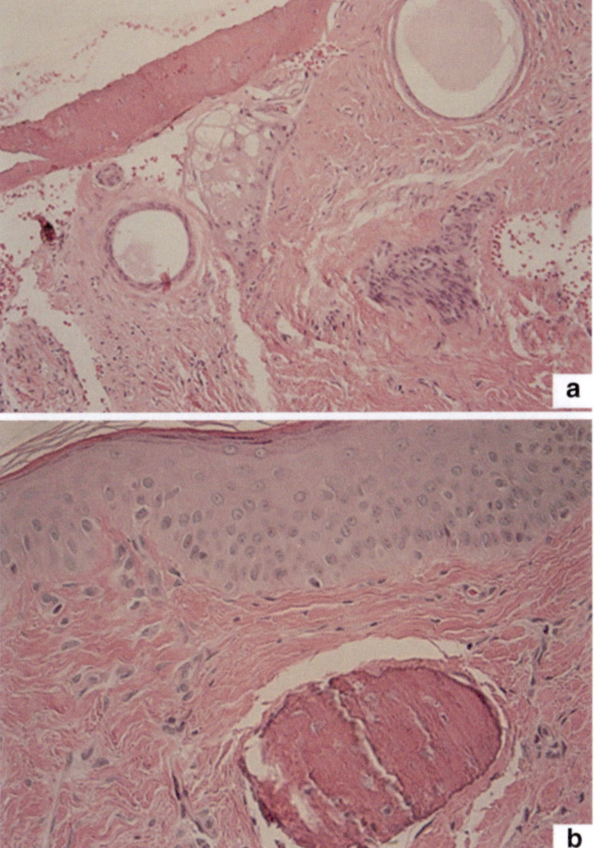

Fig. 39.4 Pathology shows small spicules to large masses of mature bone in the dermis. HE × 200 (**a**) & HE × 400 (**b**)

Diagnosis

Osteoma cutis.

Discussion

Osteoma cutis is a benign and rare dermatological condition characterized by bone formation in the subcutaneous tissue or the deep dermis. This condition may occur at any age and can be either primary or secondary.

The primary form occurs de novo without a preexisting disease. It is isolated or associated with syndromes such as Albright hereditary osteodystrophy, fibrodysplasia ossificans progressiva, progressive osseous heteroplasia, and Gardner's syndrome.

The secondary form represents 85% of cases and it develops in association with an underlying condition, such as inflammatory skin disease, tumors, trauma, malignancies, and scars. Acne vulgaris is the most common cause of secondary osteoma cutis.

The lesions of osteoma cutis may present as papules, plaques, nodules, or military (1–4 mm) lesions [1].

The main histopathologic feature of osteoma cutis is bone formation by the process of membranous ossification in subcutaneous tissue or the deep dermis. The bone thus forms a nodule of mature lamellar bone, containing osteoblasts, rarely osteoclasts, connective tissue, and mature fat cells. Occasionally marrow elements can be seen.

Treatment of osteoma cutis is mainly surgical excision of the lesion. Recurrences, especially in genetic forms, may occur [2].

Calcinosis cutis, or cutaneous calcification, is the differential diagnosis for this patient. In contrast to osteoma cutis, calcinosis cutis is characterized by calcium salt deposits in the absence of osteoids. The calcified lesions are presented as palpable nodules that can vary in shape and size, depending on the calcinosis cutis subtype. They can be painful leading to functional impairment. There are five subtypes of calcinosis cutis described: dystrophic, metastatic, idiopathic, iatrogenic, and calciphylaxis [3, 4].

The dystrophic type is associated with tissue damage and is the most frequent type. It is associated with various connective tissue diseases such as systemic sclerosis, dermatomyositis, mixed connective tissue disease, which induce tissue damage and creates a favorable environment for calcification.

The metastatic type is due to elevated calcium or phosphate levels.

The idiopathic type includes idiopathic calcified nodules of the scrotum, subepidermal calcified nodules, and tumoral calcinosis and has no underlying tissue damage or abnormal laboratory values.

Iatrogenic calcinosis is determined by the precipitation of calcium salts within the skin after administering calcium and phosphate-containing agents.

Calciphylaxis involves small and medium-size vessels with vascular calcification and skin necrosis, and it is associated with chronic renal failure and dialysis [2, 4].

The treatment is challenging and depends on the cause. Surgical treatment is chosen for small and localized lesions, whereas more generalized disease will require medical management [5].

Another condition that must be considered is dermoid cyst that typically presents as a discrete, subcutaneous nodule. Dermoid cysts result from the sequestration of ectodermal tissue along embryonic fusion planes during development [6]. Dermoid cysts have a diameter between 1–4 cm. They are most commonly localized around the eyes, but they can also occur on the scalp. The cyst presents a thick wall lined with stratified squamous epithelium and may contain other typical cutaneous structures such as hair, sebaceous lobules, eccrine glands, apocrine glands, and smooth muscle. Treatment is surgical. Preoperative imaging studies may be required to exclude a connection to central nervous system [7].

Pilomatrixoma, also known as calcifying epithelioma of Malherbe, is a benign tumor of the hair follicle matrix that presents as a solitary skin-colored or bluish nodule. When syndromic (myotonic dystrophy, Turner syndrome, Gardner syndrome) pilomatrixoma can present with multiple lesions. Over 70% of the tumors arise on the head and neck areas, although they may develop on any hair-bearing surface. Histopathological features of pilomatrixoma include islands of epithelial cells that contain basaloid matrical cells, shadow, ghost, or enucleated cells with eosinophilic cytoplasm, foreign body giant cells, and calcifications. Unless the lesion is symptomatic, no treatment is required [8].

Keloid scars are caused by an aberrant response of the healing process that follows a cutaneous injury or irritation that reaches the reticular dermis. Clinically, they appear as raised and firm scars, containing excessive collagen production; type III collagen is replaced by type I collagen, usually after four to eight weeks from the injury. Keloids extend beyond the original wound's borders, do not usually regress spontaneously, and tend to recur after excision [9].

Key Points
- Osteoma cutis refers to bone formation in the dermis and/or subcutis.
- It can be primary, but more often is secondary.
- Most common sites include the face (in female) and scalp (in male).
- It is a benign tumor with an excellent prognosis.

References

1. Ward S, Sugo E, Verge CF, Wargon O. Three cases of osteoma cutis occurring in infancy. A brief overview of osteoma cutis and its association with pseudo-pseudohypoparathyroidism. Australas J Dermatol. 2011;52(2):127–31. https://doi.org/10.1111/j.1440-0960.2010.00722.x.
2. Rongioletti F, Barnhill RL. Deposition disorders. In: Barnhill RL, Crowson AN, Magro CM, Piepkorn MW, editors. Dermatopathology. 3th ed. New York: McGraw Hill Education; 2010. p. 362–86.
3. Kroshinski D, Fairley JA. Calcifying and ossifying disorders of the skin. In: Bolognia J, Schaffer J, Cerroni L, editors. Dermatology. 4th ed. Philadelphia, PA: Elsevier; 2018. p. 784–92.
4. Le C, Bedocs PM. Calcinosis cutis. In: StatPearls. Treasure Island (FL): StatPearls Publishing; 2020.
5. Valenzuela A, Chung L. Calcinosis: pathophysiology and management. Curr Opin Rheumatol. 2015;27(6):542–8. https://doi.org/10.1097/BOR.0000000000000220.
6. Antaya RJ, Schaffer J. Developmental anomalies. In: Bolognia J, Schaffer J, Cerroni L, editors. Dermatology. 4th ed. Philadelphia, PA: Elsevier; 2018. p. 1055–73.
7. Stone MS. Cysts. In: Bolognia J, Schaffer J, Cerroni L, editors. Dermatology. 4th ed. Philadelphia, PA: Elsevier; 2018. p. 1917–29.
8. McCalmont TH, Pincus LB. Adnexal neoplasms. In: Bolognia J, Schaffer J, Cerroni L, editors. Dermatology. 4th ed. Philadelphia, PA: Elsevier; 2018. p. 1930–52.
9. Berman B, Maderal A, Raphael B. Keloids and hypertrophic scars: pathophysiology, classification, and treatment. Dermatol Surg. 2017;43(Suppl 1):S3–S18. https://doi.org/10.1097/DSS.0000000000000819.

Chapter 40
An Elderly Female Presenting with an Acute Headache and Jaw Pain

Jianbo Tong, Zhibin Zhang, Qingqing Huang, Zhezhang Liu, Wenshan Huang, Li Chen, and Xianwei Cao

A 73-year-old woman presented with a three-week history of an acute headache and jaw pain. Tha patient was treated with oral ibuprofen, but it did not relieve the pain. The patient had a history of cerebral infarction which was diagnosed four years before presentation.

A physical examination revealed a temperature of 37 °C, a pulse rate of 62 beats/min, and a blood pressure of 108/64 mmHg. Bilateral temporal arteries were enlarged and tender on palpation (Fig. 40.1).

The initial laboratory tests showed a white cell count of 12.06×10^9/L (neutrophils 83.2%, lymphocytes 6.7%, monocytes 7.7%, and eosinophils 2.3%), a hemoglobin of 101 g/L, and a platelet count of 307×10^9/L. The erythrocyte sedimentation rate and C-reactive protein concentration were 102 mm/h and 225.34 mg/L, respectively. Serum cytokine levels revealed: IL-6 of 106.14 pg/mL and γ-Interferon of 35.40 pg/mL. Superficial Color Doppler Ultrasound of temporal arteries revealed uneven thickening of the arterial wall (Fig. 40.2). Cranial Magnetic Resonance Imaging revealed mild cerebral ischemia.

J. Tong · Z. Zhang · Q. Huang · Z. Liu · W. Huang · X. Cao (✉)
Department of Dermatology, First Affiliated Hospital of Nanchang University, Nanchang University, Nanchang, P.R. China

Institute of Dermatology, Jiangxi Academy of Clinical Medical Sciences, Nanchang, P.R. China

L. Chen
Department of Medical Ultrasonics, First Affiliated Hospital of Nanchang University, Nanchang University, Nanchang, P.R. China

A. Waśkiel-Burnat et al. (eds.), *Clinical Cases in Scalp Disorders*, Clinical Cases in Dermatology, https://doi.org/10.1007/978-3-030-93426-2_40

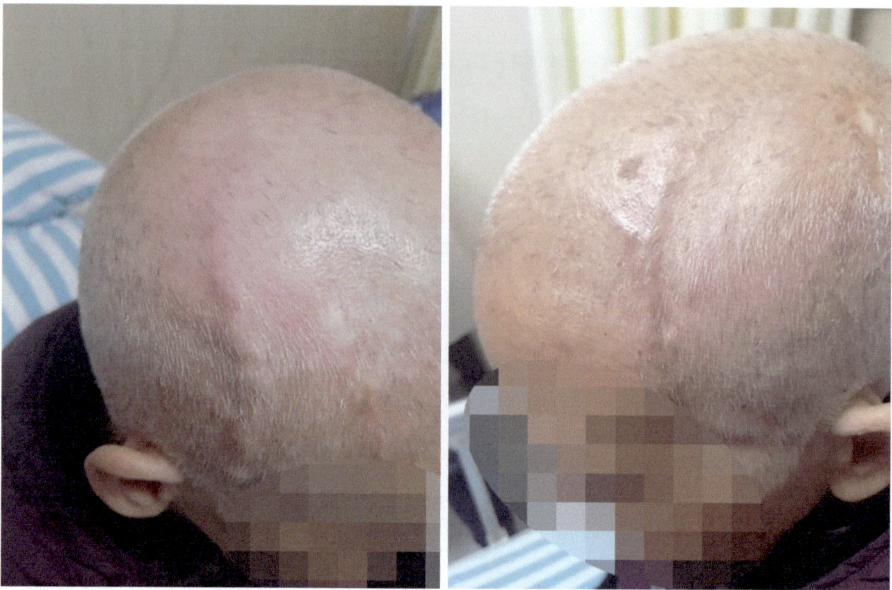

Fig. 40.1 An 73-year-old woman with enlarged, bilateral temporal arteries

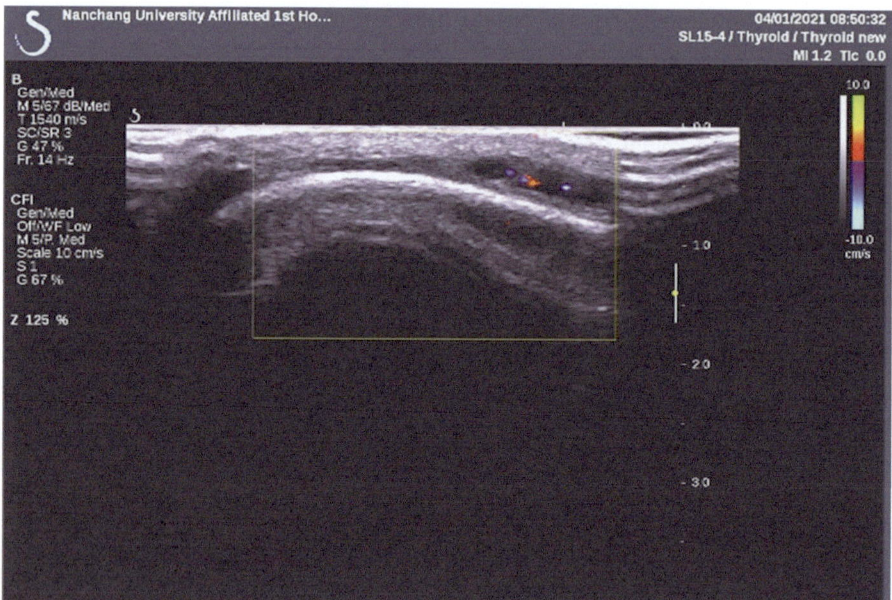

Fig. 40.2 Color doppler ultrasound of the left temporal artery with the thickening of the arterial wall

Based on the case description and the photographs, what is your diagnosis?

Differential Diagnoses
1. Giant cell arteritis.
2. Neuralgia.
3. Herpes zoster.

Diagnosis
Giant Cell Arteritis.

Discussion

Giant cell arteritis is asystematic granulomatous vasculitis which typically affects the elderly persons above 50 years of age [1]. The disease is very rare among Asians. Classic features of giant cell arteritis include headache, fever, vision loss and myalgia [2, 3].

The diagnosis of giant cell arteritis is usually made on the basis of clinical symptoms, laboratory or imaging examination, and histologic findings. The American College of Rheumatology in 1990 established diagnostic criteria for giant cell arteritis [4]. Patients should meet three of the following: age $\geq$ 50 years; new onset of localized headache; tenderness or decreased pulse in the temporal artery; erythrocyte sedimentation rate $\geq$50 mm/h; a positive biopsy of the temporal artery showing mononuclear cell infiltrates or a granulomatous process with multinucleate giant cells. However, biopsy is the gold standard diagnostic method for giant cell arteritis, it is not necessary to establish the diagnosis.

When giant cell arteritis is suspected, clinical guidelines recommend rapid initiation of corticosteroid treatment.

The presented patient was diagnosed with giant cell arteritis. She was treated with intravenous methylprednisolone 60 mg daily for seven days with a decrease of inflammatory markers. Control laboratory tests showed a white cell count of 10.32 $\times$ 10^9/L (neutrophils 72%, lymphocytes 12.7%, monocytes 6%, and eosinophils 0.4%), a hemoglobin of 95 g/L, and a platelet count of 406 $\times$ 10^9/L. The erythrocyte sedimentation rate and C-reactive protein concentration were 93 mm/h and 34.75 mg/L, respectively. Serum cytokine levels revealed IL-6 - 20.73 pg/mL and γ-Interferon - 1.16 pg/mL. Treatment with oral prednisone 60 mg daily was continuated. The patient had complete resolution of headache and jaw pain.

Key Points
- Giant cell arteritis is characterized by headache, fever, vision loss and myalgia.
- In case of giant cell arteritis, rapid initation of corticosteroid treatment is neccessary.

References

1. Zarar A, et al. Internal carotid artery stenosis associated with giant cell arteritis: case report and discussion. J Vasc Interv Neurol. 2014;7(5):24–7.
2. Pereira LS, et al. Giant cell arteritis in Asians: a comparative study. Br J Ophthalmol. 2011;95(2):214–6.
3. Kale N, Eggenberger E. Diagnosis and management of giant cell arteritis: a review. Curr Opin Ophthalmol. 2010;21(6):417–22.
4. Hunder GG, et al. The American College of Rheumatology 1990 criteria for the classification of giant cell arteritis. Arthritis Rheum. 1990;33(8):1122–8.

Chapter 41
A Bleeding Nodule on the Scalp

Uwe Wollina

An 88-year-old male patient was referred to the Department of Dermatology with an exophytic, bleeding nodule on the scalp. His medical history was positive for cutaneous squamous cell carcinoma with field cancerization on the scalp, diabetes mellitus type 2, renal insufficiency, atrioventricular block with pacemaker implantation, hypertension, hypothyreosis, gonarthrosis, and partial pulmonary resection during World War II.

On physical examination we observed a firm large scalp tumor with bleeding (Fig. 41.1). We performed a wide complete excision with 2 cm safety margins. The defect was closed with a meshed skin graft. Healing was uneventful (Fig. 41.2). A histological examination demonstrated a connective tissue derived tumor with spindle cells (Fig. 41.3). The tumor thickness was 18 mm. The spindle shaped lesion demonstrated nuclear polymorphism and atypia. The tumor cells expressed vimentin, CD68, and partially smooth-muscle actin. Numerous mitoses including typical were seen. The tumor was well vascularized. There was no relapse during 24 months of follow-up.

Based on the case description and the photographs, what is your diagnosis?

Differential Diagnoses
1. Merkel cell carcinoma.
2. Basal cell carcinoma.
3. Atypical fibroxanthoma.
4. Pleomorphic dermal sarcoma.
5. Squamous cell carcinoma.

Diagnosis
Atypical fibroxanthoma.

U. Wollina (✉)
Department of Dermatology and Allergology, Municipal Hospital of Dresden, Academic
Teaching Hospital, Dresden, Germany
e-mail: Uwe.Wollina@klinikum-dresden.de

A. Waśkiel-Burnat et al. (eds.), *Clinical Cases in Scalp Disorders*, Clinical
Cases in Dermatology, https://doi.org/10.1007/978-3-030-93426-2_41

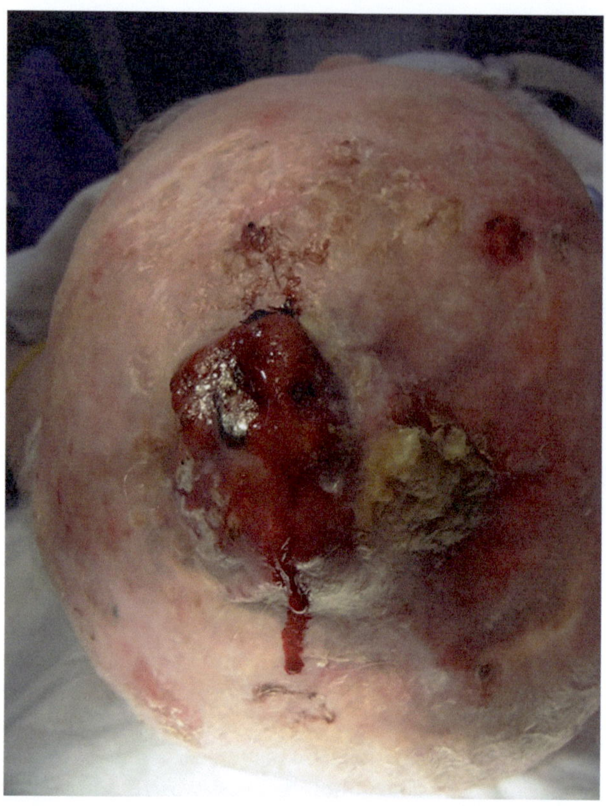

Fig. 41.1 A bleeding, exophytic nodule surrounded by field cancerization on the scalp

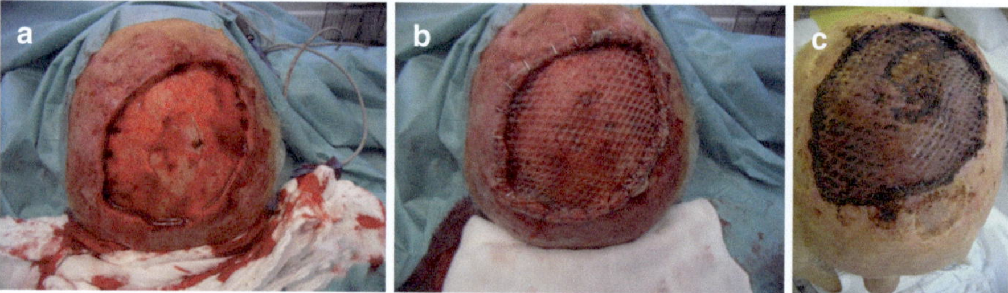

Fig. 41.2 A surgical excision of the nodule on the scalp. (**a**) Defect after wide excision. (**b**) Meshed graft transplantation. (**c**) Seven days after surgery, stable transplant with 100% take rate

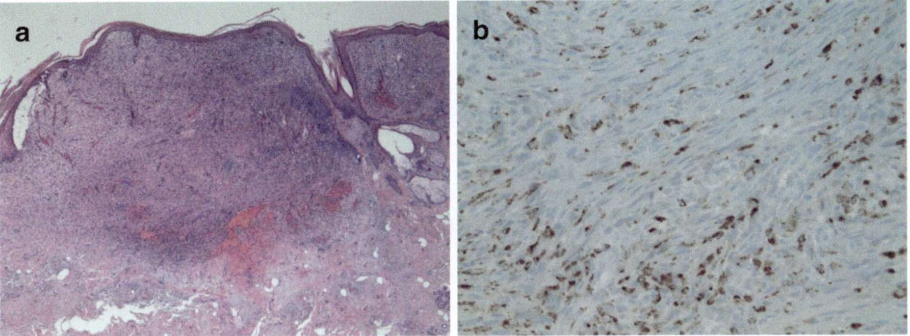

Fig. 41.3 Histology of atypical fibroxanthoma. (**a**) Dermal tumor without infiltration of the sub-cutaneous tissue (hematoxylin-eosin, ×2). (**b**) Immuno-peroxidase stain for CD68 (×20)

Discussion

The presented patient had been treated for years by dermatologists due to his field cancerization the scalp. Most lesions were classified as actinic keratoses or carcinoma in situ. Two years ago, the first squamous cell carcinoma was surgically removed. Therefore, the primary suspicion in the patient was squamous cell carcinoma [1].

However, histology showed a connective tissue tumor with the presence of spindle cells (Fig. 41.3). The tumor thickness was 18 mm. Spindle cells demonstrated both, cell and nuclear, polymorphism. The tumor cells expressed vimentin, CD68, and partially smooth-muscle actin. Numerous mitoses were seen. The tumor was well-vascularized. Based on the histology, the diagnosis of atypical fibroxanthoma was established.

Atypical fibroxanthoma is a rare mesenchymal neoplasia characterized by a rapid and exophytic growth with frequent ulceration of the overlying epidermis. The mean age of patients with atypical fibroxanthoma is about 80 years. The tumor typically occurs on the sun-exposed body areas. Men are more often affected than women. Histologically, atypical fibroxanthoma is well-circumscribed, dermal-based neoplasm composed of a variable amount of large histiocytoid cells, enlarged spindled and epithelioid cells, and multinucleated giant cells [2, 3].

Treatment of choice for atypical fibroxanthoma is complete surgical excision with a safety margins of 2 cm. Alternatively, Mohs surgery can be used [4].

Key Points
- Atypical fibroxanthoma is a rare mesenchymal tumor of the elderly.
- It is usually localized on the head and neck areas.
- Rapid growth and ulceration/bleeding are commonly presented, however clinical features of atypical fibroxanthoma are non-specific.
- Treatment of choice is complete surgical excision.
- Patient with atypical fibroxanthoma often develop other skin cancers thus follow-up is recommended.

References

1. Leibovitch I, Huilgol SC, Selva D, Hill D, Richards S, Paver R. Cutaneous squamous cell carcinoma treated with Mohs micrographic surgery in Australia I. Experience over 10 years. J Am Acad Dermatol. 2005;53(2):253–60.
2. Mentzel T, Requena L, Brenn T. Atypical fibroxanthoma revisited. Surg Pathol Clin. 2017;10(2):319–35.
3. Bitel A, Schönlebe J, Krönert C, Wollina U. Atypical fibroxanthoma: an analysis of 105 tumors. Dermatol Ther. 2020;33(6):e13962.
4. Wollina U, Schönlebe J, Ziemer M, Friedling F, Koch A, Haroske G, Kaatz M, Simon JC. Atypical fibroxanthoma: a series of 56 tumors and an unexplained uneven distribution of cases in southeast Germany. Head Neck. 2015;37(6):829–34.

Chapter 42
Bleeding Scalp Ulcer in a Patient with Multiple Neoplasias

Uwe Wollina

A 90-year-old male patient was referred to the Emergency Unit because of a malodorous, bleeding scalp ulcer. His medical history was positive for colon carcinoma, B-cell chronic lymphocytic leukemia treated with bendamustin, field cancerization on the head, tumor-associated anemia, thrombopenia, gluteal pressure sores grade III and acute urinary tract infection.

On physical examination we observed a large scalp ulcer with living organisms (Fig. 42.1). After mechanical removal of the maggots a clean ulcerated tumor was presented (Fig. 42.2).

Based on the case description and the photographs, what is your diagnosis?

Differential Diagnoses
1. Myiasis.
2. Neuropathic ulcer.
3. Leishmaniasis.
4. Ulcerated squamous cell carcinoma.
5. Secondary cutaneous B-cell chronic lymphocytic leukemia.

Diagnosis
Myiasis on squamous cell carcinoma.

U. Wollina (✉)
Department of Dermatology and Allergology, Municipal Hospital of Dresden, Academic
Teaching Hospital, Dresden, Germany
e-mail: Uwe.Wollina@klinikum-dresden.de

A. Waśkiel-Burnat et al. (eds.), *Clinical Cases in Scalp Disorders*, Clinical
Cases in Dermatology, https://doi.org/10.1007/978-3-030-93426-2_42

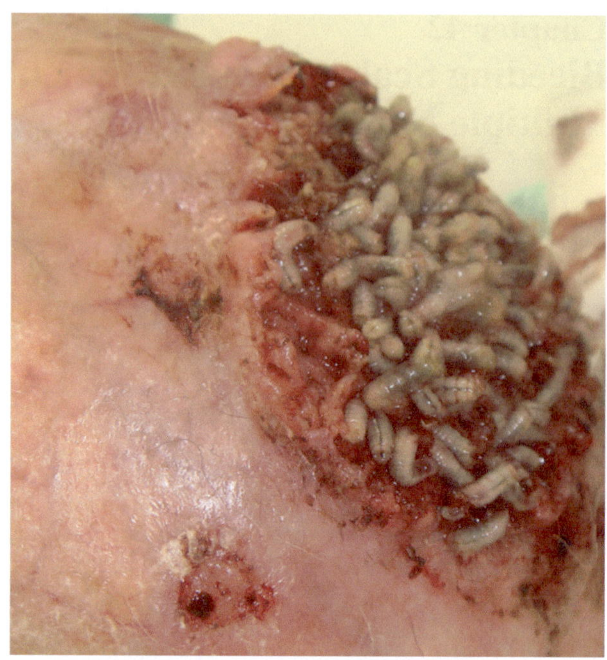

Fig. 42.1 A scalp ulceration with living animals

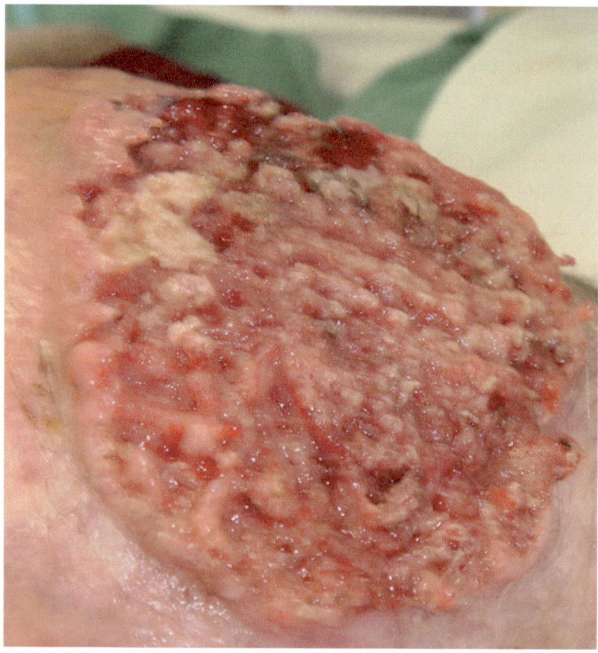

Fig. 42.2 A clean wound after maggots' removal

Discussion

Maggot therapy or biosurgery has become a regular medical treatment at the beginning of the last century but was forgotten after invention of antibiotics. The treatment has gained a renaissance around the turn of the last century to clean necrotic wounds with biofilms, such as diabetic foot ulcers or pressure sores [1].

In the present patient, infestation with maggot was accidental. This is called myiasis. Myiasis with maggots bears a risk of secondary bacterial infections including sepsis and bleeding. Maggots that feed from vital tissue can cause significant tissue damage, inflammation and pain [2]. Myiasis of skin cancer has rarely been reported [3]. The maggots should be removed mechanically to avoid further bleeding and infection [4, 5].

Due to the bad general condition of the presented patient, no treatment for squamous cell carcinoma was introduced and the further treatment was palliative only.

Key Points
- Myiasis is an infestation with maggots.
- Maggots may cause bleeding, inflammation and secondary bacterial infections. Therefore, they should be mechanically removed.

References

1. Wollina U, Karte K, Herold C, Looks A. Biosurgery in wound healing—the renaissance of maggot therapy. J Eur Acad Dermatol Venereol. 2000;14(4):285–9.
2. Bernhardt V, Finkelmeier F, Verhoff MA, Amendt J. Myiasis in humans—a global case report evaluation and literature analysis. Parasitol Res. 2019;118(2):389–97.
3. Lysaght TB, Wooster ME, Jenkins PC, Koniaris LG. Myiasis-induced sepsis: a rare case report of *Wohlfahrtiimonas chitiniclastica* and *Ignatzschineria indica* bacteremia in the continental United States. Medicine (Baltimore). 2018;97(52):e13627.
4. Wollina U. Myiasis on squamous cell carcinoma of skin. Wien Med Wochenschr. 2015;165(3-4):79–82.
5. Lo SY, Teah MK, Ho YZ, Yeap TB. Perioperative challenges in managing a patient with COVID-19 undergoing debridement for massive scalp myiasis. BMJ Case Rep. 2021;14(2):e241189.

Chapter 43
A Chronic Erosive and Pustular Lesion on the Scalp

Uwe Wollina

An 88-year-old female patient was referred to the Department of Dermatology because of a chronic ulcerative lesion on the scalp (Fig. 43.1). The lesion was painless, and no itch was reported. The patient lived in nursing home since 10 years.

On physical examination, an ill-defined ulcerated scalp lesion with alopecia was observed. The lesion was about 5.4 cm of maximum diameter. The ulcer was surrounded by atrophic skin.

A complete excision of the tumor with rotation skin flap was performed (Fig. 43.2). Healing was unremarkable. Histology showed no evidence of an invasive carcinoma. However, subcorneal pustules, epidermal atrophy and erosions were noted.

Based on the case description and the photographs, what is your diagnosis?

Differential Diagnoses
1. Squamous cell carcinoma.
2. Basal cell carcinoma.
3. Skin picking syndrome.
4. Chronic atrophic dermatosis of the scalp.
5. Ulcerated herpes zoster.

Diagnosis
Chronic atrophic dermatosis of the scalp.

U. Wollina (✉)
Department of Dermatology and Allergology, Städtisches Klinikum Dresden, Academic Teaching Hospital of the Technical University, Dresden, Germany
e-mail: Uwe.Wollina@klinikum-dresden.de

A. Waśkiel-Burnat et al. (eds.), *Clinical Cases in Scalp Disorders*, Clinical Cases in Dermatology, https://doi.org/10.1007/978-3-030-93426-2_43

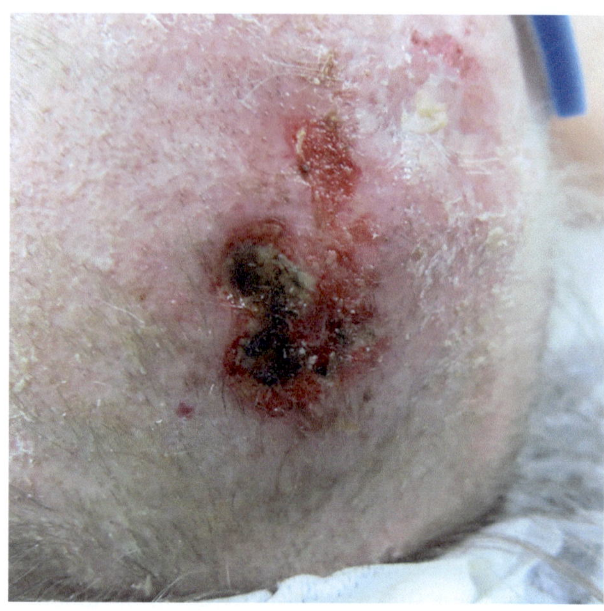

Fig. 43.1 A chronic ulcerated, ill-defined lesion on the scalp. Hair loss and atrophy is also presented

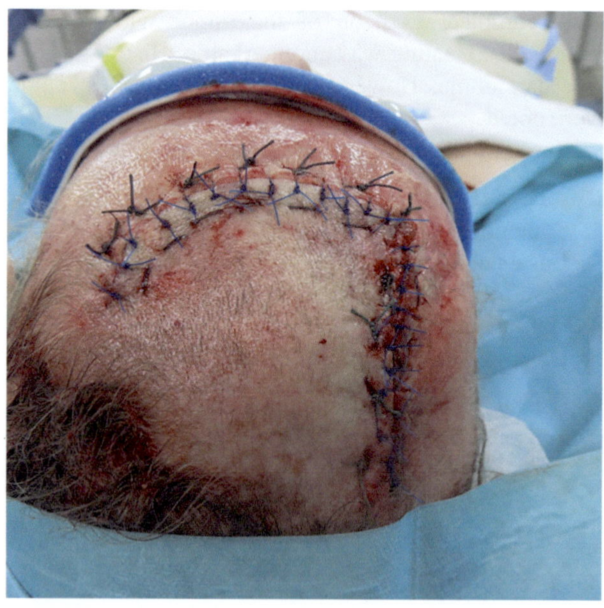

Fig. 43.2 A complete surgical removal of the lesion with rotation skin flap

Discussion

Chronic atrophic dermatosis of the scalp, also known as erosive pustular dermatosis of the scalp, is a rare non-infectious, inflammatory disorder. The disease was first described in 1979 by Pye et al. [1]. It is most common in elderly people, but certain drugs and trauma may induce similar lesions in younger patients.

The clinical presentation consists of pustular, crusted and eroded scalp lesions with scarring alopecia. Main differential diagnoses include squamous cell carcinoma and other skin malignancies.

The first-line treatment consists of high-potency topical corticosteroids, often used in combination with topical antibiotics. Topical tacrolimus may be an alternative, but its use would be off label. Furthermore, topical tacrolimus applied on open wounds may lead to unexpected high systemic concentrations with the risk of renal failure [2]. Photodynamic therapy may be beneficial, however it was also described as a trigger factor [3].

In case of recalcitrant lesions and uncertain histology, a complete surgical excision is recommended [4].

Key Points
- Chronic atrophic dermatosis of the scalp is a rare non-infectious inflammatory disorder.
- The disease is most common in elderly patients.
- The first choice treatment are high-potency topical corticosteroids.

References

1. Pye RJ, Peachey RD, Burton JL. Erosive pustular dermatosis of the scalp. Br J Dermatol. 1979;100(5):559–66.
2. Wollina U. Letter to the editor: temporary renal insufficiency associated with topical tacrolimus treatment of multilocal pyoderma gangrenosum. J Dermatol Case Rep. 2013;7(3):106–7.
3. Starace M, Alessandrini A, Baraldi C, Piraccini BM. Erosive pustular dermatosis of the scalp: challenges and solutions. Clin Cosmet Investig Dermatol. 2019;12:691–8.
4. Semkova K, Tchernev G, Wollina U. Erosive pustular dermatosis (chronic atrophic dermatosis of the scalp and extremities). Clin Cosmet Investig Dermatol. 2013;6:177–82.

Chapter 44
Cradle Cap in a Child with Cerebral Palsy

Ni Luh Putu Ratih Vibriyanti Karna, Prima Sanjiwani Saraswati Sudarsa, and Marrietta Sugiarti Sadeli

A three-year-old Asian boy was referred to the Department of Dermatology and Venereology because of the scalp erythema with oily, thick, white to yellowish scales. The patient was diagnosed with cerebral palsy spastic type and global developmental delay. Treatment with topical corticosteroids and antifungal drugs was beneficial, however relapses occured.

On physical examination, multiple well-defined, varying is size, erythematous patches mostly covered with oily, thick, white to yellowish scales were detected (Fig. 44.1). Dermoscopy showed arborizing vessels, atypical red vessels, and thick, white to yellowish scales (Fig. 44.2). In potassium hydroxide (KOH) examination, spores as the fungal element were found.

Based on the case description and the photographs, what is your diagnosis?

Differential Diagnoses
1. Tinea capitis.
2. Seborrheic dermatitis.
3. Sebopsoriasis.
4. Atopic dermatitis.
5. Irritant contact dermatitis.

Diagnosis
Seborrheic dermatitis.

N. L. P. R. V. Karna (✉) · P. S. S. Sudarsa · M. S. Sadeli
Faculty of Medicine Universitas Udayana, Department of Dermatology and Venereology,
Sanglah Hospital, Indonesian Society of Dermatology and Venereology,
Denpasar-Bali, Indonesia
e-mail: vibriyanti@unud.ac.id; primasanjiwani@unud.ac.id

A. Waśkiel-Burnat et al. (eds.), *Clinical Cases in Scalp Disorders*, Clinical Cases in Dermatology, https://doi.org/10.1007/978-3-030-93426-2_44

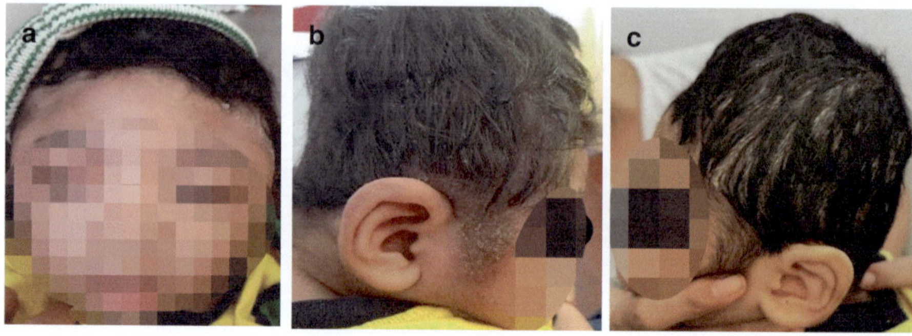

Fig. 44.1 (**a–c**) Red patches and scales all over the scalp

Fig. 44.2 Dermoscopy with the presence of erythema and yellowish and whitish scales

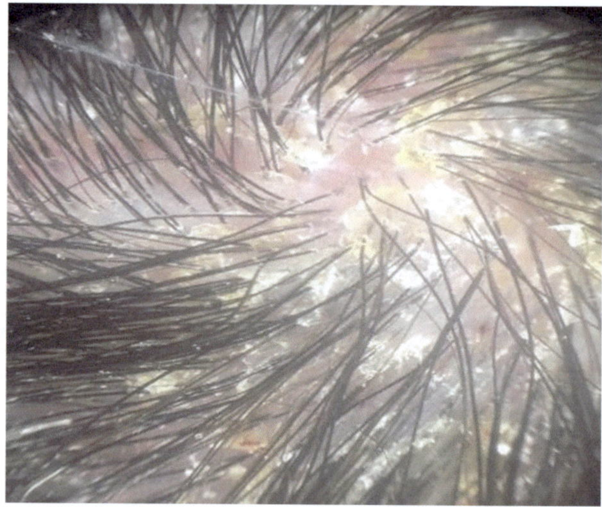

The final diagnosis was seborrheic dermatitis. Treatmement with ketoconazole 2% shampoo twice a week and desoximetasone 0.25% + ketoconazole 2% mixed cream twice daily was started. After improvement (two weeks), the treatment was changed to ketoconazole 2% shampoo topically once a week and hydrocortisone 2.5% + ketoconazole 2% mixed cream twice daily.

Discussion

Seborrheic dermatitis affects up to 42% of general population. It is mainly observed in three age groups: in infants between two weeks and 12 months of age; in adolescent; and in adults in the age between of 30 and 60 years [1, 2]. Men are more frequently affected compared to women (3.0%: 2.6%) in all age groups, suggesting that seborrheic dermatitis may be related to sex hormones such as androgens [3, 4]. In infants up to three months of age, seborrheic dermatitis mainly affects the scalp (termed "cradle cap"), face, and diaper area [5–8].

Several risk factors are thought to play a role in the development of serborrheic dermatitis. The exact etiopathogenesis of the disease has not been fully elucidated, but it is thought to be associated with *Malassezia* yeast, immunological abnormalities, sebaceous gland activity and individual susceptibility [2, 5].

Seborrheic dermatitis is associated with neurological and psychiatric diseases. The neurological disorders that cause facial immobility and accumulation of sebum are associated with serborrheic dermatitis [6, 7]. The pathophysiology of this coexistence is complex. Neuroendocrine activity has an important influence on sebaceous glands and seborrheic dermatitis [9, 10]. Furthermore, dysregulation of sympathetic flow may change the immune response and thus result in favorable conditions for the growth of *Malassezia* spp [11].

Seborrheic dermatitis is usually diagnosed based on the clinical mainifestation. If cradle cap persists longer than 12 months, other diagnoses should be excluded. A microscopic examination for *Malassezia* shows the budding form of yeast and spores; hyphae is not presented [12].

Therapy for seborrheic dermatitis includes antimycotic and anti-inflammatory drugs. The azole antifungal agents are effective in Malassezia spp. growth inhibition and have an anti-inflammatory effect [3]. Low or moderate potency topical corticosteroids can be used in severe cases [13].

The presented patient was diagnosed with seborrheic dermatitis in association with cerebral palsy.

Key Points
- Seborrheic dermatitis is a common chronic disease that affects both adults and infants.
- Cradle cap is a subset of infantile seborrheic dermatitis.
- Cradle cap is self-limited condition; if the lesions still persist after 12 months of age, alternative diagnoses should be excluded.

References

1. Suh DH. Seborrheic dermatitis. In: Kang S, Amagai M, Bruckner AL, Enk AH, Margolis DJ, McMichael AJ, Orringer JS, editors. Fitzpatrick's dermatology in general medicine. 9th ed. New York: McGraw Hill Companies; 2019. p. 428–37.
2. Wikramanayake TC, Borda LJ, Miteva M, Paus R. Seborrheic dermatitis—looking beyond Malassezia. Exp Dermatol. 2019;28:991–1001.
3. Sampaio AL, Mameri AC, Vargas TJ, Ramos-e-Silva M, Nunes AP, et al. Seborrheic dermatitis. An Bras Dermatol. 2011;86:1061–71.
4. Naldi L, Rebora A. Clinical practice. Seborrheic dermatitis. N Engl J Med. 2009;360:387–96.
5. Borda LJ, Wikramanayake TC. Seborrheic dermatitis and dandruff: a comprehensive review. J Clin Investig Dermatol. 2015;3(2):1–22.

6. Schwartz RA, Janusz CA, Janniger CK. Seborrheic dermatitis: an overview. Am Fam Physician. 2006;74:125–30.
7. Dessinioti C, Katsambas A. Seborrheic dermatitis: etiology, risk factors, and treatments: facts and controversies. Clin Dermatol. 2013;31:343–51.
8. Foley P, Zuo Y, Plunkett A, Merlin K, Marks R. The frequency of common skin conditions in preschool-aged children in Australia: seborrheic dermatitis and pityriasis capitis (cradle cap). Arch Dermatol. 2003;139:318–22.
9. Mastrolonardo M, Diaferio A, Logroscino G. Seborrheic dermatitis, increased sebum excretion, and Parkinson's disease: a survey of (im) possible links. Med Hypotheses. 2003;60:907–11.
10. Bilgili SG, Akdeniz N, Karadag AS, Akbayram S, Calka O, et al. Mucocutaneous disorders in children with down syndrome: case-controlled study. Genet Couns. 2011;22:385–92.
11. Ijaz N, Fitzgerald D. Seborrhoeic dermatitis. Br J Hosp Med. 2017;78(6):C88–91.
12. Thayikkannu AB, Kindo AJ, Veeraraghavan M. Malassezia-can it be ignored? Indian J Dermatol. 2015;60(4):332–9.
13. Gary G. Optimizing treatment approaches in seborrheic dermatitis. J Clin Aesthet Dermatol. 2013;6(2):44–9.

Chapter 45
A Disfiguring Scalp Lesion

Amr M. Ammar, Shady M. Ibrahim, and Mohamed L. Elsaie

A 65-year-old woman presented with a five-year history of a disfigured lesion with coexisted hair loss on the scalp.

A physical examination revealed ill-defined, erythematous area with hair loss and scaling (Fig. 45.1).

On dermoscopy, large keratotic yellow dots with radial, thin arborizing vessels emerging from the dot (also known as "red spider in yellow dot"), fine interfollicular scaling, and white areas lacking od follicular openings were observed (Fig. 45.2). A dermoscopy-guided biopsy was performed (Fig. 45.3).

Based on the case description, clinical and dermoscopic photographs, what is your diagnosis?

Differential Diagnoses
1. Alopecia areata.
2. Lichen planopilaris.
3. Discoid lupus erythematosus.
4. Dissecting cellulitis.

Diagnosis
Discoid lupus erythematosus.

A. M. Ammar · S. M. Ibrahim
Department of Dermatology and Venerology, Al-Azhar University, Cairo, Egypt

M. L. Elsaie (✉)
Department of Dermatology and Venereology, National Research Center, Giza, Egypt

A. Waśkiel-Burnat et al. (eds.), *Clinical Cases in Scalp Disorders*, Clinical Cases in Dermatology, https://doi.org/10.1007/978-3-030-93426-2_45

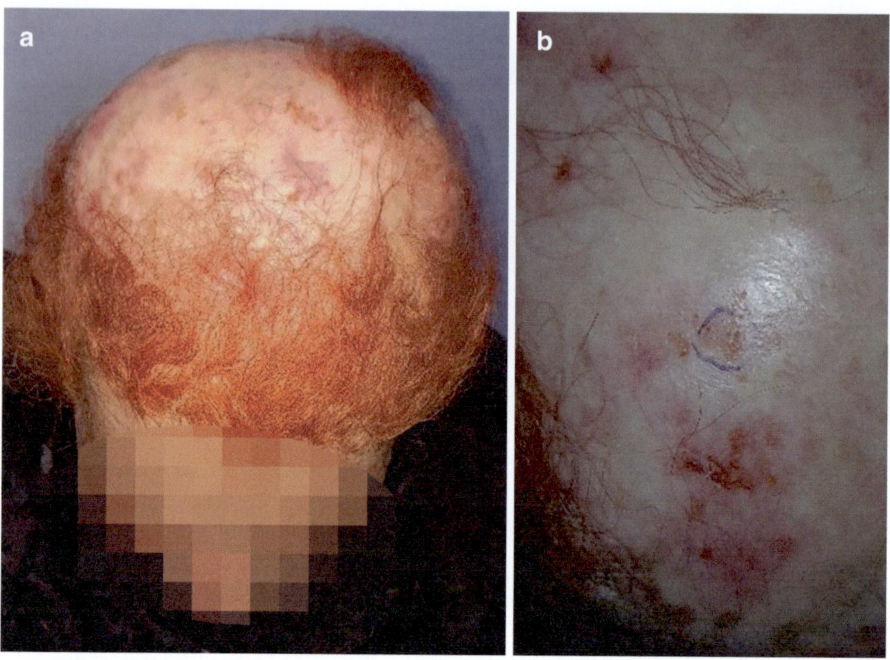

Fig. 45.1 An Ill-defined erythematous area of hair loss with coexisted scaling

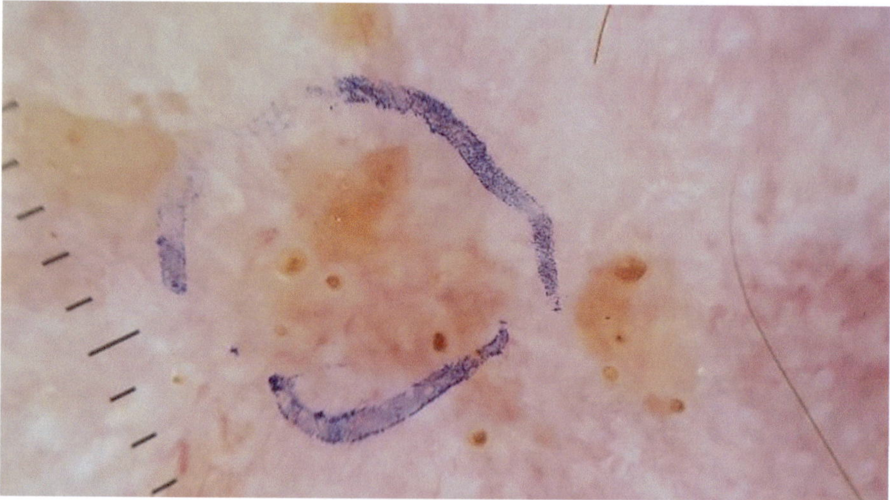

Fig. 45.2 Large keratotic yellow dots with radial, thin arborizing vessels emerging from the dot. Red dots are also presented

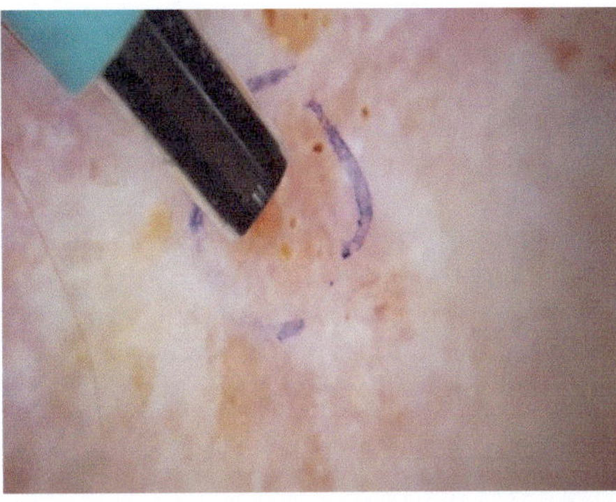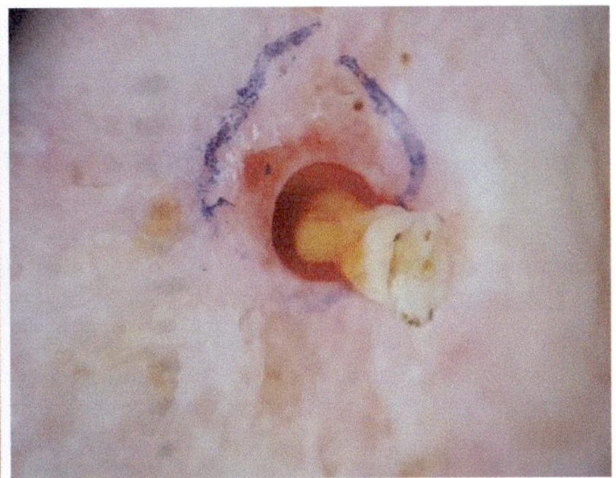

Fig. 45.3 A dermoscopy-guided biopsy

Discussion

Discoid lupus erythematosus represents the most common subtype of cutaneous lupus erythematosus. The disease is usually diagnosed based on the clinical presentation. However, in some cases, biopsy is required to distuinguish discoid lupus erythematosus from other inflammatory, infectious or neoplastic diseases [1].

Dermoscopy is a useful tool that improves diagnostic accuracy in the preoperative evaluation of pigmented skin tumours [2]. It is also used in diagnosing nonpigmented tumours and inflammatory skin disorders [3]. Dermoscopy and videodermoscopy have been shown as helpful methods in differentation between disoid lupus erythematosus and other scarring alopecias such as lichen planopilaris [4, 5].

Perifollicular whitish halo, follicular keratotic plugs and telangiectasias are the most common dermoscopic criteria for discoid lupus erythematosus. In advanced lesions white areas lacking of follicular openings are observed [6, 7].

Dermoscopy is helpful in selecting the best site for the biopsy. A biopsy should not be performed from area of scarring [8]. In the presented patient, the initital diagnosis of discoid lupus erythematosus was confirmed in histopathological examination.

Key Points
- Discoid lupus erythematosus represents the most common subtype of cutaneous lupus erythematosus.
- Dermoscopy is a useful tool that improves diagnostic accuracy in discoid lupus erythematosus.
- In case of cicatricial alopecia, a biopsy should not be performed from area of scarring.

References

1. James WD, Berger T, Elston D. Psoriasis. In: Odom RB, James WD, Berger T, editors. Andrews' diseases of the skin. Clinical dermatology. 10th ed. Amsterdam: Elsevier, WB Saunders; 2006. p. 157–60.
2. Argenziano G, Soyer HP, Chimenti S, et al. Dermoscopy of pigmented skin lesions: results of a consensus meeting via the internet. J Am Acad Dermatol. 2003;48:679–93.
3. Lallas A, Kyrgidis A, Tzellos T, et al. Accuracy of dermoscopic criteria for the diagnosis of psoriasis, dermatitis, lichen planus and pityriasis rosea. Br J Dermatol. 2012;166:1198–205.
4. Ross EK, Vincenzi C, Tosti A. Videodermoscopy in the evaluation of hair and scalp disorders. J Am Acad Dermatol. 2006;55:799–806.
5. Tosti A, Torres F, Misciali C, et al. Follicular red dots: a novel dermoscopic pattern observed in scalp discoid lupus erythematosus. Arch Dermatol. 2009;145:1406–9.
6. Elston DM, McCollough ML, Warschaw KE, Bergfeld WF. Elastic tissue in scars and alopecia. J Cutan Pathol. 2000;27:147–52.
7. Fabbri P, Amato L, Chiarini C, et al. Scarring alopecia in discoid lupus erythematosus: a clinical, histopathologic and immunopathologic study. Lupus. 2004;13:455–62.
8. Miteva M, Tosti A. Dermoscopy guided scalp biopsy in cicatricial alopecia. J Eur Acad Dermatol Venereol. 2013;27(10):1299–303.

Chapter 46
Dissecting Folliculitis of the Scalp

Qaira Anum, Tofrizal, Dwi Sabtika Julia, and Sherly Birawati

A 17-year-old Indonesian male was referred to the Department of Dermatology and Venereology with painful nodules with coexisted scarring alopecia on the scalp. The lesions started on the vertex and spread to the occipitial area. The patient suffered from acne conglobata and obesity. He was a smoker.

On physical examination painful, multiple, fluctuating, confluent nodules on the vertex and occipital scalp with coexisted scarring alopecia were observed (Fig. 46.1). Bacterial culture showed that *Staphylococcus epidermidis*. In histopathological examination, an extensive inflammatory reaction at the subcutaneous plane, causing disruption of subcutaneous adipose tissue, as well as at the perifollicular area in the upper dermis and around the sebaceous glands was observed (Fig. 46.2).

Based on the case description, clinical picture, histopathological examination and bacterial culture the presented patient was diagnosed with dissecting cellulitis. He was initially treated with intralesional triamcinolone acetonide injections 10 mg/mL every four weeks and oral ciprofloxacin at 500 mg twice a day. After three months of treatment, clinical examination revealed a good clinical improvement, with hair regrowth (Fig. 46.3). Treatment was well tolerated, and no adverse effects were noted on the follow-up visits.

Q. Anum (✉) · D. S. Julia · S. Birawati
Faculty of Medicine, Department of Dermatology and Venereology, Universitas Andalas, Dr M Djamil Hospital, Indonesian Society of Dermatology and Venereology, Padang, Indonesia

Tofrizal
Histopathology Department of Faculty of Medicine, Universitas Andalas, Dr M Djamil Hospital, Padang, Indonesia

A. Waśkiel-Burnat et al. (eds.), *Clinical Cases in Scalp Disorders*, Clinical Cases in Dermatology, https://doi.org/10.1007/978-3-030-93426-2_46

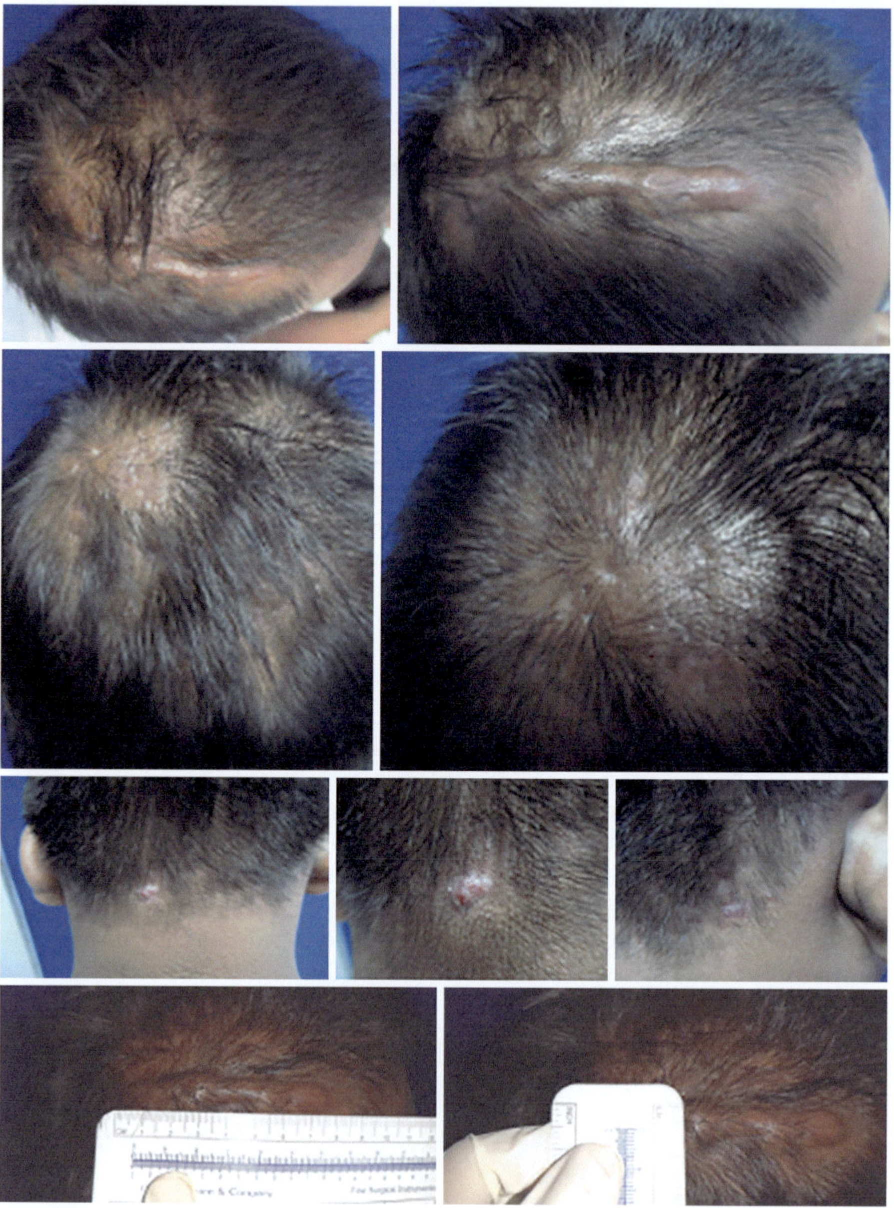

Fig. 46.1 Multiple, fluctuating, confluent nodules on the vertex and occipital scalp with coexisted scarring alopecia

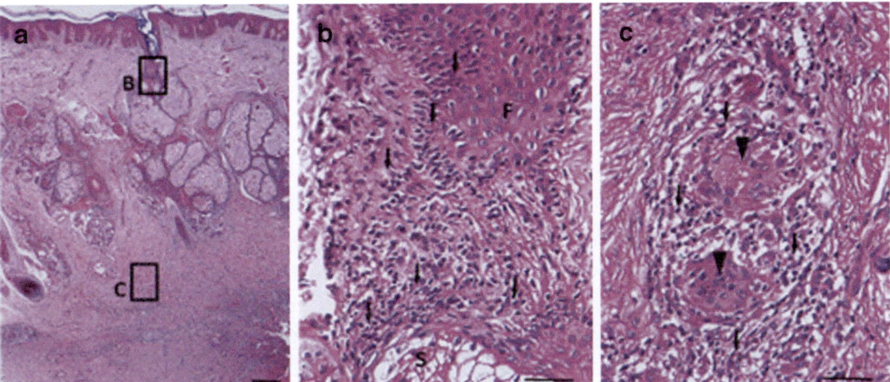

Fig. 46.2 Histology shows an extensive inflammatory reaction at the subcutaneous plane (C), causing disruption of subcutaneous adipose tissue, as well as at the perifollicular area in the upper dermis (B) and around the sebaceous glands: (**a**) Inflammatory infiltrate consists mainly of lymphocytes (arrow) mixed with neutrophils and some plasma cells; inflammatory cells infiltrate the follicular epithelium (F) and are around sebaceous gland (S): (**b**) Granulomas containing histiocytes as well as giant cells (arrow head) (**c**) Box B and C in (**a**) indicates area of (**b**) and (**c**), respectively. Haematoxylin-eosin, bars (**a**) 500 μm, (**b** and **c**) 100 μm

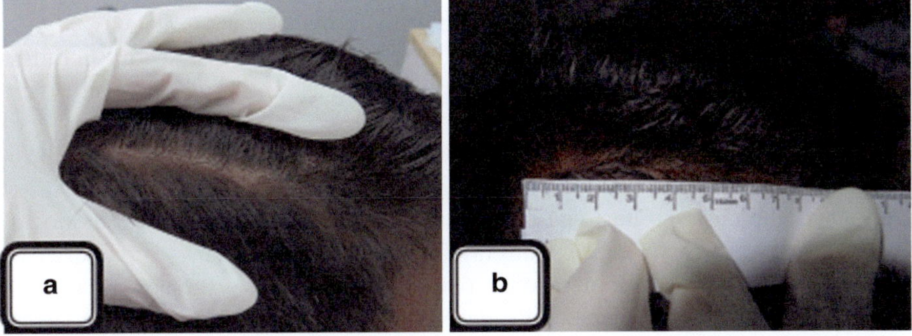

Fig. 46.3 A clinical improvement (**a**) 2 months after the treatment initation (**b**) 3 months after the treatment initation

Differential Diagnoses

1. Dissecting folliculitis.
2. Folliculitis decalvans.
3. Keloid.
4. Cylindroma.

Diagnosis
Dissecting cellulitis.

Discussion

Dissecting cellulitis is a rare, chronic, suppurative disease which predominantly occurs in black young men with the age range between 10 and 17 years. The disease belongs to the follicular occlusion triad. Follicular occlusion, androgens, seborrhea, secondary bacterial infections and abnormal host response to bacterial antigens seem to play an important role in pathogenesis of dissecting cellulitis. Moreover, the role of environmental factors including smoking, obesity, high carbohydrate diet, and humidity is also suggested [1–4].

Dissecting cellulitis is mostly found on the vertex and occipital areas. It is characterized by painful fluctuating and suppurative nodules, abscesses and sinuses with purulent discharge. Chronic and relapsing courses result in cicatricial alopecia [1–6].

Characteristic histopathological features of early stages of dissecting cellulitis include an intra- and perifollicular neutrophilic infiltrate with follicular occlusion along with lymphocytes, plasmocytes, eosinophils and giant cells [1, 6]. At more advanced stages the typical findings are sinus tracts lined by squamous epithelium, follicular perforation and perifollicular and deep dermal abscesses [1].

There is no consensus regarding the optimal management of dissecting cellulitis [6]. Chaw-Ning et al. proposed the therapeutic algorithm based on severity and activity of the disease (Fig. 46.4) [7].

The first-line therapy includes topical and systemic antibiotics (such as erythromycin, tetracyclines, clindamycin, minocycline, cloxacillin, cephalosporin with or without rifampicin), intralesional corticosteroids, and oral prednisolone. In moderate to severe refractory disease, isotretinoin at a dose of 0.5–1 mg/kg/day, may be considered [1, 8–11]. Biologic agents, photodynamic or laser therapy are considered as the second-line therapeutic options in patients with moderate to severe refractory disease [10]. A X-ray epilation and surgical excision should be considered in patients with very severe disease [10].

Key Points
- Dissecting folliculitis belongs to the follicular occlusion triad.
- The role of environmental factors such as smoking, obesity, high carbohydrate diet, humidity in pathogenesis of dissecting cellulitis is suggested.
- Dissecting cellulitis is mostly found on the vertex and occipital scalp and it is characterized by painful, fluctuating and suppurative nodules, abscesses and sinuses with purulent discharge.

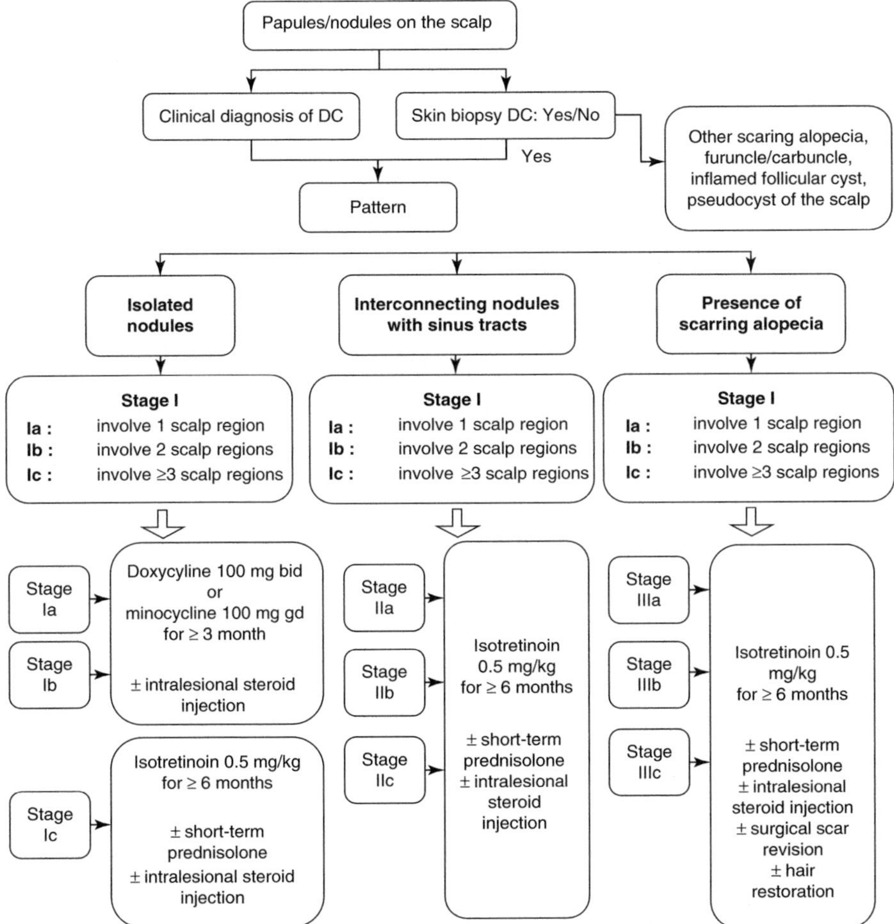

Fig. 46.4 The therapeutic algorithm for dissecting cellulitis according to Chaw-Ning et al. [7]. *DC* dissecting cellulitis

References

1. Otberg N, Shapiro J. Fitzpatrick's dermatology, vol. 2. 9th ed. New York: McGraw-Hill; 2019. p. 524–1536.
2. Branisteanu DE, Molodoi A, Ciobanu D, Badescu A, Stoica LE, Tolea I. The importance of histopathologic aspects in the diagnosis of dissecting cellulitis of the scalp. Rom J Morphol Embryol. 2009;50(4):719–24.
3. Oakley A, Marrison C. Follicular occlusion syndrome. DermNet New Zealand Trust (online serial). April 2014. Available from https://dermnetnz.org/topics/follicular-occlusion-syndrome
4. Diaz-Perez LM, Ramirez KE, Sanchez-Duenas LE. A new familial presentation of dissecting cellulitis: the genetic implications on scarring alopecias. JAAD Case Rep. 2020;6:705–7.

5. Plewig G. Hidradenitis Suppurativa/Acne Inversa/Dissecting Terminal Hair Folliculitis. Plewig and Kligman's Acne and Rosacea. Cham: Springer Mature Switzerland AG; 2019. p. 1–46.
6. Elder DE, Elenitsas R, Johnson BL, Murphy GF. Lever's histopathology of the skin. 9th ed. Philadelphia: Lippincott Williams and Wilkins; 2005. p. 493–7.
7. Chaw-Ning L, Chen W, Chao-Kai H, Tzu-Teng W, Yu-Yun LJ, Chao-Chun Y. Dissecting folliculitis (dissecting cellulitis) of The scalp: a 66-patient case series and proposal of classification. J Dtsch Dermatol Ges. 2018;16:1–8.
8. Hintze JM, Howard BE, Donald C, Hayden RE. Surgical management and reconstruction of Hoffman's disease (dissecting cellulitis of the scalp). Hindawi Publishing Corporation; 2016. p. 1–4.
9. Navarro-Trivino FJ, Almazan-Fernandez FM. Rodenas-Herranz T, Ruiz-Villaverde R. Dissecting cellulitis of the scalp successfully treated with topical resorcinol 15%. Wiley Online Library; 2020. p. 1–6.
10. Thomas J, Aguh C. Approach to treatment of refractory dissecting cellulitis of the scalp-systematic review. J Dermatolog Treat. 2019:1471–753.
11. Guo W, Zhu C, Stevens G, Silverstein D. Analyzing the efficacy of isotretinoin treating dissecting cellulitis: a literature review and meta-analysis. Drug R D. 2021;21(1):1–9.

Chapter 47
An Elderly Man with a Nodular Lesion on the Scalp

Erdinc Terzi, Aliye Ceyla Ozdemir, Umit Türsen, and Sedat Altın

A 83-year-old man presented with a two-year history of a gradually enlarging nodulo-ulcerative mass on the left parietal region of the scalp. He had no history of sunburns or and precancerous lesions. He had a significant alopecia with chronic actinic damage (Fig. 47.1).

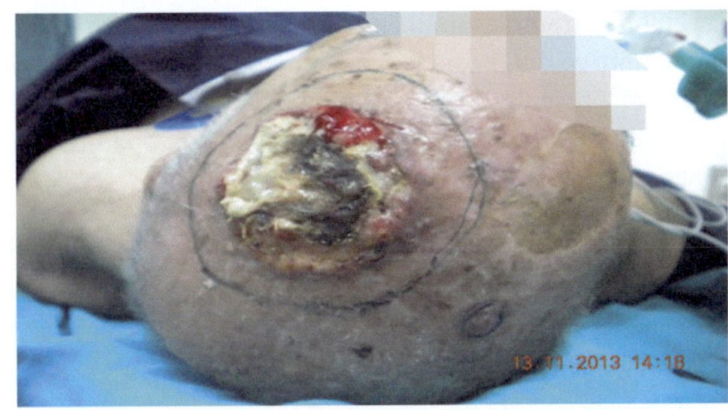

Fig. 47.1 A large nodulo-ulcerative mass on the parietal region of the scalp

E. Terzi (✉)
Faculty of Dentistry, Altınbaş University, Bakırkoy, Istanbul, Turkey

A. C. Ozdemir
Department of Plastic and Reconstructive Surgery, Private Yalova Hospital, Yalova, Turkey

U. Türsen
Faculty of Medicine, Department of Dermatology, Mersin University, Mersin, Turkey

S. Altın
Department of Pathology, Yalova State Hospital, Yalova, Turkey

© The Author(s), under exclusive license to Springer Nature
Switzerland AG 2022
A. Waśkiel-Burnat et al. (eds.), *Clinical Cases in Scalp Disorders*, Clinical
Cases in Dermatology, https://doi.org/10.1007/978-3-030-93426-2_47

On physical examination, a large nodulo-ulcerative mass on the parietal region of the scalp was observed. There was no lympadenopathy on the neck, preauricular, and postauricular regions. An ultrasonography and computed tomography of the neck were normal.

Based on the case description and the photographs, what is your diagnosis?

1. Squamous cell carcinoma.
2. Basal cell carcinoma.
3. Melanoma.
4. Sebaceous carcinoma.
5. Tricholemmal carcinoma.

Diagnosis
Squamous cell carcinoma.

Discussion

Squamous cell carcinoma is the second common skin cancer [1]. Differential diagnoses of squamous cell carcinoma include basal carcinoma, melanoma, sebaceous carcinoma, tricholemmal carcinoma and keratoacanthoma [2]. Among these tumors, the definitive diagnosis is made based on histopathological examination.

In the presented patient, the tumor was totally excised and a split thickness skin graft taken from the leg was applied. A histopathologic examination revealed features of squamous cell carcinoma (Fig. 47.2).

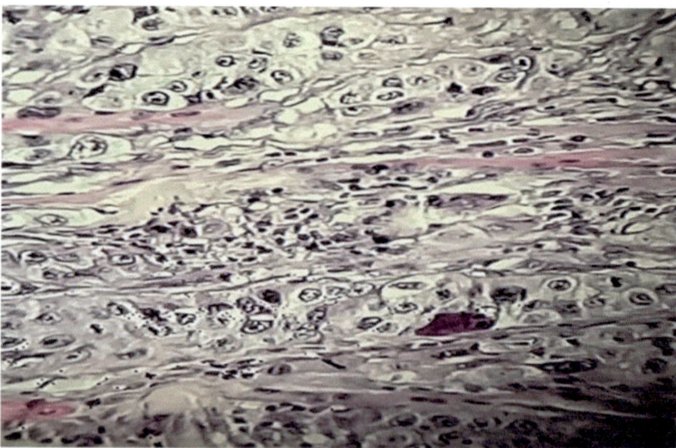

Fig. 47.2 Histology shows different sized and shaped bizarre giant cells (H&E ×40)

References

1. García-Sancha N, Corchado-Cobos R, Pérez-Losada J, Cañueto J. MicroRNA Dysregulation in Cutaneous Squamous Cell Carcinoma. Int Mol Sci. 2019;20:2181.
2. Smolyannikova VA, Nefedova MA. Trichilemmal carcinoma in a patient with squamous cell skin cancer. Arch Dermatol. 2019;81:31–5.

Chapter 48
Erythematous and Desquamative Lesions Treated with Larval Secretions

Erdal Polat, Defne Özkoca, Burhan Engin, and Zekayi Kutlubay

A 45-year-old woman presented with a three-year history of scaling and itching of the scalp. The patient had been treated with topical corticosteroids and antifungal creams, lotions and shampoos without improvement. No other dermatological or non-dermatological diseases were reported.

A physical examination of the scalp revealed an erythema, diffuse, yellow, thick scales and longitudinal yellow hair casts (Fig. 48.1). No other skin lesions were presented.

Based on the case description and the photographs, what is your diagnosis?

Differential Diagnoses
1. Seborrheic dermatitis.
2. Scalp psoriasis.

E. Polat
Cerrahpaşa Medical Faculty, Department of Microbiology and Alternative Medicine, İstanbul University-Cerrahpaşa, Istanbul, Turkey

D. Özkoca · B. Engin
Cerrahpaşa Medical Faculty, Department of Dermatology and Venerology, İstanbul University-Cerrahpaşa, Istanbul, Turkey

Z. Kutlubay (✉)
Cerrahpaşa Medical Faculty, Department of Dermatology and Venerology, İstanbul University-Cerrahpaşa, Istanbul, Turkey

Cerrahpaşa Tıp Fakültesi, Deri ve Zührevi Hastalıkları Anabilim Dalı, İstanbul Üniversitesi-Cerrahpaşa, İstanbul, Turkey

A. Waśkiel-Burnat et al. (eds.), *Clinical Cases in Scalp Disorders*, Clinical Cases in Dermatology, https://doi.org/10.1007/978-3-030-93426-2_48

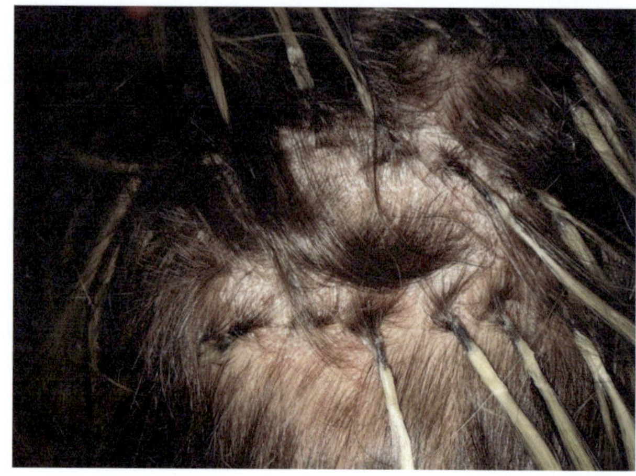

Fig. 48.1 A 45-year-old woman with an erythema and diffuse yellow, thick scales. Moreover, longitudinal yellow hair casts are presented

Diagnosis

Seborrheic dermatitis treated with *Lucilia sericata* larval secretions.

Discussion

Seborrheic dermatitis is a common eczamatous disorder that has a relapsing nature. It affects 1–3% of the immunocompetent individuals; and is more common in males compared to females. The disease is common in infants less than three months of age, adolescents, young adults and elderly. The frequency of the disease increases in the patients infected with Human Immunodeficiency Virus or who suffer from parkinsonism [1].

Malessezia furfur has a key role in the pathogenesis of seborrheic dermatitis; therefore the treatment concentrates on topical antifungal and anti-inflammatory agents [2]. The conventional treatment modalities are topical selenium sulphide/sulphur, zinc pyrithione, tar, bifonazole, lithium succinate, miconazole, benzoyl peroxide, ketoconazole, propylene glycol, fluconazole, corticosteroids, metronidazole, ciclopirox and terbinafine; and oral ketoconazole, itraconazole and terbinafine [3].

The secretions of *Lucilia sericata* larvae have been used in the treatment of ulcers and debriment of soft tissue wounds and necrotic debris for 20 years [4].

The presented patient was diagnosed with seborrheic dermatitis. She did not want to use topical formulations; therefore she was consulted in the Microbiology Department. *Lucilia sericata* larval secretions were used to treat the patient. The

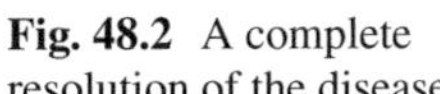

Fig. 48.2 A complete resolution of the disease

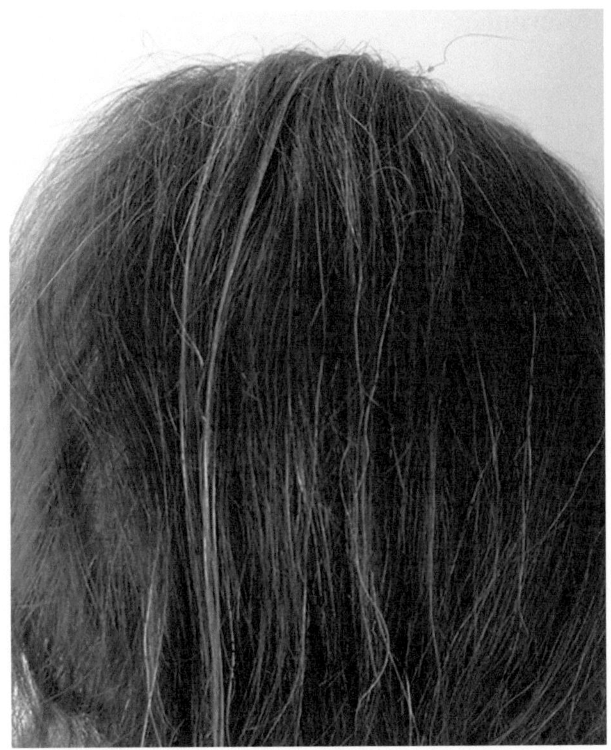

oxygen injection headpiece of the Beauty Instrument-Hydra Facial was used to spray sterile larval secretions on to the scalp with an atmospheric pressure of 4–5 units. The treatment was applied once a day for 20 days. A complete resolution of the skin lesions was achieved (Fig. 48.2).

Key Points
- Seborrheic dermatitis is a common eczamatous disorder that has a relapsing nature.
- The conventional treatment modalities for seborrheic dermatitis are topical selenium sulphide/sulphur, zinc pyrithione, tar, bifonazole, lithium succinate, miconazole, benzoyl peroxide, ketoconazole, propylene glycol, fluconazole, corticosteroids, metronidazole, ciclopirox and terbinafine; and oral ketoconazole, itraconazole and terbinafine.

References

1. Dessinioti C, Katsambas A. Seborrheic dermatitis: etiology, risk factors, and treatments: facts and controversies. Clin Dermatol. 2013;31(4):343–51. https://doi.org/10.1016/j.clindermatol.2013.01.001.
2. Borda LJ, Perper M, Keri JE. Treatment of seborrheic dermatitis: a comprehensive review. J Dermatolog Treat. 2019;30(2):158–69. https://doi.org/10.1080/09546634.2018.1473554.
3. Gupta AK, Bluhm R. Seborrheic dermatitis. J Eur Acad Dermatol Venereol. 2004;18(1):13–26.; quiz 19-20. https://doi.org/10.1111/j.1468-3083.2004.00693.x.
4. Polat E, Cakan H, Aslan M, Sirekbasan S, Kutlubay Z, Ipek T, Ozbilgin A. Detection of anti-leishmanial effect of the *Lucilia sericata* larval secretions in vitro and in vivo on Leishmania tropica: first work. Exp Parasitol. 2012;132(2):129–34. https://doi.org/10.1016/j.exppara.2012.06.004.

Chapter 49
Hyperkeratotic Plaques on the Scalp and Outer Ears

Uwe Wollina

Introduction

An 84-year-old male patient presented with multiple asymptomatic hyperkeratotic plaques on the scalp, outer ears, nose and cheeks (Figs. 49.1 and 49.2). He had been working in building trade for more than 40 years. His medical history was remarkable for hypertensive cardiac disease.

On physical examination we observed multiple verrucous and hyperkeratotic plaques on sun-exposed areas. The hyperkeratosis was variable in thickness and morphology. An erosive lesion was noted on the left cheek. The surrounding skin was atrophic with telangiectasias and pigmentary changes. His Fitzpatrick phototype was II. A calculation of lifetime ultraviolet radiation (UVR) exposure and profession-related UVR-exposure was performed. The professions–related exposure was >40% of lifetime exposure.

Based on the case description and the photographs, what is your diagnosis?

Differential Diagnoses
1. Seborrheic keratoses.
2. Basal cell carcinomas.
3. Field cancerization.
4. Actinic porokeratosis.
5. Human papilloma virus-induced warty keratomas.

Diagnosis
Field cancerization.

U. Wollina (✉)
Department of Dermatology and Allergology, Städtisches Klinikum Dresden, Academic
Teaching Hospital of the Technical University, Dresden, Germany
e-mail: Uwe.Wollina@klinikum-dresden.de

A. Waśkiel-Burnat et al. (eds.), *Clinical Cases in Scalp Disorders*, Clinical
Cases in Dermatology, https://doi.org/10.1007/978-3-030-93426-2_49

Fig. 49.1 (**a**) Multiple hyperkeratotic plaques on the scalp. (**b**) Multiple hyperkeratotic plaques on the scalp

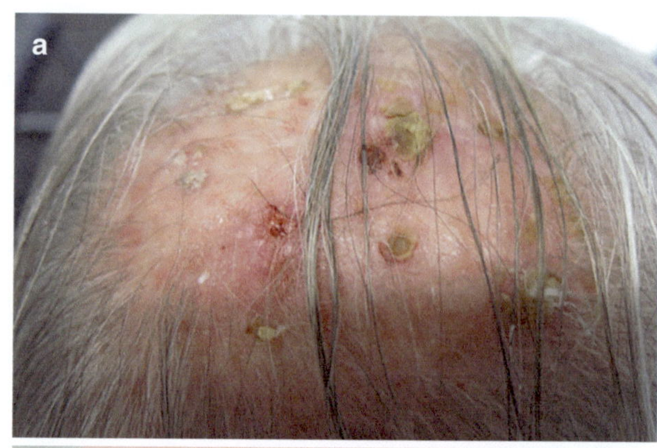

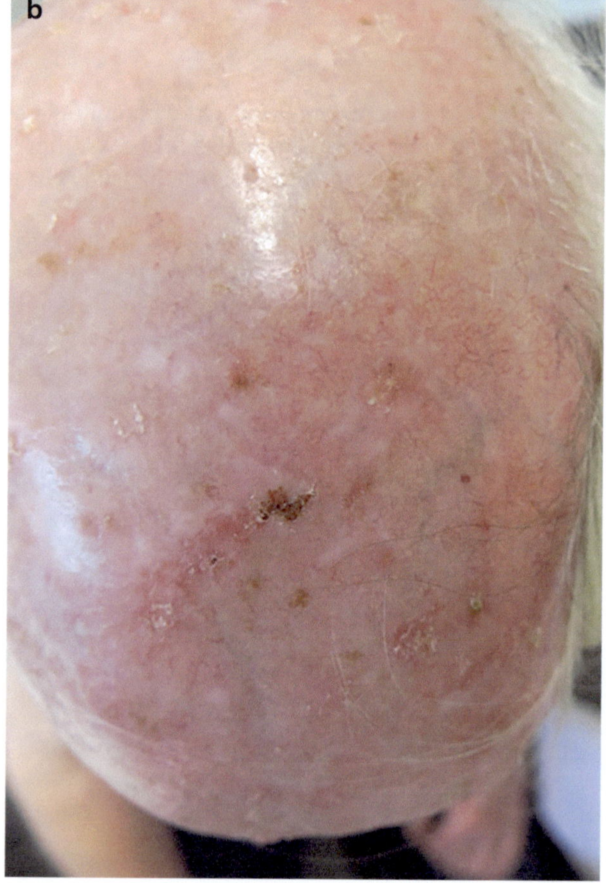

Fig. 49.2 Hyperkeratotic plaques and verruciform lesions on the outer ear

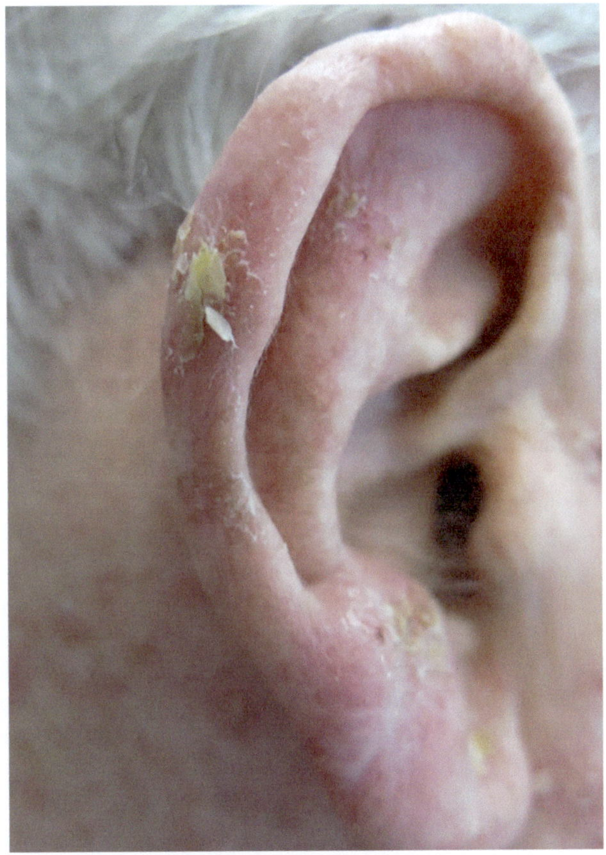

The ulcerated lesion on the cheek was surgically removed by delayed Mohs surgery. Histology showed features of SCC stage Ib which was completely removed. Defect closure was realized by skin advancement flap and two layered sutures.

For the field cancerization of the scalp with actinic keratoses Olsen grade I to II [1], photodynamic therapy was performed. The session started with roughing of the skin with a mono-filamentous fiber pad and disinfection. Thereafter, a gel containing 78 mg 5-aminolevulinic acid in a nanoemulsion was applied. The area was covered by aluminum foil for 3 hours. Irradiation was performed with a BF-RHODO LED® (Biofrontera) device emitting red light with a peak wavelength of 635 nm for 10 min (37 J/cm^2). During irradiation, the skin surface was treated by cooled air and ice-spray. After photodynamic therapy, we recommended skin care with a cream containing an extract of *Mahonia aquifolium* for at least two weeks [2]. In the presented patient, the occurrence of multiple actinic keratoses on UVR-exposed skin, outdoor profession and ≥40% lifetime UVR-exposure by outdoor profession justify the recognition of occupational skin cancer [3].

Discussion

Actinic keratoses are common lesions of UVR-exposed skin in humans of Fitzpatrick type I or II. Their prevalence increases with age. In Central Europe, the prevalence is about 3% of the general population, while in Australia the prevalence increases from 7 to 74% with the age. A higher UVR-exposure leads to earlier development and more severe course of actinic keratoses [4].

Actinic keratosis is a potential precursor of squamous cell carcinoma. Therefore, treatment is recommended. Currently, the percentage of transformation from actinic keratosis to squamous cell carcinoma is unknown.

Single lesions can be removed by shaving, cryotherapy or ablative laser.

In case of field cancerization topical therapy with 3.75% or 5%, imiquimod 0.5% 5-fluorouracil with 10% salicylic acid, 5% 5-fluorouracil, 3% diclofenac in 2.5% hyaluronic acid is approved by the European Medical Association (EMA). Treatment time varies between two and 12 weeks.

Photodynamic therapy is approved for treatment of field cancerization. The following photosensitizers are available: methyl aminolaevulinic acid cream, 5-aminolaevulinic acid patch or nanoemulsified gel. Narrow-band irradiation was shown to be more effective than broad band light sources. Meta-analyses have shown that photodynamic therapy with narrow-band irradiation is more effective than all topical drugs except 5% 5-fluorouracil. PDT is also characterized by good cosmetic outcome [5]. The ulcerated lesion on the cheek was surgically removed by delayed Mohs surgery. Histology showed features of SCC stage Ib which was completely removed. Defect closure was realized by skin advancement flap and two layered sutures. For the field cancerization with actinic keratoses Olsen grade I to II on the scalp [1], PDT was performed. The session started with roughing of the skin with a mono-filamentous fiber pad and disinfection. Thereafter, a gel containing 78 mg 5-aminolevulinic acid in a nanoemulsion (Ameluz®, Biofrontera AG, Leverkusen, Germany) was applied. The area was covered by aluminum foil for 3 h. Irradiation was performed with a BF-RHODO LED® (Biofrontera) device emitting red light with a peak wavelength of 635 nm for 10 min (37 J/cm^2). During irradiation, the skin surface was treated by cooled air and ice-spray. After PDT, we recommended skin care with a cream containing an extract of *Mahonia aquifolium* for at least two weeks [2].

Key Points
- Actinic keratosis is caused by chronic ultraviolet irradiation.
- It is potential precursor of squamous cell carcinoma.

References

1. Olsen EA, Abernethy ML, Kulp-Shorten C, Callen JP, Glazer SD, Huntley A, McCray M, Monroe AB, Tschen E, Wolf JE Jr. A double-blind, vehicle-controlled study evaluating masoprocol cream in the treatment of actinic keratoses on the head and neck. J Am Acad Dermatol. 1991;24(5 Pt 1):738–43.
2. Wollina U, Gaber B, Koch A. Photodynamic treatment with nanoemulsified 5-aminolevulinic acid and narrow band red light for field cancerization due to occupational exposure to ultraviolet light irradiation. Georgian Med News. 2018;274:138–43.
3. Diepgen TL, Brandenburg S, Aberer W, Bauer A, Drexler H, Fartasch M, John SM, Krohn S, Palfner S, Römer W, Schuhmacher-Stock U, Elsner P. Skin cancer induced by natural UV-radiation as an occupational disease—requirements for its notification and recognition. J Dtsch Dermatol Ges. 2014;12(12):1102–6.
4. Lai V, Cranwell W, Sinclair R. Epidemiology of skin cancer in the mature patient. Clin Dermatol. 2018;36(2):167–76.
5. Vegter S, Tolley K. A network meta-analysis of the relative efficacy of treatments for actinic keratosis of the face or scalp in Europe. PLoS One. 2014;9(6):e96829.

Chapter 50
An Infectious Scalp Disorder

Purwita Sari, Monica, Yosep Ferdinand Rahmat Sugianto, Holy Ametati, Novi Kusumaningrum, and Liza Afriliana

A seven-year-old Japanese girl was referred to the Department of Dermatology and Venerology with severe pruritus and scaly patch on the scalp since two months. The patient had a cat. She denied pulling her hair. No family members had similar skin lesions.

On physical examination, we found an ill-defined area of hair loss approximately six cm in diameter. Short and dull hairs with coexisted whitish, fine scales in the center and around the lesion were observed. A Wood's lamp examination revealed blue-green fluorescence (Fig. 50.1). Her body weight was 17 kg.

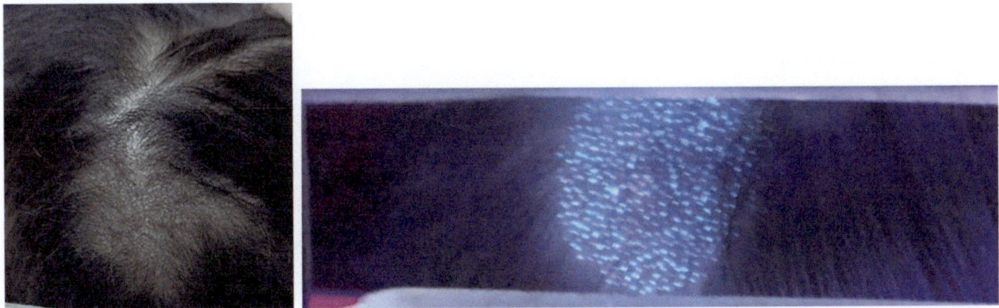

Fig. 50.1 An grayish, ill-defined patch of hair loss with the presence of short and dull hairs. Moreover, whitish, fine scaling is observed. A Wood's lamp examination of the scalp revealed bright blue-green fluorescence

P. Sari (✉) · Monica (✉) · Y. F. R. Sugianto · H. Ametati · N. Kusumaningrum · L. Afriliana
Department of Dermatology and Venereology, Faculty of Medicine Universitas Diponegoro, Dr. Kariadi General Hospital, Semarang, Indonesia

Indonesian Society of Dermatology and Venereology, Jakarta, Indonesia

A. Waśkiel-Burnat et al. (eds.), *Clinical Cases in Scalp Disorders*, Clinical Cases in Dermatology, https://doi.org/10.1007/978-3-030-93426-2_50

Based on the case description and the photographs, what is your diagnosis?

Differential Diagnoses
1. Gray patch tinea capitis.
2. Seborrheic dermatitis.
3. Alopecia areata.
4. Trichotillomania.

Diagnosis
Tinea capitis.

Discussion

The diagnosis of tinea capitis is mainly established based on patient's history and clinical features supported by Wood's lamp examination, direct mycological examination with potassium hydroxide and fungal culture. Fungal culture still remains as a gold standard diagnostic method [1, 2].

Treatment of choice for tinea capitis in children is microsized griseofulvin 20–25 mg/kg/day [1, 3]. Ketokonazol 2% shampoo two–four times weekly for two–four weeks is recommended as adjuvant therapy [1]. The differential diagnoses for the presented patient included seborrhoeic dermatitis, alopecia areata and tinea capitis. In seborrheic dermatitis, no broken hairs are presented [4]. Alopecia areata is characterized by the presence of well-defined areas of hair loss within the skin remains normal [5]. The patient did not have habit of hair pulling, thus trichotillomania was excluded [6].

In the presented patient, a direct mycological examination showed an ectothrix invasion on the hair shaft (Fig. 50.2). In fungal culture, *Microsporum canis* was isolated (Fig. 50.3). The patient was treated with oral micronized griseofulvin 375 mg daily and topical ketoconazole 2% shampoo three times a week for eight weeks. Complete resolution of the skin lesions was observed. A follow-up mycological examination was negative.

Key Points
- Tinea capitis is a superficial fungal infection commonly seen in children and caused by *Microsporum* and *Trichophyton*.
- Tinea capitis typically requires oral treatment.

Fig. 50.2 A direct
mycological examination
shows ectothrix invasion
on the hair shaft

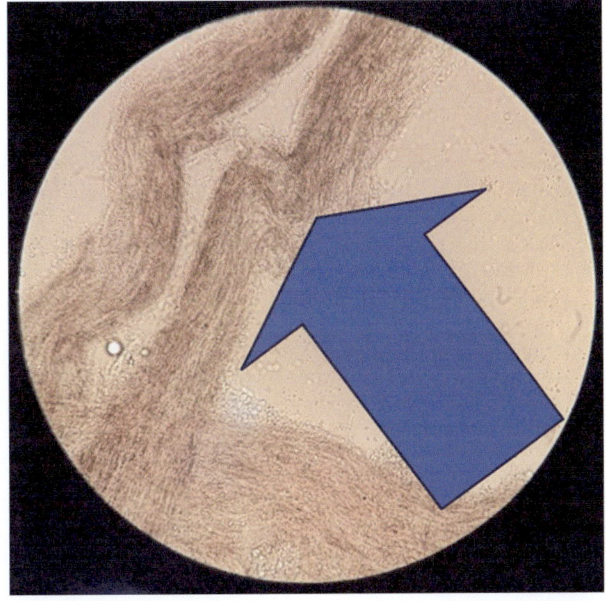

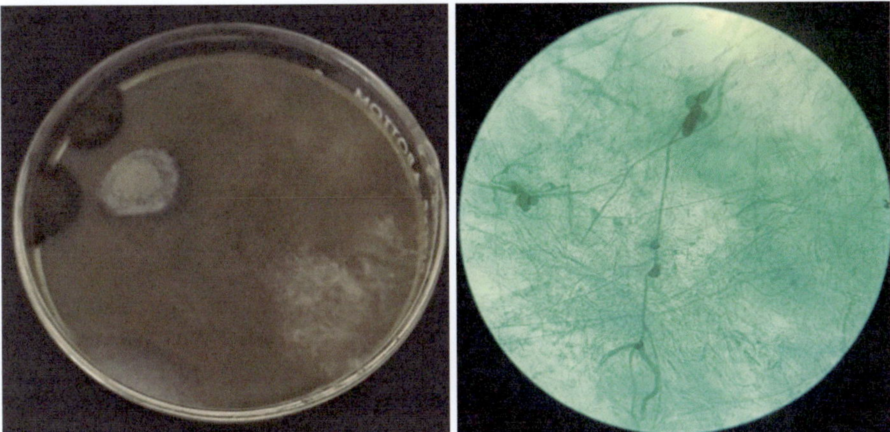

Fig. 50.3 Fungal culture with the growth of *Microsporum canis*. A microscopic examination
revealed macroconidia consistent with *Microsporum canis*

References

1. Craddock LN, Schieke SM. Superficial fungal infection. In: Kang S, Amagai M, Bruckner AL, Enk AH, Margolis DJ, McMichael AJ, et al., editors. Fitzpatrick's dermatology. 9th ed. New York: McGraw Hill; 2019. p. 2923–51.
2. Shemer A, Grunwald MH, Gupta AK, Lyakhovetsky A, Daniel CR, Amichai B. Griseofulvin and fluconazole reduce transmission of tinea capitis in schoolchildren. Pediatr Dermatol. 2015;32(5):696–700.
3. Chen X, Jiang X, Yang M. Systemic antifungal therapy for tinea capitis in children (Review). Cochrane Library. 2016:3–39.
4. Suh DH. Seborrheic dermatitis. In: Kang S, Amagai M, Bruckner AL, editors. Fitzpatrick's Dermatology, vol. 1. 9th ed. New York: McGraw-Hill Education; 2019. p. 428–37.
5. Islam N, Leung PSC, Huntley AC, Eric Gershwin M. The autoimmune basis of alopecia areata: a comprehensive review. Autoimmun Rev. 2015;14(2):81–9.
6. Grant JE, Redden SA, Leppink EW, Chamberlain SR. Trichotillomania and co-occurring anxiety. Compr Psychiatry. 2017;72:1–5.

Chapter 51
Itchy Scalp

Amr Mohammad Ammar, Shady M. Ibrahim, and Mohamed L. Elsaie

A 30-year-old woman presented with a three-month history of the scalp pruritus.

On physical examination, multiple white nodes attached to hairs at different lengths were observed (Fig. 51.1).

Dermoscopy showed multiple, white, shiny structures attached to hairs at different lengths, some with convex border (viable nit) others with concave borders (empty nits) (Figs. 51.2 and 51.3).

Based on the case description and the photographs, what is your diagnosis?

Differential Diagnoses
1. Seborrheac dermatitis.
2. White piedra.
3. Pediculosis humanus capitis.
4. Trichorrhexis nodosa.

A. M. Ammar · S. M. Ibrahim
Department of Dermatology and Venerology, Al-Azhar University, Cairo, Egypt

M. L. Elsaie (✉)
Department of Dermatology and Venereology, Medical Research and Clinical Studies Institute, National Research Centre, Cairo, Egypt

A. Waśkiel-Burnat et al. (eds.), *Clinical Cases in Scalp Disorders*, Clinical Cases in Dermatology, https://doi.org/10.1007/978-3-030-93426-2_51

Fig. 51.1 Multiple white nodes attached to hairs at different lengths

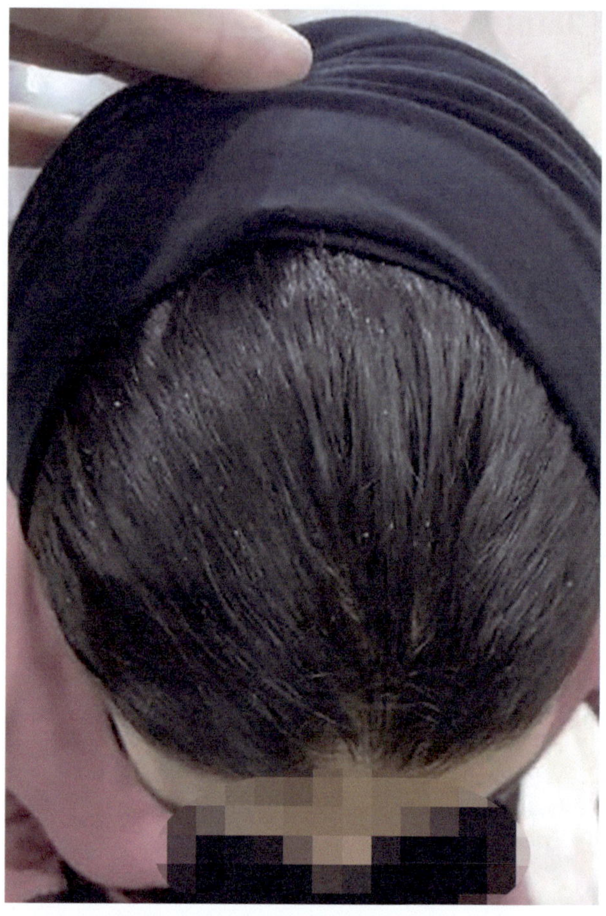

Fig. 51.2 Multiple, white, shiny structures attached to hairs at different lengths

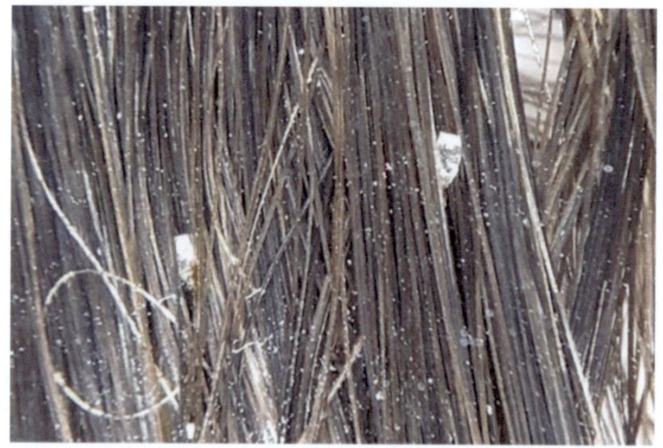

Fig. 51.3 Some structures
are with convex border
(viable nit) others with
concave borders (empty
nits)

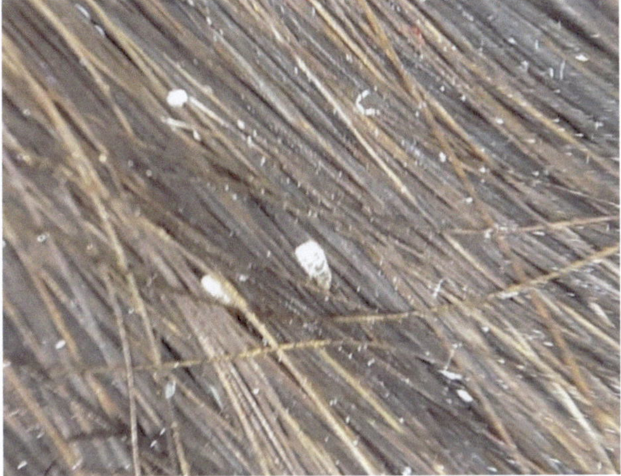

Diagnosis
Pediculosis humanus capitis.

Discussion

The head louse, Pediculus humanus capitis, is an important hematophagous ecto-parasite of humans. An infestation with this obligate ectoparasite constitutes one of the most serious public health problems worldwide [1]. Dermatitis, fatigue, psycho-logical irritability, paranoia, and weakness are the most common allergic reactions caused by pediculosis capitis.

This louse has been associated with humans for thousand years and is dispersed throughout the world due to human migration [2, 3].

Head lice infestation also known as pediculosis capitis is the infestation of human hair and scalp cause by head louse (Pediculus humanus capitis) [1, 2]. Head lice are obligate blood-feeding human ectoparasites. They are connected to human hosts during all life stage and feed on only human blood, do not occur on pets or other animals and do not have wings and can not jump [1–6]. However, head lice are generally spread through direct transmission via head-to-head contact with an infected person, they may also spread through indirect transmission by sharing clothing, hairbrushes, hats, towels or other personal items. Head lice infestation is usually detected by three type of evidence; itching and inflammation of the scalp and neck, sighting of lice and detection of eggs attached to hair shafts [4–6].

The clinical symptoms, of head lice infestation are pruritus, lymphadenopathy, con-junctivitis, and allergic reaction. A chronic severe infestation among children may lead to anemia [1–7]. In addition, head lice infestation causes not only physical symptoms but also psychological stress because patients believe that head lice infestation is a result of being dirty [8]. However, head lice are a common infection in school-age children worldwide [8, 9].

Dermoscopy is a noninvasive technique that gained popularity for the evaluation of pigmented skin lesions, particularly for the early detection of melanoma [10]. Despite this main application, dermoscopy has also been described as an aid in the diagnosis and follow-up of human parasitosis, such as scabies, tungiasis, cutaneous larva migrans, and pediculosis. New generations of hand-held dermoscopes using polarized light no longer require direct contact, which prevents the possible risk of transfection in the latter cases [11–14].

Key Points

- The head louse, Pediculus humanus capitis, is an important hematophagous ectoparasite of humans; an infestation with this obligate ectoparasite constitutes one of the most serious public health problems worldwide.
- Head lice infestation is usually detected by three type of evidence; itching and inflammation of the scalp and neck, sighting of lice and detection of eggs attached to hair shafts.

References

1. Durden LA. Lice (Phthiraptera). In: Mullen GR, Durden LA, editors. Medical and veterinary entomology. 3rd ed. London: Academic Press; 2019. p. 79–106.
2. Light JE, Allen JM, Long JM, Carter TM, Barrow L, Suren G, et al. Geographic distribution and origins of human head lice (Pediculus humanus capitis) based on mitochondrial data. J Parasitol. 2008;94:1275–81.
3. Drali R, Mumcuoglu KY, Raoult D. Human lice in paleoentomolog and paleomicrobiology. Paleomicrobiol Humans. 2016;15:181–90.
4. Nutanson I, Steen CJ, Schwartz RA, Janniger CK. Pediculus humanus capitis: an update. Acta Dermatlv. 2008;17:147.
5. Frankowski BL, Bocchini JA. Clinical report: head lice. Pediatrics. 2010;126:392–403.
6. Guenther L, Cunna BA. Pediculosis (lice). Asian Pac J Trop Biomed. 2012;2:901–4.
7. Frey RJ, Alic M. Lice infestation. 2011. http://www.Healthofchildren.com. Accessed 9 May 2011.
8. Diamantis SA, Morrell DS, Burthart CN. Treatment of head lice. Dematol Ther. 2009;22:273–8.
9. Gur I, Schneeweiss R. Head lice treatments and school policies in the US in an era of emerging resistance: a cost effectiveness analysis. Pharm Econ. 2009;27:725–34.
10. Bush SE, Rock AN, Jones SL, Malenke JR, Clayton DH. Efficacy of the LouseBouster, a new medicaldevice for treating head lice (Anoplura: Pediculidae). J Med Entomol. 2011;48:67–72.
11. Argenziano G, Soyer HP, Chimenti S, Talamini R, Corona R, Sera F, et al. Dermoscopy of pigmented skin lesions: results of a consensus meeting via the Internet. J Am Acad Dermatol. 2003;48:679–93.
12. Argenziano G, Fabbrocini G, Delfino M. Epiluminescence microscopy. A new approach to in vivo detection of Sarcoptes scabiei. Arch Dermatol. 1997;133:751–3.
13. Bauer J, Forschner A, Garbe C, Röcken M. Dermoscopy of tungiasis. Arch Dermatol. 2004;140:761–3.
14. Elsner E, Thewes M, Worret WI. Cutaneous larva migrans detected by epiluminescent microscopy. Acta Derm Venereol. 1997;77:487–8.

Chapter 52
Keloids on the Scalp

Piotr Brzeziński, César Bimbi, and Katarzyna Borowska

A 44-year-old man presented with keloids. The patient reported multiple nonpruritic scalp abscesses for the last 10 years. He also complained of intermittent fever and joint pain. The lesions often oozed a serosanguinous discharge and bled occasionally. The abscesses were drained several times. Moreover, the patient was treated with several antibiotics and prednisone without significant improvement. Family history was negative. He did not take any medications or supplements.

On physical examination, flesh-colored, tender, fluctuant nodules with scarring alopecia on the scalp were noted (Fig. 52.1a, b). The nodules formed intercommunicating sinuses that expressed a serosanguinous discharge when palpated. No nuchal lymph nodes were palpable. Fungal and bacteriological cultures were negative. On trichoscopy, broken hair shafts of variable length, black dots, yellow dots and 3D yellow dots (soap bubble), empty follicular openings, peri- and interfollicular scales, and erythema (Fig. 52.2a, b). In histopathology, a superficial and deep perifollicular suppurative and granulomatous infiltrate around a cystically dilated, partially disrupted hair follicle was observed. Gram-positive cocci within the hair follicle were presented.

P. Brzeziński (✉)
Department of Physiotherapy and Medical Emergency, Faculty of Health Sciences, Pomeranian Academy, Slupsk, Poland

Department of Dermatology, Provincial Specialist Hospital in Slupsk, Ustka, Poland

C. Bimbi
Brazilian Society of Dermatology, Porto Alegre, Brazil

K. Borowska
Department of Histology and Embryology with Experimental Cytology Unit, Medical University of Lublin, Lublin, Poland

A. Waśkiel-Burnat et al. (eds.), *Clinical Cases in Scalp Disorders*, Clinical Cases in Dermatology, https://doi.org/10.1007/978-3-030-93426-2_52

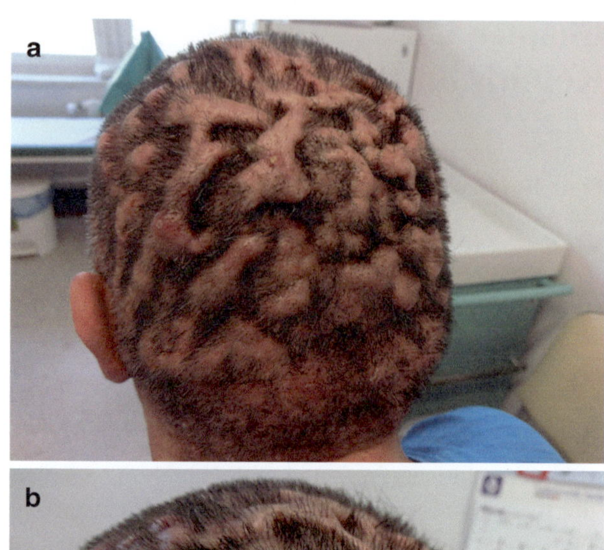

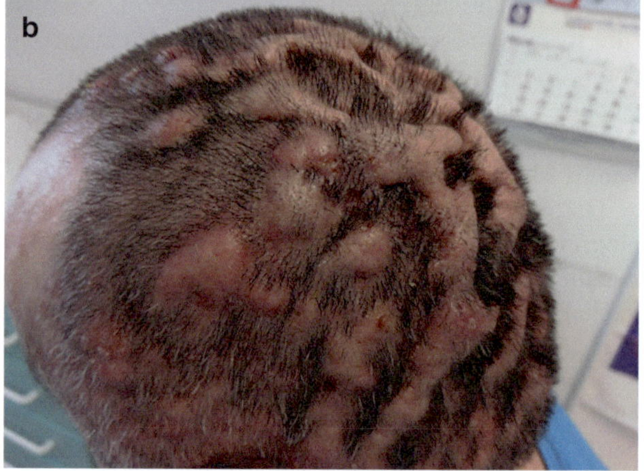

Fig. 52.1 (a, b) A 44-year-old man with multiple nodular lesions on the scalp. Multiple purulent. Erythematous, interconnecting plaques, some boggy with dried and yellow crusts on the scalp are presented

Based on the case description and the photograph, what is your diagnosis?

Differential Diagnoses
1. Acne keloidalis.
2. Dissecting cellulitis.
3. Folliculitis decalvans.
4. Pseudopelade of Brocq.
5. Discoid lupus erythematosus.
6. Kerion.

Diagnosis
Dissecting cellulitis.

Fig. 52.2 Trichoscopy: (**a**) "3D" yellow dot (blue arrow), yellow areas (green arrow), diffuse erythema (red arrow), short regrowing hairs (yellow arrow), follicular pustules (black arrow), empty follicular openings (gray arrow), exclamation mark hair (violet arrow); (**b**) "3D" yellow dot (blue arrow), amorphous area (yellow arrow), diffuse erythema (green arrows), perifollicular scales (red arrow), short regrowing hairs (gray arrow), skin clefts with emergent hairs (black arrow)

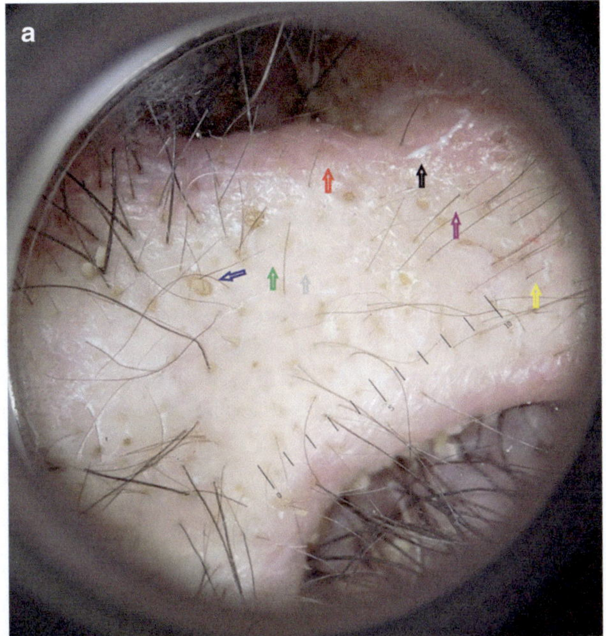

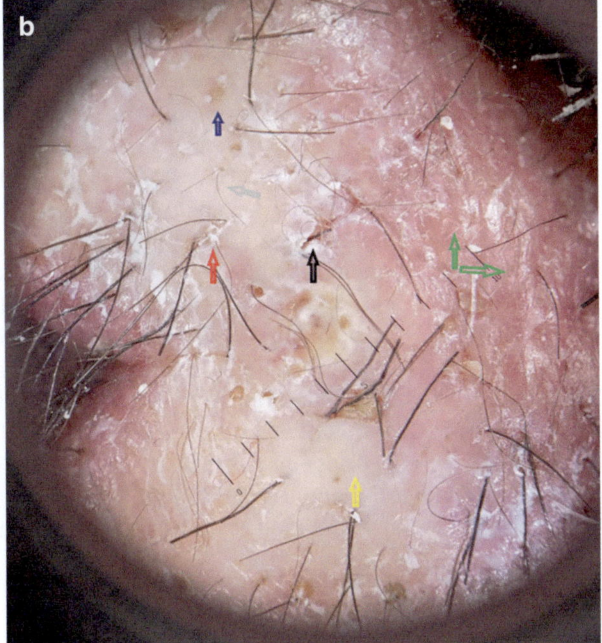

Discussion

Dissecting cellulitis (DC), also known as perifolliculitis capitis abscedens et suffodiens (Hoffman), manifests with perifollicular pustules, nodules, abscesses and sinuses that evolve into scarring alopecia [1]. DC has been reported worldwide. However, the incidence of DC is likely under-reported. In the U.S., it predominantly occurs in African American men between 20 and 40 years of age. DC more rarely occurs in other races and women [2]. DC is likely a reaction pattern, as is shown by its varied therapeutic successes and failures [1, 3]. The etiology of DC remains enigmatic. The disease is distinct from hidradenitis suppurativa, which is shown by their varied responses to therapies and their histologic differences. Like hidradenitis suppurativa, DC likely involves both follicular dysfunction and an aberrant cutaneous immune response to commensal bacteria, such as coagulase negative staphylococci [1, 3, 4]. It is described that DC can coexist with keratitis-ichthyosis-deafness syndrome, Crohn disease and pyoderma gangrenosum, arthritis and keratitis [3, 5, 6]. The literature suggests that most cases of DC can be treated effectively. However, the lack of clinical studies regarding DC prevents full understanding of the disease and limits the ability to define a consensus treatment algorithm. Medical therapies include antibiotic soap (chlorhexidine and benzoyl peroxide), dapsone, intralesional triamcinolone, zinc supplements, topical and oral isotretinoin, oral antibiotics (tetracycline and doxycycline), and oral corticosteroids. Simple incision and drainage and wide excision with split-thickness skin grafting have been used to treat severe cases when medical therapy has failed [3, 7].

Older therapeutic options include: low dose oral zinc, isotretinoin, minocycline, sulfa drugs, tetracycline, prednisone, intralesional triamcinolone, incision and drainage, dapsone, antiandrogens (in women), topical clindamycin, topical isotretinoin, X-ray epilation and ablation, ablative CO_2 lasers, hair removal lasers (800 nm and 694 nm), and surgical excision.

Newer therapies include tumor necrosis factor blockers, quinolones, macrolide antibiotics, rifampin, alitretinoin, metronidazole, and high dose zinc sulphate (135–220 mg TID). Isotretinoin seems to provide the highest chance of remission, but the number of reports is small, dosing schedules variable, and the long term follow up beyond a year is negligible; moreover, treatment failures have been reported. Tumor necrosis factor inhibitors can succeed when isotretinoin fails, either as monotherapy, or as a bridge to aggressive surgical treatment, but long term data is lacking. Non-medical therapies noted in the last decade include: the 1064 nm laser, photodynamic therapy, and modern external beam radiation therapy [8–10].

Key Points
- Dissecting cellulitis is a chronic inflammatory dermatosis that results in disfiguring and painful, purulent lesions.
- Isotretinoin seems to provide the highest chance of remission.

References

1. Scheinfeld N. Dissecting cellulitis (Perifolliculitis Capitis Abscedens et Suffodiens): a comprehensive review focusing on new treatments and findings of the last decade with commentary comparing the therapies and causes of dissecting cellulitis to hidradenitis suppurativa. Dermatol Online J. 2014;20(5):22692.
2. Zerrouki N, Omahsan L, Zizi N, Dikhaye S. Cellulite disséquante du cuir chevelu [Dissecting cellulitis of the scalp]. Rev Prat. 2019;69(1):63. French.
3. Thomas J, Aguh C. Approach to treatment of refractory dissecting cellulitis of the scalp: a systematic review. J Dermatolog Treat. 2019:1–6. https://doi.org/10.1080/09546634.2019.1642441. Epub ahead of print.
4. Lee CN, Chen W, Hsu CK, Weng TT, Lee JY, Yang CC. Dissecting folliculitis (dissecting cellulitis) of the scalp: a 66-patient case series and proposal of classification. J Dtsch Dermatol Ges. 2018;16(10):1219–26. https://doi.org/10.1111/ddg.13649. Epub 2018 Aug 31.
5. Bimbi C, Brzeziński P. Combined treatment of keloids and scars with Nd:YAG 1064 nm laser and cryotherapy: Report of clinical cases. Our Dermatol Online. 2020;11(2):149–53. https://doi.org/10.7241/ourd.20202.8.
6. Hassan I, Bhat T, Altaf H, Sameem F, Masood Q. Role of oral zinc sulphate in warts-a placebo controlled, single-blinded study. Our Dermatol Online. 2013;4(1):24–7. https://doi.org/10.7241/ourd.20131.04.
7. Puri N, Puri A. A clinical and histopathological study of cicatricial alopecia. Our Dermatol Online. 2013;4(3):311–5. https://doi.org/10.7241/ourd.20133.75.
8. Abreu Velez AM, Smoller BR, Howard MS. Central centrifugal cicatricial alopecia amalgamated with alopecia areata: immunologic findings. Our Dermatol Online. 2014;5(3):287–91. https://doi.org/10.7241/ourd.20143.72.
9. Melo DF, Slaibi EB, Siqueira TMFM, Tortelly VD. Trichoscopy findings in dissecting cellulitis. An Bras Dermatol. 2019;94(5):608–11. https://doi.org/10.1016/j.abd.2019.09.006. Epub 2019 Sep 30. PMID: 31777364; PMCID: PMC6857556.
10. Sung KY, Lee S, Jeong Y, Lee SY. Dissecting cellulitis of the scalp: a diagnostic challenge. Arch Plast Surg. 2020;47(6):631–2. https://doi.org/10.5999/aps.2020.00633. Epub 2020 Nov 15. PMID: 33238356; PMCID: PMC7700848.

Chapter 53
Kerion in Pediatric Age

I. G. A. A. Dwi Karmila, Anak Agung Gde Putra Wiraguna, and Putu Dyah Sawitri

A 6-year-old boy was referred to the Dermatology and Venereology with a reddish nodules on the back of the scalp since three weeks. A severe pruritus and the presence of brittle hairs were reported. Moreover, one week ago, a nodules appeared on the left side of the neck.

A physical examination of the scalp showed well–defined erythematous plaques and nodules with multiple pustules and erosions. Moreover, within the skin lesions multiple broken hairs 0.2–0.5 cm long were present (Fig. 53.1).

Based on the case description and the photographs, what is your diagnosis?

Differential Diagnoses
1. Kerion.
2. Furunculosis.
3. Carbuncles.
4. Seborrhoeic dermatitis.

Diagnosis
Kerion.

On Wood's lamp examination, a yellow-green fluorescence was found. A direct mycological examination with 10% potassium hydroxide showed spores outside the hair shaft (ectothrix). In fungal culture, *Microsporum canis* was isolated.

I. G. A. A. D. Karmila (✉) · A. A. G. P. Wiraguna · P. D. Sawitri
Department of Dermatology and Venereology, Faculty of Medicine Universitas Udayana, Sanglah Hospital, Denpasar-Bali, Indonesia

Indonesian Society of Dermatology and Venereology, Jakarta, Indonesia
e-mail: karmila@unud.ac.id; wiraguna@unud.ac.id

A. Waśkiel-Burnat et al. (eds.), *Clinical Cases in Scalp Disorders*, Clinical Cases in Dermatology, https://doi.org/10.1007/978-3-030-93426-2_53

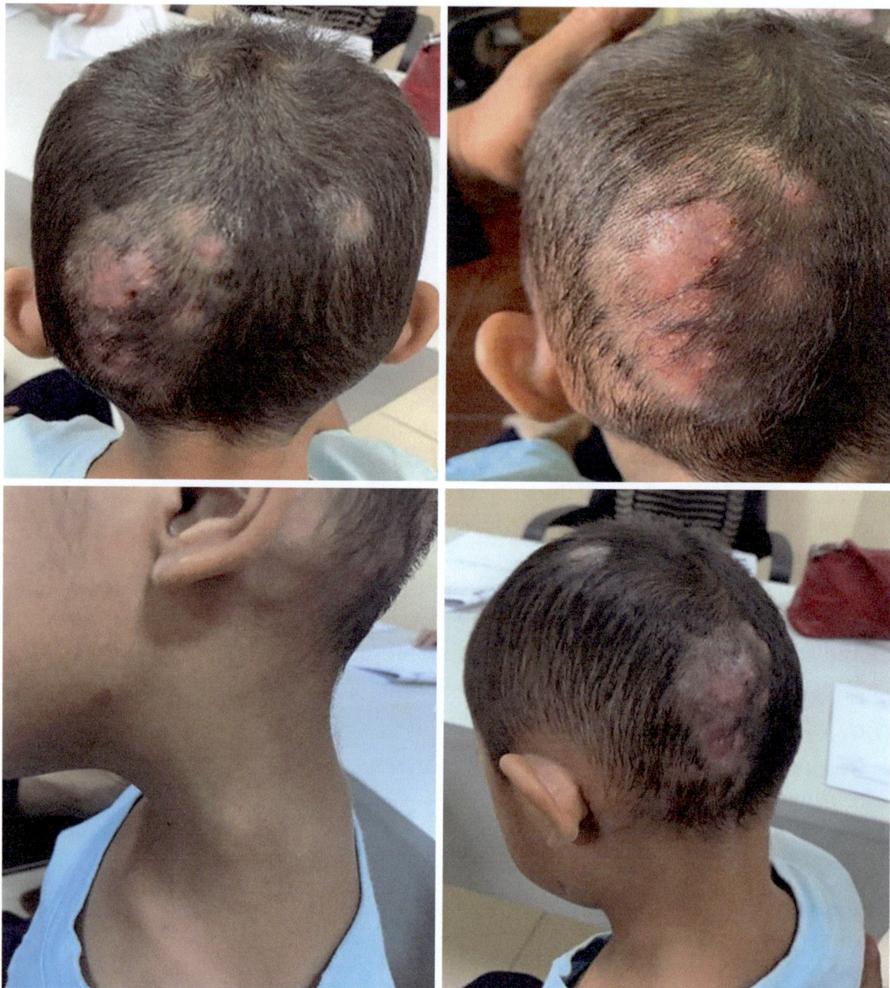

Fig. 53.1 A six-year-old boy with lesions on the scalp and enlarged lymh nodes

The patient was diagnosed with kerion. He was treated with systemic microsize griseofulvin 400 mg daily for eight weeks and ketoconazole shampoo 2% two to three times a week.

Discussion

Tinea capitis is often found in children, especially at prepubertal age. Most of the cases (93.3%) occurred below 14 years of age. Symptoms of tinea calitis include itching, fever and pain. The pattern of tinea capitis is divided into:

non-inflammatory and inflammatory. Inflammatory tinea capitis is often associated with posterior cervical lymphadenopathy. The lesions may show the kerion form, nodules, broken hair and pustular discharge. The condition can lead to scarring alopecia [1, 2].

In tinea capitis, the source of transmission is an important aspect that needs to be explored. Therefore, it is important to inquire about the history of contact with both humans and animals [3].

A Wood's lamp examiantion is helpful in diagnosing tinea capitis. A yellow-green fluorescence indicated the presence of *Microsporum canis*. Dermoscopy is a frequently used method for diagnosing pigmented lesions. In recent years many studies have shown the usefulness of dermoscopy in the evaluation of hair and scalp abnormalities including tinea capitis [4].

Griseofulvin is still recommended for the treatment of tinea capitis in patients over four years of age. It is still the drug of choice because of its safety profile and good tolerance in children. The recommended dose of microsize griseofulvin in children is 20–25 mg/kg/day and ultramicrosize griseofulvin 15 mg/kg/day for six to 12 weeks [5].

Key Points
- Tinea capitis is a common dermatophyte infection found mainly in children.
- The diagnosis of tinea capitis is established based on the patient's history, clinical picture, as well as Wood's lamp and dermoscopic examination. Griseofulvin is the first-line treatment for tinea capitis in children.

References

1. Leung AK, Hon KL, Leong KF, Barankin B, Lam JM. Tinea capitis: an update review. Recent Patents Inflamm Allergy Drug Discov. 2020;14:58–68.
2. Fuller LC, et al. British association of dermatologists guidelines for the management of tinea capitis. BJD. 2014;171:454–63.
3. Sajjan AG, Mangalgi SS. Clinicomycological profile of tinea capitis in children residing in orphanages. Int J Biol Med Res. 2012;3(4):2405–7.
4. Hernandez-Bel P, Malvehy J, Crocker A, Sanchez-Carazo JL, Febrer I, Alegre V. Comma hairs: a new dermoscopic marker for tinea capitis. Actas Dermosifilogr. 2012;103(9):836–7.
5. Craddock LN, Schieke SM. Superficial fungal infection: mycoses, dermatophytes, dermathophytoses. In: Kang S, Amagai M, Bruckner AL, Enk AH, Margolis DJ, McMichael AJ, Orringer JS, editors. Fitzpatrick's dermatology in general medicine. 9th ed. New York: McGraw-Hill; 2019. p. 2925–51.

Chapter 54
A Red Nodule on the Scalp

Cahit Yavuz and Umit Türsen

Introduction

A 47-year-old male presented with a three-year history of a nodular lesion on the scalp. The patient reported a rapid growth of the lesion for the last month. There was no history of systemic disease, drug use or malignancy.

On physical examination, a non-sensitive, 2 cm in diamater, reddish-brown, fixed nodule with polypoid protrusion on the left temporal area was presented (Fig. 54.1).

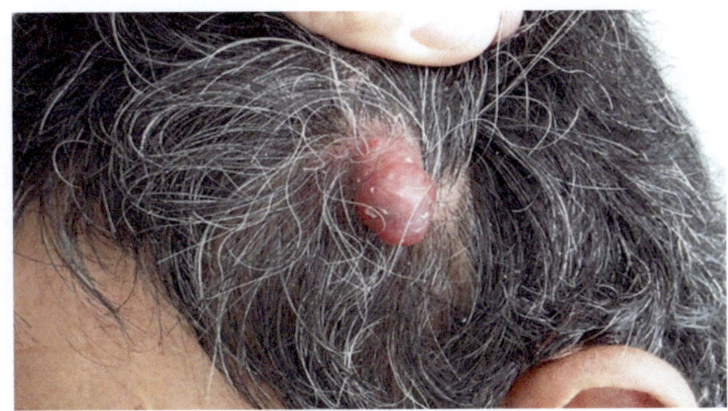

Fig. 54.1 A solitary, reddish-brown nodule on the left temporal region of the scalp

C. Yavuz (✉)
Department of Dermatology, Konya City Hospital, Konya, Turkey

U. Türsen
Mersin University Faculty of Medicine, Department of Dermatology, Mersin, Turkey

© The Author(s), under exclusive license to Springer Nature Switzerland AG 2022
A. Waśkiel-Burnat et al. (eds.), *Clinical Cases in Scalp Disorders*, Clinical Cases in Dermatology, https://doi.org/10.1007/978-3-030-93426-2_54

Based on the case description and the photograph, what is your diagnosis?

Differential Diagnoses
1. Trichilemmal cyst.
2. Dermoid cyst.
3. Langerhans cell histiocytosis.
4. Cutaneous metastasis.
5. Epidermoid cyst.

Diagnosis
Cutaneous metastasis.

A complete surgical excision of the lesion was performed. Histology showed a tumor in the dermis formed by polygonal-shaped cells with uniform, round nuclei and clear cytoplasm. A rich vascular network within the tumor was observed (Fig. 54.2). In the immunohistochemical staining, a positive immunoreaction with Vimentin, EMA, CK8/18, CD10 and AE1/AE3 was detected (Fig. 54.3). Based on the histopathological and immunohistochemical findings the patient was diagnosed with cutaneous metastasis from renal cell carcinoma. The patient was referred to the Urology and Oncology Clinics. He was diagnosed with renal cell carcinoma on the right kidney. Moreover, colon metastasis were detected.

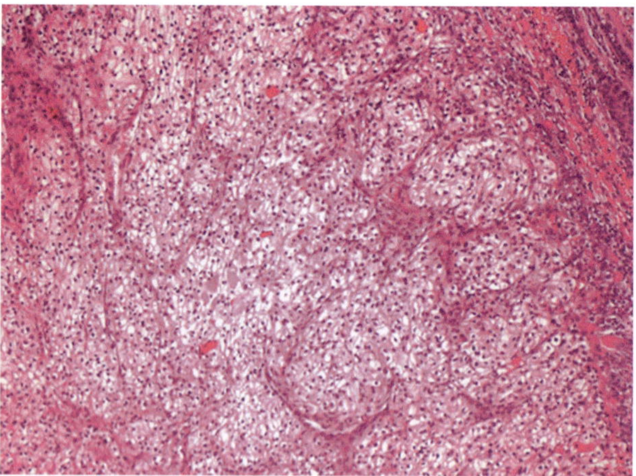

Fig. 54.2 Histology shows a tumor in the dermis formed by polygonal-shaped cells with uniform, round nuclei and clear cytoplasm

Fig. 54.3 Immounohisto-
chemical staining

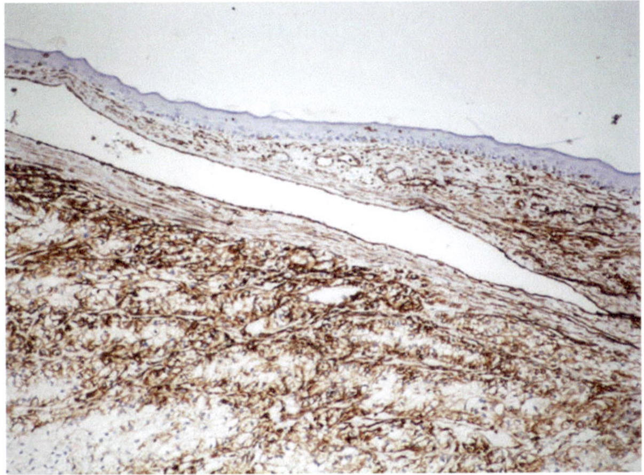

A surgical excision of primary tumor was performed. Chemotherapy was started. A regular follow up of the patient is ongoing.

Discussion

Cutaneous metastases are not common condition. Nevertheless, they may be the first sign of internal malignancy [1]. Patients with history of cancer should be aware about posibility of development of cutaneous metastasis [2].

Key Points
- Cutaneous metastases are not common condition.
- Nevertheless, they may be the first sign of internal malignancy.

References

1. Alcaraz I, Cerroni L, Rutten A, Kutzner H, Requena L. Cutaneous metastases from internal malignancies: a clinicopathologic and immunohistochemical review. Am J Dermatopathol. 2012;34:347–93.
2. Cohen HT, McGovern FJ. Renal cell carcinoma. N Engl J Med. 2005;353:2477–90.

Chapter 55
Multiple Ulcers on the Scalp in an Immunocompromised Patient

Sandra Widaty, Vashty Amanda Hosfiar, and Randy Satria Nugraha

A 20-year-old female patient was admitted to the Department of Hematology with acute lymphocytic leukemia, febrile neutropenia and pancytopenia. She was treated with vincristine and methylprednisolone. The patient was consulted in the Department of Dermatology and Venereology because of multiple nodules on the scalp. The nodules discharged yellowish fluid after being scratched by the patient. The nodules rapidly multiply, ulcerated, and then covered with brown-black crusts. The patient also complained of itching and pain.

A physical examination revealed multiple ulcerations with elevated and erythematous borders covered by black crusts (Fig. 55.1). Lymph nodes on the neck were enlarged, firm, mobile and painless. Laboratory tests showed a decreased level of hemoglobin (8.9), low platelet (23,000) and leukocyte count (1860). Moreover, low number of eosinophils (0%) and neutrophils (4.3%) as well as a high number of lymphocytes (65.6%) and monocytes (30.1%) were detected. There were also prolonged prothrombin time 16.7 (9.8–12.5), prolonged activated partial thromboplastin time 63.1 (31–47), and a high level of C-reactive protein (182.8) and procalcitonin (104.9).

Based on the case description and the photographs, what is your diagnosis?

Differential Diagnoses
1. Ecthyma gangrenosum caused by *Pseudomonas aeruginosa*.
2. Ecthyma gangrenosum caused by other Gram-negative or Gram-positive bacteria or fungi.

S. Widaty (✉) · V. A. Hosfiar · R. S. Nugraha
Department of Dermatology and Venereology, Faculty of Medicine Universitas Indonesia, Dr. Cipto Mangunkusumo Hospital, Jakarta, Indonesia

Indonesian Society of Dermatology and Venereology, Jakarta, Indonesia
e-mail: sanwidaty@ui.ac.id

A. Waśkiel-Burnat et al. (eds.), *Clinical Cases in Scalp Disorders*, Clinical Cases in Dermatology, https://doi.org/10.1007/978-3-030-93426-2_55

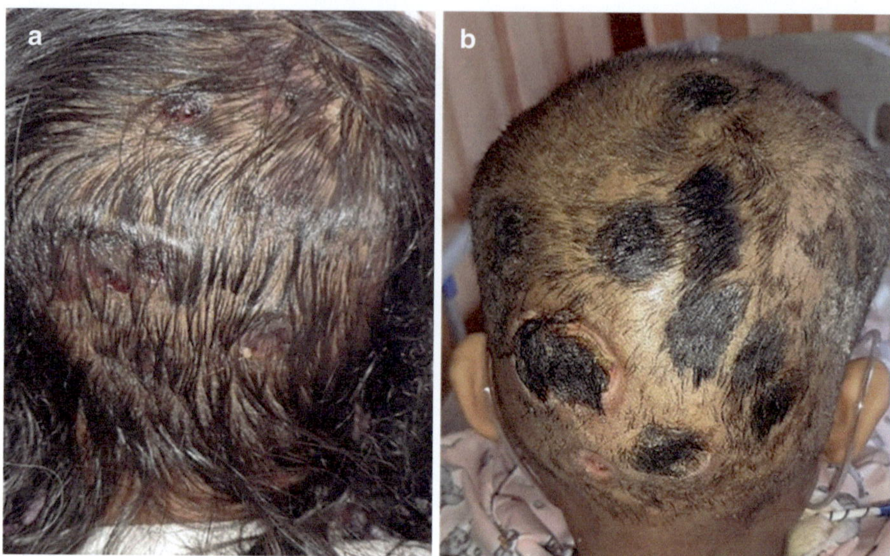

Fig. 55.1 Multiple ulcerations with overlying crusts in scalp of a 20-year-old leukemic patient (**a**) before treatment (**b**) day 10 after treatment

3. Pyoderma gangrenosum.
4. Cutaneous aspergillosis.
5. Calciphylaxis.
6. Acute meningococcemia.

Diagnosis

Ecthyma gangrenosum caused by *Pseudomonas aeruginosa*.

Culture of the patient's blood showed *Pseudomonas aeruginosa* which was sensitive to ciprofloxacin and cefepime. Culture of the ulcer showed similar organisms. Histopathological examination was not performed because the patient had thrombocytopenia and prolonged prothrombin and activated partial thromboplastin time. The patient was diagnosed with ecthyma gangrenosum caused by *Pseudomonas aeruginosa*.

The patient was given intravenous cefepime 2 g three times a day, intravenous ciprofloxacin 400 mg twice a day, fusidic acid cream twice a day, and wet compress with sodium chloride solution for 10 days. On the day 11, cefepime was switched to piperacillin with tazobactam 4.5 g four times a day. The ulcer improved, and seemed to be clean and dry. On day 13, the patient died due to an increased intracranial pressure.

Discussion

Ecthyma gangrenosum (EG) is a skin and soft tissue infection (SSTI) which is commonly found in immunocompromised patients. From a study in 2017, skin disorders e.g., ulcerations and subcutaneous diseases, contributed to 1.79% of global burden of diseases so they should be taken into account [1]. EG is diagnosed based on clinical and laboratory findings. EG commonly occurs due to bacteremia caused by Gram-negative bacteria infection, particularly *P. aeruginosa* [2]. The cause of bacteremia has not yet been elucidated but the patients are often hospitalized with immunocompromised conditions.

Establishing the diagnosis of SSTI is challenging because the result of microbiology examination from the blood takes time and it is not always the definitive cause of the skin manifestations. Similarly with the results of culture from superficial lesion; it can be misleading because it is more likely to be colonization, not the causative agent of the infection [3]. In this patient, despite no histopathological examination, the culture of blood and skin lesion showed same pathogen, which was *P. aeruginosa*. Therefore, it is suitable with the clinical finding, which was characteristic findings of EG, ulceration with overlying black crusts.

An increased number of Gram-negative bacilli infections is correlated with an increased number of other multidrug-resistant bacteria (MDR) infections. In *P. aeruginosa* infections, there were reports of MDR infections against carbapenem and other drugs; however, only 4% of the cases were resistant against piperacillin—tazobactam [4–6]. This patient showed improvement following switching of antibiotics to piperacillin—tazobactam which was shown to be sensitive from the drug susceptibility test.

This presented patient had multiple lesions on the scalp with a history of neutropenia. The management of EG resulted in improvement of the patient's condition. However, the patient died due to her comorbidities. The prognosis of EG depends on several factors, which are the number of lesions, prolonged neutropenia, and delayed treatment [7]. Therefore, the management should be comprehensive and interdisciplinary collaboration is needed.

Key Points
- Ecthyma gangrenosum is a common skin and soft tissue infection in immunocompromised patients.
- Establishing the diagnosis of ecthyma gangrenosum and other skin and soft tissue infections is challenging and we should consider the correlation of clinical and microbiological findings.
- The management of skin and soft tissue infections should be comprehensive and involve multidiscipline.

References

1. Karimkhani C, Dellavalle RP, Coffeng LE, et al. Global skin disease morbidity and mortality: an update from the global burden of disease study 2013. JAMA Dermatol. 2017;153:406–12.
2. Mordorski B., Friedman AJ. Gram-negative coccal and bacillary infections. Kang S, Amagai M, Bruckner AL, Enk AH, Margolis DJ, McMichael AJ, et al., editors. Fitzpatrick's dermatology. 9th ed. New York, MacGraw Hill 2019. p. 2789 -2796.
3. Poulakou G, Lagou S, Tsiodras S. What's new in the epidemiology of skin and soft tissue infections in 2018? Curr Opin Infect Dis. 2019;32:77–86. https://doi.org/10.1097/QCO.0000000000000527.
4. Jabbour JJ, Kanj SS. Gram-negative skin and soft tissue infections. Infect Dis Clin N Am. 2020; https://doi.org/10.1016/j.idc.2020.10.008. Article In Press.
5. Wu DC, Chan WW, Metelista AL, et al. *Pseudomonas* skin infection. Am J Clin Dermatol. 2011;12(3):157–69.
6. Zilberberg MD, Shorr AF. Prevalence of multidrug resistant *Pseudomonas aeruginosa* and carbapenem-resistant *Enterobacteriaceas* among specimens from hospitalized patients with pneumonia and blood-stream infections in the United States from 2000 to 2009. J Hosp Med. 2013;8(10):559–63.
7. Agger WA, Mardan A. *Pseudomonas aeruginosa* infections of intact skin. Clin Infect Dis. 1995;20(2):302–8.

Chapter 56
Nodular Alopecic Lesions

Ayşe Nilhan Atsü, Nazlı Caf, Zafer Türkoğlu, and Zekayi Kutlubay

An otherwise healthy five-year-old girl was presented with a six-week history of a painful lesions and hair loss. The lesions started as a small area of hair loss with coexisted erythema, folliculitis and scaling. Pruritus was reported. The patient was previously treated with oral amoxicilin combined with clavulanic acid and topical fucidic acid with no improvement. With time, edema and pain occured. Moreover, the progression of hair loss was reported. The patient's family lived in rural areas and carried out cattle and ovine breeding. Moreover, numerous contacts with stray dogs and cats were reported. Siblings, parents, and other family members did not have similar symptoms or signs.

A physical examination of the patient revealed red-colored five alopecic plaques (5×5, 3×2, 0.5×0.3, 0.5×0.2, and 1×1 cm) on the right temporal region and a solitary plaque (1×1 cm) on the frontal area of her scalp. All the plaques were covered with yellow adherent crusts. The lesions were filled with pus and discharge was observed (Fig. 56.1). The presence of multiple pustules especially within the largest plaque was detected (Fig. 56.2). A dermatological examination of other body parts was normal. Enlarged and painful right cervical and occipital lymph nodes

A. N. Atsü
Faculty of Health Sciences, Istanbul Kent University, Istanbul, Turkey
e-mail: nilhan.atsu@kent.edu.tr

N. Caf (✉) · Z. Türkoğlu
Department of Dermatology, Başakşehir Çam ve Sakura City Hospital, Istanbul, Turkey

Z. Kutlubay
Cerrahpaşa Faculty of Medicine, Department of Dermatology, Istanbul University-Cerrahpaşa, Istanbul, Turkey

A. Waśkiel-Burnat et al. (eds.), *Clinical Cases in Scalp Disorders*, Clinical Cases in Dermatology, https://doi.org/10.1007/978-3-030-93426-2_56

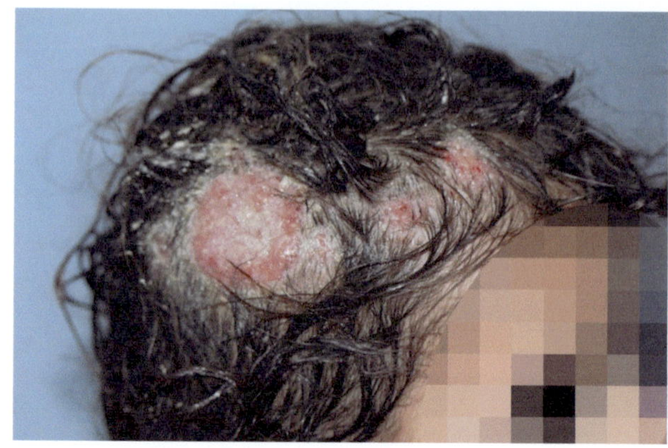

Fig. 56.1 Five alopecic plaques (5 × 5, 3 × 2, 0.5 × 0.3, 0.5 × 0.2, and 1 × 1 cm) on the right temporal area. On the frontal region, a solitary plaque (1 x 1 cm) is observed. All the plaques are covered with yellow adherent crusts

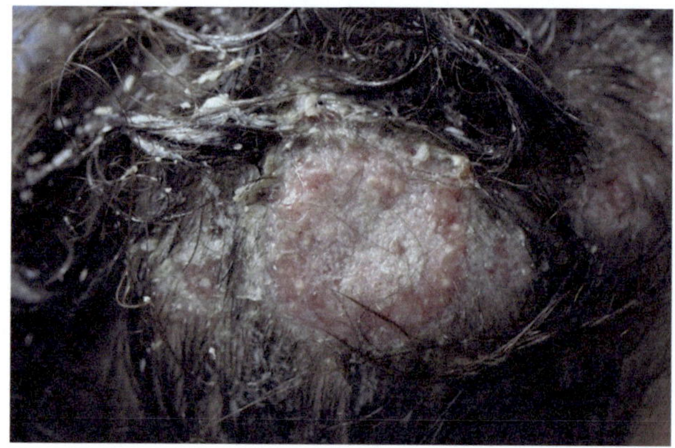

Fig. 56.2 An erythematous and inflammatory patch on the right temporal region. Multiple pustules are observed

(approximately 1 × 1.5 cm in diameter) and were palpated. Hepatosplenomegaly was not detected. Dermoscopy revealed comma hairs, pustules, bent hairs, scales, crusts, and erythema. A Wood's lamp examination showed green fluorescence. A direct mycological examination was negative.

Complete blood count showed mild anemia and leukocytosis (11.19 × 10³ μL). C-reactive protein and erythrocyte sedimentation rate were increased (7.6 mg/L and 65 mm/h, respectively). There were no other noticeable abnormalities. Viral Hepatitis and HIV serology were negative. In fungal culture, the growth of Microsporum canis was observed.

Based on the case description and the photographs, what is your diagnosis?

1. Scalp abscess.
2. Kerion celsi.
3. Alopecia areata.
4. Discoid lupus erythematosus.

Diagnosis
Kerion celsi.

Discussion

Tinea capitis is the most common infection in prepubertal individuals and it is most frequent in children aged three to seven years. An increased incidence of tinea capitis in this age group is associated with the absence of sebum secretion. The disease is not expected in infants and adults, but it can be rarely seen. There is a relation between the disease with low socioeconomic status and poor hygiene. Several pathogens may lead to tinea capitis such as *Microsporum canis*, *Trichophyton verrucosum*, *Trichophyton mentagrophytes*, *Trichophyton tonsurans*, and *Trichophyton schoenleinii*. Clinical presentation of T.capitis may be divided into two subtypes: inflammatory and non-inflammatory. Living in rural areas and immune system disorders may facilitate the development of kerion. Zoophilic dermatophytes are more prominent in kerion formation [1]. Kerion celsi is an inflammatory or suppurative form of tinea capitis which occurs as a result of an increased hypersensitivity to dermatophyte infection. It presents as a painful and erythematous, inflammatory crusted nodule(s). Pustules may be observed. Although the lesion is mostly solitary, multiple plaques may also be present. Purulent drainage and regional lymphadenopathy usually accompany. The hair is easily pulled in the infected area.

If the disease is not diagnosed early and treatment is not started quickly, the infection may result in fibrosis and cicatricial alopecia. *Trichophyton mentagrophytes*, *Trichophyton verrucosum*, *Trichophyton megnininii*, and *Trichophyton tonsurans* can be listed as the causing factors of kerion. Besides, *Microsporum canis* and *Microsporum gypseum* infections may also lead to the formation of kerion celsi [2]. Clinical examination and fungal culture are very essential in diagnosing tinea capitis. Skin biopsy should be avoided in pediatric population. In direct mycology test with 10–30% potassium hydroxide, fungal elements such as hyphae and spores may be observed [1]. A Wood's lamp examination may be utilized in the diagnosis. In infections caused by *Microsporum canis*, a Wood's lamp investigation reveals green fluorescence due to ectothrix infections. Trichophyton verrucosum may also lead to ectothrix infections. Endothrix type of infection caused by *Trichophyton tonsurans*, *Trichophyton soudanense*, *Trichophyton rubrum*, *Trichophyton violaceum*, or *Trichophyton rubrum* does not reflect any color under Wood's light [3]. Dermoscopic evaluation is also valuable in the process of diagnosis. Broken hairs, scales, follicular keratosis, black dots, bent hairs, erythema, comma hairs, crusts, forked hairs, bar code-like hairs, follicular pustules, V-shaped hairs may be observed in patients with kerion celsi [4].

Skin abscess refers to collection of pus in the epidermis, dermis, and/or deeper layers. A more superficial form is called a furuncle. Carbuncles are deeply located skin abscesses formed by the fusion of multiple furuncles. Gram-positive bacteria such as *Staphylococcus aures* and *Streptococci* cause more than 90% of skin abscesses, while Gram-negative bacteria are isolated in <10% of cases. Skin abscesses can be induced by trauma, insect bites, animal scratches and bites, poor hygiene, atopic dermatitis, and immune disorders and may occur on any skin surface. On clinical examination, erythematous and sensitive induration can be palpated, and a central pustule usually accompanies. Besides, the lesion may fluctuate during palpation. Skin abscesses can vary in size but are usually 1–3 cm. Fever and fatigue may be accompanied in larger skin abscesses. In addition, leukocytosis and an increase in inflammatory markers can be observed in the peripheral blood. Lymphadenopathy may also be observed. Spontaneous drainage generally occurs. Diagnosis is made mainly by clinical examination. Ultrasound, tissue material culture, PCR, and hemoculture can be utilized in the diagnosis [5].

Alopecia areata is a common inflammatory hair loss. This disease can occur in people of all ages, sexes, and ethnic backgrounds. Although the exact pathophysiological mechanism of the disease is still unknown, autoimmune attack and other immune alterations are emphasized. The frequency of the disease is higher in patients with autoimmune disease and personal atopy history. In alopecia areata, small round alopecic areas (patchy alopecia areata) are usually observed. However, a complete scalp hair loss (alopecia totalis) to complete scalp and body hair loss (alopecia universalis) may be present [6]. Although alopecia areata generally shows an asymptomatic course, some patients may experience burning and stinging sensation, itch, or pain [7]. There is no obvious inflammation or scar. Nail findings such as pitting and brittleness in patients with alopecia areat may be detected [6]. In addition to dermatological examination, dermoscopy is also important. Characteristic dermoscopic findings of alopecia areata are exclamation mark hairs, yellow dots, and dystrophic hairs.

Discoid erythematosus among the pediatric population is rare. The disease causes alopecic scarring plaques on the scalp with ill-defined borders. Adherent scales cover the alopecic surfaces and follicular plugs may be observed macroscopically when the scale is removed [8]. In general, the lesions are characterized by skin atrophy, telangiectasia, changes in pigmentation, follicular plugging, and scarring [9]. Diagnosis of discoid lupus erythematosus may be difficult; the lesions can mimic bacterial and fungal infections. Characteristic dermoscopic features of discoid lupus erythematosus are loss of follicular ostia, follicular keratotic plugs, arborizing vessels, honeycomb pigmented network, dyschromia, scaling, and follicular red dot pattern [10]. A direct immunofluorescence test shows complement or immunoglobulin deposits in the dermo-epidermal junction [8].

Key Points
- Kerion celsi is an inflammatory or suppurative form of tinea capitis which occurs as a result of increased hypersensitivity to dermatophyte infection.
- Kerion celsi presents as a painful and inflammatory crusted nodule. Although the lesion is mostly solitary, multiple plaques may also be present.
- If the diagnosis is not made early and treatment is not started quickly, the infection may result in fibrosis and cicatricial alopecia.
- A clinical examination, dermoscopy, direct mycology test with 10–30% potassium hydroxide, Wood's lamp examination, and fungal culture are valuable in the diagnosis of kerion celsi.

References

1. John AM, Schwartz RA, Janniger CK. The kerion: an angry tinea capitis. Int J Dermatol. 2016;57(1):3–9. https://doi.org/10.1111/ijd.13423.
2. Arenas R, Toussaint S, Isa-Isa R. Kerion and dermatophytic granuloma. Mycological and histopathological findings in 19 children with inflammatory tinea capitis of the scalp. Int J Dermatol. 2006;45(3):215–9. https://doi.org/10.1111/j.1365-4632.2004.02449.x.
3. Hay RJ. Tinea capitis: current status. Mycopathologia. 2016;182(1–2):87–93. https://doi.org/10.1007/s11046-016-0058-8.
4. Aqil N, BayBay H, Moustaide K, Douhi Z, Elloudi S, Mernissi FZ. A prospective study of tinea capitis in children: making the diagnosis easier with a dermoscope. J Med Case Rep. 2018;12(1):383. https://doi.org/10.1186/s13256-018-1914-6. PMID: 30591075; PMCID: PMC6309099.
5. Galli L, Venturini E, Bassi A, Gattinara GC, Chiappini E, Defilippi C, et al. Common community-acquired bacterial skin and soft-tissue infections in children: an intersociety consensus on impetigo, abscess, and cellulitis treatment. Clin Ther. 2019; https://doi.org/10.1016/j.clinthera.2019.01.010.
6. Strazzulla LC, Wang EHC, Avila L, Lo Sicco K, Brinster N, Christiano AM, Shapiro J. Alopecia areata. J Am Acad Dermatol. 2018;78(1):1–12. https://doi.org/10.1016/j.jaad.2017.04.1141.
7. Alkhalifah A. Alopecia areata update. Dermatol Clin. 2013;31(1):93–108. https://doi.org/10.1016/j.det.2012.08.010.
8. Miettunen PM, Bruecks A, Remington T. Dramatic response of scarring scalp discoid lupus erythematosus (DLE) to intravenous methylprednisolone, oral corticosteroids, and hydroxychloroquine in a 5-year-old child. Pediatr Dermatol. 2009;26(3):338–41. https://doi.org/10.1111/j.1525-1470.2009.00916.x.
9. Arkin LM, Ansell L, Rademaker A, Curran ML, Miller ML, Wagner A, Paller AS. The natural history of pediatric-onset discoid lupus erythematosus. J Am Acad Dermatol. 2015;72(4):628–33. https://doi.org/10.1016/j.jaad.2014.12.028.
10. Tosti A, Torres F, Misciali C, Vincenzi C, Starace M, Miteva M, Romanelli P. Follicular red dots. Arch Dermatol. 2009;45(12) https://doi.org/10.1001/archdermatol.2009.277.

Chapter 57
A Nodular Scalp Lesion

Amr Mohammad Ammar, Shady M. Ibrahim, and Mohamed L. Elsaie

A 61-year-old man presented with an asymptomatic lesion on the scalp since two years.

A physical examination revelaed a well-defined erythematous multilobulated nodule with oozing, ulceration and crustation on the right temporal area (Fig. 57.1).

On dermoscopy, well-demarcated, round to oval, varied in size, reddish areas were observed (Fig. 57.2).

Based on the case description, clinical and dermoscopic photographs, what is your diagnosis?

Differential Diagnoses
1. Basal cell carcinoma.
2. Pyogenic granuloma.
3. Acquired capillary hemangioma.
4. Kaposi's sarcoma.

Diagnosis
Acquired capillary hemangioma.

A. M. Ammar · S. M. Ibrahim
Department of Dermatology and Venerology, Al-Azhar University, Cairo, Egypt

M. L. Elsaie (✉)
Department of Dermatology and Venereology, Medical Research and Clinical Studies
Institute, National Research Centre, Cairo, Egypt

A. Waśkiel-Burnat et al. (eds.), *Clinical Cases in Scalp Disorders*, Clinical
Cases in Dermatology, https://doi.org/10.1007/978-3-030-93426-2_57

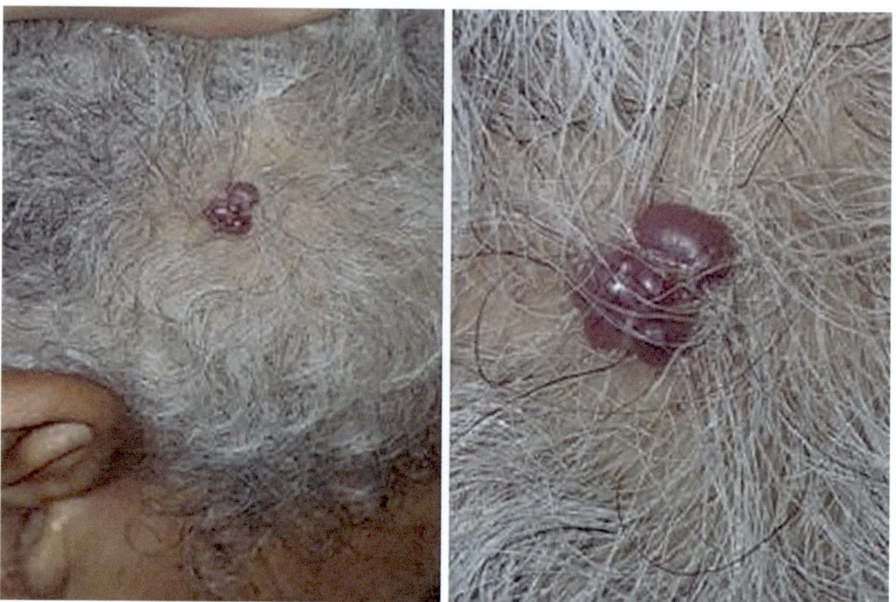

Fig. 57.1 A single erythematous nodule on right temporal area

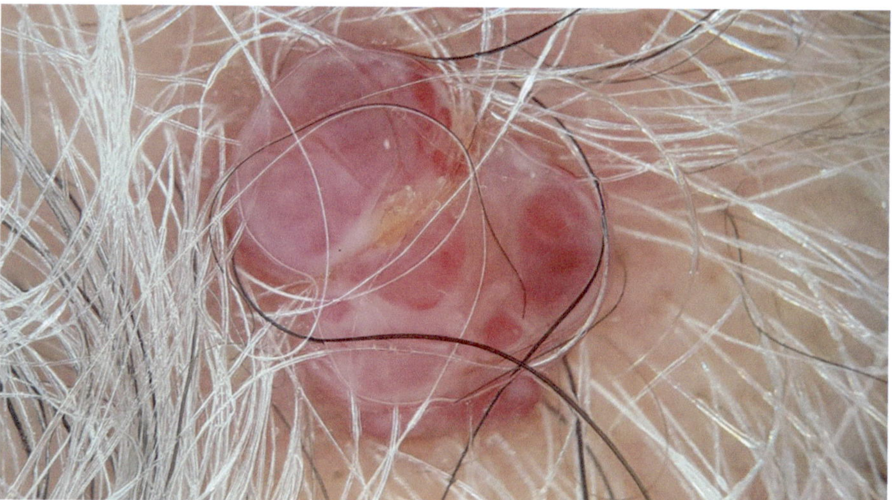

Fig. 57.2 Dermoscopy shows well-demarcated, round to oval, varied in size, reddish areas (lacunae). No vascular structures are seen inside the lacunae

Discussion

Vascular anomalies pose a diagnostic challenge due to inconsistent classification systems, poor understanding of natural history, and overlapping clinical and histological features [1]. The currently used classification, proposed by Mulliken and Glowacki, was adopted by the International Society for the Study of Vascular Anomalies in 1996 [1]. Accordingly, vascular anomalies are classified into vascular tumors (lesions characterized by endothelial hyperplasia) and malformations (lesions characterized by dysmorphogenesis and normal endothelial turnover) [1–3].

Hemangiomas are the most common vascular tumors [2]. They rarely present at birth, show a rapid growth during the first six months of life, and spontaneously involute with time [2]. Vascular malformations, on the other hand, are present at birth, show proportionate growth throughout the life of the individual, and are infiltrative in nature [2, 4]. The hemangioma feels firm and rubbery and is difficult to compress as compared to a malformation which is readily compressible [5].

Hemangiomas are further classified according to the time of presentation as "congenital" or "infantile" [2]. Congenital hemangiomas are rare and present at birth [2]. They either rapidly involute in infancy (rapidly involuting congenital hemangioma) or never involute (noninvoluting congenital hemangioma) [2]. Infantile hemangiomas are the most common tumor in infancy and occur in around 4–10% of the population [2]. Hemangiomas can also be classified depending on their depth as superficial, deep, and compound [1]. The superficial hemangioma extends into the superficial dermis and appears red and nodular [2, 5]. A deep hemangioma involves the lower dermis or subcutaneous tissue and presents as a protrusion with an overlying bluish hue [2, 5]. Compound hemangiomas have both deep and superficial components [2].

Acquired capillary hemangiomas appear to be true capillary neoplasms and need to be carefully differentiated from neoplastic conditions such as Kaposi's sarcoma, angiosarcoma, acquired tufted angioma, and intravascular papillary endothelial hyperplasia [6, 7]. A close differential is pyogenic granuloma, a common cutaneous vascular tumor, which grows rapidly and is commonly confused with a hemangioma [3]. It occurs at any age with a slight female predilection, affecting 1% of pregnant women. These lesions, however, are of smaller size (average diameter 6.5 mm) often associated with crusting of the surface epithelium followed by sloughing of the distal tissue [3]. Repeated and copious bleeding episodes are the rule [3]. Histologically, it is a perithelial, rather than an endothelial, tumor and consists of loose and vascular granulation tissue with an ulcerated or eroded surface epithelium and inflammatory cells [4, 8].

Acquired capillary hemangioma of the eyelid, periocular region and scalp are a very rare phenomenon [7]. The exact etiology is unknown. It has been associated with hormonal changes and increased estrogen levels during puberty and pregnancy [9, 10]. Overexpression of angiogenic growth factors, including vascular endothelial growth factor (VEGF), has been associated with capillary hemangiomas [11]. Adult or acquired "hemangiomas" do not involute like their infantile counterparts [12]. No

regressive nature of the lesion, cosmesis, visual obstruction, and prevention of accidental trauma and bleeding are the main reasons for seeking treatment [11].

There is, however, no standard treatment modality for the management of adult capillary hemangiomas, though many treatment options have been tried successfully. These lesions have been managed using intralesional corticosteroids and cutting diathermy without any evidence of recurrence.

Key Points

- Hemangiomas are the most common vascular tumors. They rarely present at birth, show a rapid growth during the first six months of life, and spontaneously involute with time.
- Overexpression of angiogenic growth factors, including vascular endothelial growth factor (VEGF), has been associated with capillary hemangiomas.
- Adult or acquired "hemangiomas" do not involute like their infantile counterparts.

References

1. Theologie-Lygidakis N, Schoinohoriti OK, Tzerbos F, Iatrou I. Surgical management of head and neck vascular anomalies in children: a retrospective analysis of 42 patients. Oral Surg Oral Med Oral Pathol Oral Radiol. 2014;117:e22–31.
2. Richter GT, Friedman AB. Hemangiomas and vascular malformations: current theory and management. Int J Pediatr. 2012;2012:645678.
3. Mulliken JB, Fishman SJ, Burrows PE. Hemangiomas and other vascular tumors. In: Wells SA, editor. Current problems in surgery: vascular anomalies. Boston: Mosby; 2000. p. 529–51. [Google Scholar].
4. Rachappa MM, Triveni MN. Capillary hemangioma or pyogenic granuloma: a diagnostic dilemma. Contemp Clin Dent. 2010;1:119–22. [PMC free article] [PubMed] [Google Scholar].
5. McGill T, Mulliken J. Otolaryngology head and neck surgery. In: Vascular anomalies of the head and neck. Baltimore: Mosby; 1993. p. 333–46. [Google Scholar].
6. Brannan S, Reuser TQ, Crocker J. Acquired capillary haemangioma of the eyelid in an adult treated with cutting diathermy. Br J Ophthalmol. 2000;84:1322.
7. Leroux K, den Bakker MA, Paridaens D. Acquired capillary hemangioma in the lacrimal sac region. Am J Ophthalmol. 2006;142:873–5.
8. Oda D. Soft-tissue lesions in children. Oral Maxillofac Surg Clin North Am. 2005;17:383–402.
9. Pushker N, Bajaj MS, Kashyap S, Balasubramanya R. Acquired capillary haemangioma of the eyelid during pregnancy. Clin Exp Ophthalmol. 2003;31:368–9.
10. Garg R, Gupta N, Sharma A, Jain R, Beri S, D'Souza P, et al. Acquired capillary hemangioma of the eyelid in a child. J Pediatr Ophthalmol Strabismus. 2009;46:118–9.
11. Steeples LR, Bonshek R, Morgan L. Intralesional bevacizumab for cutaneous capillary haemangioma associated with pregnancy. Clin Exp Ophthalmol. 2013;41:413–4.
12. Connor SE, Flis C, Langdon JD. Vascular masses of the head and neck. Clin Radiol. 2005;60:856–68.

Chapter 58
A Pigmented Scalp Lesion

Amr Mohammad Ammar, Shady M. Ibrahim, and Mohamed L. Elsaie

A 35-year-old women presented with an asymptomatic scalp lesion since three years.

A physical examination revealed a well-defined localized area of alopecia with crustation (Fig. 58.1).

On dermoscopy, a localized area of alopecia with multiple erosions, crustations, blue grey dots, globules, and leaf-like structures at the periphery of lesion were detected. Moreover, there were thin arborizing vessels crossing the midline (Fig. 58.2).

Based on the case description, clinical and dermoscopic photographs, what is your diagnosis?

Differential Diagnoses
1. Basal cell carcinoma.
2. Discoid lupus erythematosus.
3. Angiokeratoma.
4. Kaposi's sarcoma.

Diagnosis
Basal cell carcinoma.

A. M. Ammar · S. M. Ibrahim
Department of Dermatology and Venerology, Al-Azhar University, Cairo, Egypt

M. L. Elsaie (✉)
Department of Dermatology and Venereology, Medical Research and Clinical Studies Institute, National Research Centre, Cairo, Egypt

A. Waśkiel-Burnat et al. (eds.), *Clinical Cases in Scalp Disorders*, Clinical Cases in Dermatology, https://doi.org/10.1007/978-3-030-93426-2_58

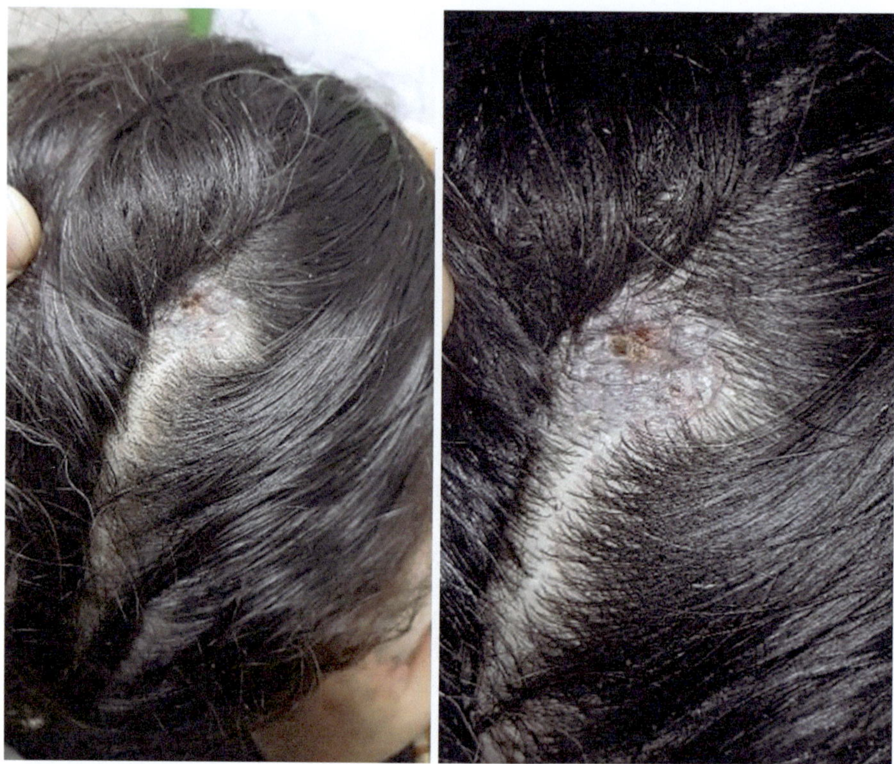

Fig. 58.1 A well-defined localized area of alopecia with crustation

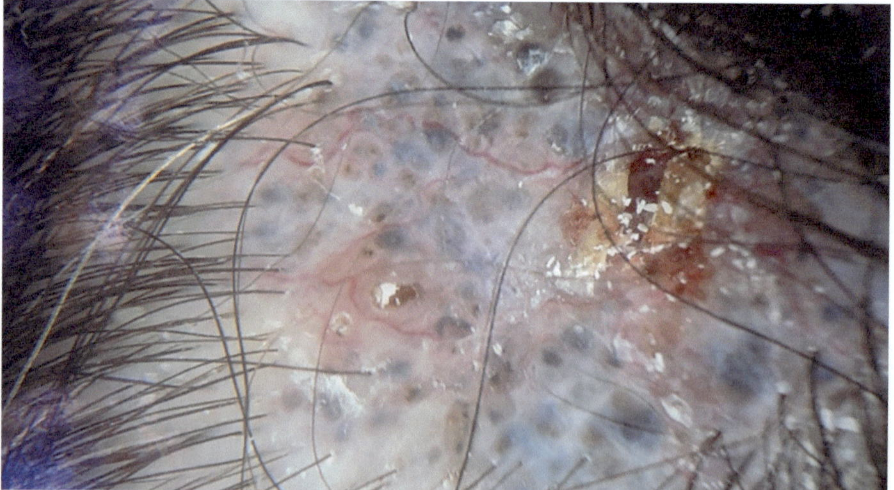

Fig. 58.2 Dermoscopy shows a localized area of alopecia with multiple erosions, crustations, blue grey dots, globules, and leaf-like structures at the periphery of the lesion. Moreover, there are thin arborizing vessels crossing the midline are present

Discussion

Basal cell carcinoma (BCC) is a neoplastic proliferation of basaloid cells probably originating from basal cells of follicular origin. It may appear on any nonglabrous site though it is commonly seen on sun-exposed areas particularly the face. Involvement of palm and sole is very rare except in nevoid BCC syndrome [1].

BCC is the most frequent malignant neoplasm in white-skinned individuals [1]. It is a slow-growing tumor, a neoplastic proliferation of follicular basal cells [2] that is typically locally invasive with virtually no metastatic risk [1]. It has been proposed that BCC precursor cells are keratinocytes, as is the case with squamous cell carcinoma (SCC) [1]. In most countries, for statistical purposes, SCC and BCC have been commonly considered under the same denomination of non-melanoma skin cancer (NMSC) for several years due to misleading oncologic records that have not discriminated SCC from BCC [3–5]. Nevertheless, according to Andrade et al. (2012) [1], BCC and SCC represent different clinical entities resulting from different etiopathological pathways, so they should always be considered separately.

Despite the high prevalence of BCC, its etiopathogenesis is still unclear, and previous studies have indicated a multifactorial basis for this pathology [5].

BCCs develop in different body areas, including the scalp, which represents a unique anatomical region in which pilosebaceous follicles are concentrated, and the area is protected from the sun. Considering that sun exposure is one of the main BCC risk factors, it is uncertain as to why BCCs develop on the scalp. Moreover, BCCs on the scalp have been described as more aggressive [5, 6].

In <0.5% of all BCC cases [6], the tumor reaches a diameter larger than 5 cm and then is called giant BCC. In most of the giant BCCs, the risk factors are the lack of awareness and self-negligence [7, 8]. In more than 50% of the cases, there is a strong association with smoking [9]. Most of the giant BCC are locally or distally metastatic at the time of presentation [10]. Due to the late presentation and larger size many giant BCCs may not maintain the morphological characteristic of the original tumor and mimic squamous cell carcinoma.

Key Points
- Basal cell carcinoma is a neoplastic proliferation of basaloid cells probably originating from basal cells of follicular origin.
- It is the most frequent malignant neoplasm in white-skinned individuals.
- Despite the high prevalence of basal cell carcinoma, its etiopathogenesis is still unclear.

References

1. Andrade P, Brites MM, Vieira R, Mariano A, Reis JP, Tellechea O, Figueiredo A. Epidemiology of basal cell carcinomas and squamous cell carcinomas in a Department of Dermatology: a 5 year review. An Bras Dermatol. 2012;87(2):212–9.
2. Sarkar S, Kunal P, Kishore B, Ghosh K. Neglected basal cell carcinoma on scalp. Indian J Dermatol. 2016;61(1):85–7.
3. Dessinioti C, Antoniou C, Katsambas A, Stratigos AJ. Basal cell carcinoma: what's new under the sun? Photochem Photobiol. 2010;86(3):481–91.
4. Ferrandiz C, Fuente MJ, Ferrandiz L, Carrascosa JM. Basal cell carcinoma. Cancer Treat Res. 2009;146:263–78.
5. Heller ER, Gor A, Wang D, Hu Q, Lucchese A, Kanduc D, Sinha AA. Molecular signatures of basal cell carcinoma susceptibility and pathogenesis: a genomic approach. Int J Oncol. 2013;42(2):583–96.
6. Takemoto S, Fukamizu H, Yamanaka K, Nakayama T, Kora Y, Mineta H. Giant basal cell carcinoma: improvement in the quality of life after extensive resection. Scand J Plast Reconstr Surg Hand Surg. 2003;37:181–5. [PubMed] [Google Scholar].
7. Lorenzini M, Gatti S, Giannitrapani A. Giant basal cell carcinoma of the thoracic wall: a case report and review of the literature. Br J Plast Surg. 2005;58:1007–10. [PubMed] [Google Scholar].
8. Manstein CH, Gottlieb N, Manstein ME, Manstein G. Giant basal cell carcinoma: a series of seven T3 tumors without metastasis. Plast Reconstr Surg. 2000;106:653–6. [PubMed] [Google Scholar].
9. Smith JB, Randle HW. Giant basal cell carcinoma and cigarette smoking. Cutis. 2001;67:73–6. [PubMed] [Google Scholar].
10. Scanlon EF, Volkmer DD, Oviedo MA, Khandekar JD, Victor TA. Metastatic basal cell carcinoma. J Surg Oncol. 1980;15:171–80.

Chapter 59
A Scaly Scalp in a Child

Amr Mohammad Ammar, Shady M. Ibrahim, and Mohamed L. Elsaie

A 10-year-old child presented with a localized area of hair loss since two months.

A physical examination revealed diffuse scaling of the scalp with no hair loss (Fig. 59.1).

On dry trichoscopy diffuse white scaling of the scalp without hair loss was observed. On trichoscopy with immersion fluid, multiple morse code, zigzag hairs, cork screw hairs, coma hairs and Z hairs were detected (Figs. 59.2 and 59.3).

Based on the case description and the photographs, what is your diagnosis?

Differential Diagnoses
1. Psoriasis.
2. Tinea capitis.
3. Seborrheac dermatitis.
4. Alopecia areata.

Diagnosis
Tinea capitis.

A. M. Ammar · S. M. Ibrahim
Department of Dermatology and Venerology, Al-Azhar University, Cairo, Egypt

M. L. Elsaie (✉)
Department of Dermatology and Venereology, Medical Research and Clinical Studies Institute, National Research Centre, Cairo, Egypt

A. Waśkiel-Burnat et al. (eds.), *Clinical Cases in Scalp Disorders*, Clinical Cases in Dermatology, https://doi.org/10.1007/978-3-030-93426-2_59

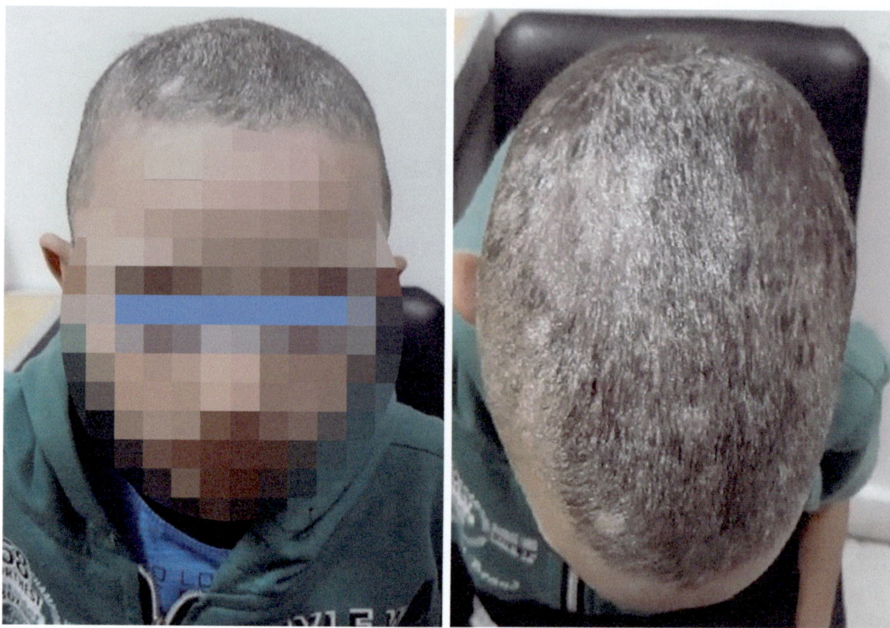

Fig. 59.1 Diffuse scaling of the scalp with no hair loss

Fig. 59.2 Wet trichoscopy shows diffuse white scaling of the scalp without hair loss

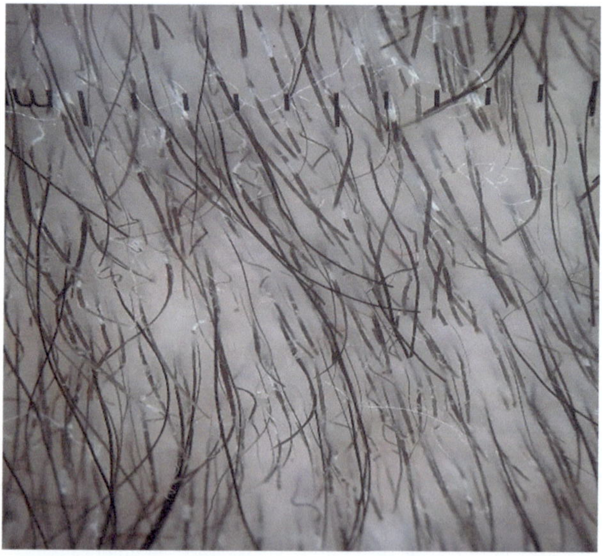

Fig. 59.3 Dry trichoscopy
with immersion fluid
shows multiple morse
code, zigzag hairs, cork
screw hairs, coma hairs
and Z hairs

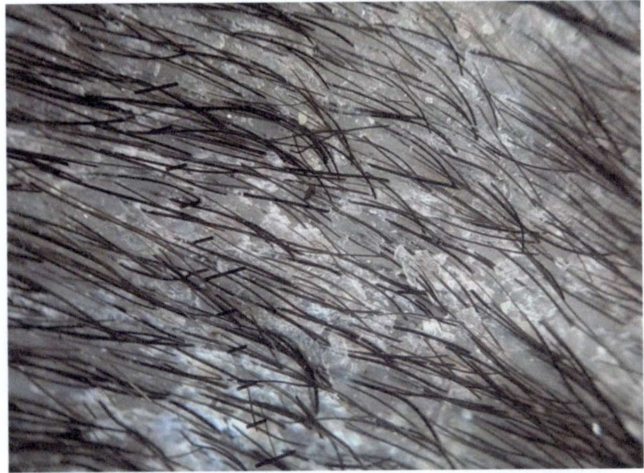

Discussion

Tinea capitis is caused by superficial fungal infection of the scalp, eyebrows and eyelashes with a propensity for attacking hair shafts and follicles. The disease is considered to be a form of superficial mycosis or dermatophytosis [1].

Causative agents of tinea capitis include keratinophilic fungi termed dermatophytes. These fungi usually are present in non-living cornified layers of the skin and its appendages. They are sometimes capable of invading the outermost layer of skin, stratum corneum, or other keratinized skin appendages derived from epidermis, such as hair and nails [2].

Dermatophytic fungi causing tinea capitis can be divided into anthropophilic and zoophilic organisms. Anthropophilic fungi grow preferentially on humans. The most common type of anthropophilic fungi forms large conidia of approximately 3–4 μm in diameter within the hair shaft. Zoophilic fungi are acquired through direct contact with infected animals. In this case, smaller conidia of approximately 1–3 μm in diameter are typically present, extending around the exterior of the hair shaft [3]. In Egypt, tinea capitis is the most common form of dermatophyte infection. The most frequently isolated dermatophyte species is *Trichophyton violaceum*, followed by *Microsporum canis*, *Trichophyton rubrum*, and *Microsporum boullardii*. *Epidermophyton floccosum* and *Trichophyton tonsurans* are rarely isolated [4–6].

Trichoscopy is a simple, fast, and inexpensive method for diagnosing and monitoring tinea capitis in children. However, mycology remains the gold standard diagnostic method. In 2008, Slowinska et al. for the first time descibed comma hairs in two children with tinea capitis [3]. In 2011, Hughes et al. reported the presence of corkscrew hairs in six dark-skinned children with tinea capitis, especially in cases of Trichophyton soudanense infection [7]. The authors suggested that corkscrew hair could be a variant of comma hair in dark-skinned patients, or a characteristic feature of Trichophyton soudanense infection [7].

Key Points
- Tinea capitis is caused by superficial fungal infection of the scalp.
- Dermatophytic fungi causing tinea capitis can be divided into anthropophilic and zoophilic organisms.
- Trichoscopy is a simple, fast, and inexpensive method for diagnosing and monitoring tinea capitis in children.

References

1. Seebacher C, Bouchara JP, Mignon B. Updates on the epidemiology of dermatophyte infections. Mycopathologia. 2008;166(5–6):335.
2. Bonifaz A, Isa-Isa R, Araiza J, Cruz C, Hernández MA, Ponce RM. Cytobrushculture method to diagnose tinea capitis. Mycopathologia. 2007;163(6):309–13.
3. Slowinska M, Rudnika L, Schwartz RA, Kowalska-Oledzka E, Rakowska A, Sicinska J, et al. Comma hairs: a dermoscopic marker for tinea capitis: a rapid diagnostic method. J Am Acad Dermatol. 2008;59:S77–9.
4. Zaki S-M, Ibrahim N, Shetaia YM, Abdel-Ghany K. Dermatophyte infections in Cairo, Egypt. Mycopathologia. 2008;167(3):133–7.
5. Younes AEKH, Mohamed E-EM, Tawfik KM, Ezzat AA. Tinea capitis in Assiut (Egypt). AAMJ. 2012;10(1)
6. Aqil N, BayBay H, Moustaide K, Douhi Z, Elloudi S, Aqil FZM, et al. A prospective study of tinea capitis in children: making the diagnosis easier with a dermoscope. J Med Case Rep. 2018;12:383. https://doi.org/10.1186/s13256-018-1914-6.
7. Hughes R, Chiaverini C, Bahadorian P, et al. Corkscrew hair: a new dermoscopic sign for diagnosis of tinea capitis in black children. Arch Dermatol. 2011;147:355.

Chapter 60
An Ulcerated Plaque on the Frontal Scalp

Uwe Wollina

A 56-year-old female patient was referred to the Department of Dermatology and Allergology because of a chronic lesion on the frontal scalp presented since five years. The patient was previously treated with topical corticosteroids and antibiotics with no improvement.

Her medical history was unremarkable. No history of trauma was reported.

On physical examination we observed a single lesion partialy covered by crust on the frontal area of the scalp. After crust removal, an ulceration surrounded by an erythematous plaque and scar-like area was presented. Hair density was significantly reduced (Fig. 60.1). In bacteriological culture, *Staphylococcus aureus* was isolated.

Based on the case description and the photographs, what is your diagnosis?

Differential Diagnoses
1. Squamous cell carcinoma.
2. Neuropathic ulcer.
3. Discoid lupus erythematosus.
4. Ulcerated scar.
5. Ulcerated lichen planopilaris.

This case was presented in [6].

U. Wollina (✉)
Department of Dermatology and Allergology, Municipal Hospital of Dresden, Academic Teaching Hospital, Dresden, Germany
e-mail: Uwe.Wollina@klinikum-dresden.de

© The Author(s), under exclusive license to Springer Nature Switzerland AG 2022
A. Waśkiel-Burnat et al. (eds.), *Clinical Cases in Scalp Disorders*, Clinical Cases in Dermatology, https://doi.org/10.1007/978-3-030-93426-2_60

Fig. 60.1 An ulceration surrounded by erythematous plaque and scar-like area with hair loss

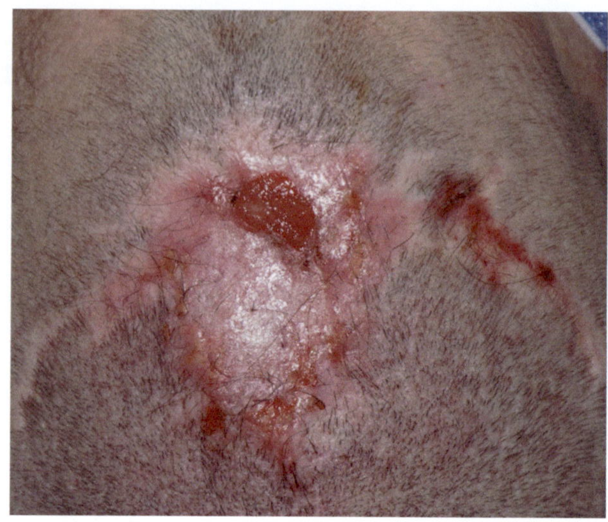

Diagnosis
Ulcerated lichen planopilaris.

Discussion

Our patient was suspected to present with a skin cancer on the scalp. Therefore, the decision for complete surgical excision was made. Surgery was performed under general anesthesia. The defect was closed by tissue advancement flap combined with bilateral extension. Healing was unremarkable (Fig. 60.2). A histologic investigation excluded a skin cancer. It demonstrated hyperkeratotic plugs in the lower portion of the infundibulum of sebaceous glands. Moreover, epidermal hypergranulosis, basal vacuolar degeneration, and a lichenoid lymphocytic infiltrate were presented. There was a significant loss of elastic fibers. A direct immunofluorescence test was positive for linear deposits of fibrin. This confirmed the diagnosis of lichen planopilaris.

Lichen planus (LP) is a common inflammatory disorder of skin and mucous membranes characterized by pruritus and erythematous papules with Wickham stripes. Follicular lichen planopilaris (LPP) affects hair bearing areas. There are three variants of LPP, including Graham-Little-Piccardi-Lasseur syndrome, frontal fibrosing alopecia, and classic LPP. Classic LPP presents as patchy progressive cicatricial alopecia mostly on the scalp. In contrast, frontal fibrosing alopecia is characterized by the recession of the fronto-temporal hair line. In Graham-Little-Piccardi-Lasseur syndrome, cicatricial alopecia of the scalp, non-cicatricial alopecia the axillae and groin, and follicular papular hyperkeratosis of the trunk and the

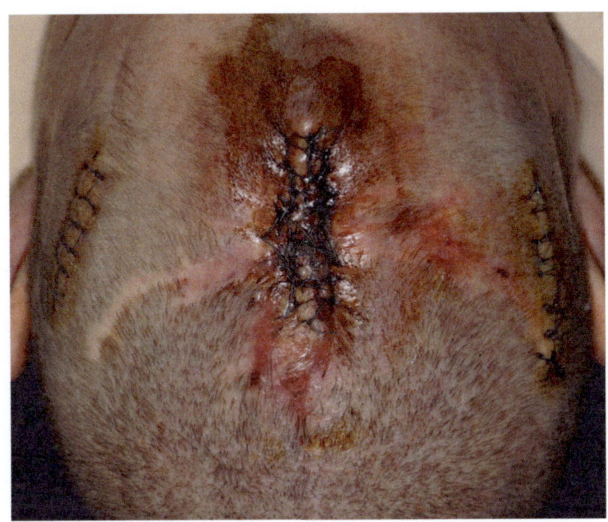

Fig. 60.2 Five days after surgery

extremities are observed. LPP shows an association with thyroid disorders [1]. Longstanding ulcerated LPP can cause secondary neoplasia such as squamous cell carcinoma [2].

Treatment of classic LPP consists of topical or intralesional corticosteroids and topical calcineurin inhibitors. Moreover, it has been described that mechlorethamine 0.016% gel daily for 24 weeks results in a significant improvement [3]. Oral minocycline, methotrexate, ciclosporin A, hydrochloroquine, mycophenylate mofetil or isotretinoin may be useful [4]. Moreover, an efficacy of tofacitinib in LPP has been reported [5]. Ulcerated LPP can be an indication for surgical treatment [6, 7].

Key Points
- Lichen planopilaris is a follicular subtype of lichen planus.
- Ulcerated LPP is rare but seems to be a risk factor for secondary squamous cell carcinoma.

References

1. Larkin SC, Cantwell HM, Imhof RL, Torgerson RR, Tolkachjov SN. Lichen planopilaris in women: a retrospective review of 232 women seen at Mayo clinic from 1992 to 2016. Mayo Clin Proc. 2020;95(8):1684–95.
2. Garrido Colmenero C, Martín Castro A, Valenzuela Salas I, Martínez García E, Blasco Morente G, Tercedor SJ. Squamous cell carcinoma in lichen planopilaris. J Dermatol Case Rep. 2013;7(3):84–7.

 3. Pincelli TP, Heckman MG, Cochuyt JJ, Sluzevich JC. Valchlor® in the treatment of lichen planopilaris and frontal fibrosing alopecia: a single arm, open-label, exploratory study. Int J Trichol. 2020;12(5):220–6.
 4. Fatemi F, Mohaghegh F, Danesh F, Saber M, Rajabi P. Isotretinoin for the treatment of facial lichen planopilaris: a new indication for an old drug, a case series study. Clin Case Rep. 2020;8(12):2524–9.
 5. Plante J, Eason C, Snyder A, Elston D. Tofacitinib in the treatment of lichen planopilaris: a retrospective review. J Am Acad Dermatol. 2020;83(5):1487–9.
 6. Wollina U, Heinig B, Koch A, Nowak A, Tchernev G, França K, Lotti T. Ulcerating lichen planopilaris – successful treatment by surgery. Open Access Maced J Med Sci. 2018;6(1):96–8.
 7. Assouly P, Reygagne P. Lichen planopilaris: update on diagnosis and treatment. Semin Cutan Med Surg. 2009;28(1):3–10.

Index